AF361658

Molecular Basis and Gene Therapies of Cystic Fibrosis

Molecular Basis and Gene Therapies of Cystic Fibrosis

Editors

John Engelhardt
Claude Ferec

MDPI • Basel • Beijing • Wuhan • Barcelona • Belgrade • Manchester • Tokyo • Cluj • Tianjin

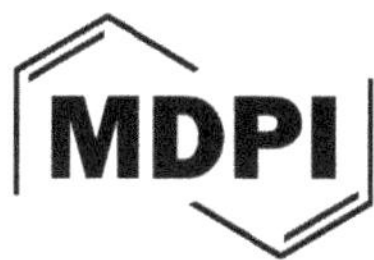

Editors

John Engelhardt
University of Iowa
USA

Claude Ferec
University of Western Brittany
France

Editorial Office
MDPI
St. Alban-Anlage 66
4052 Basel, Switzerland

This is a reprint of articles from the Special Issue published online in the open access journal *Genes* (ISSN 2073-4425) (available at: https://www.mdpi.com/journal/genes/special_issues/Cystic_Fibrosis).

For citation purposes, cite each article independently as indicated on the article page online and as indicated below:

LastName, A.A.; LastName, B.B.; LastName, C.C. Article Title. *Journal Name* **Year**, *Volume Number*, Page Range.

ISBN 978-3-03943-683-5 (Hbk)
ISBN 978-3-03943-684-2 (PDF)

Contents

About the Editors

John Engelhardt please add John Engelhardt Biographical Notes.

Claude Ferec MD-PhD, Pharm, Prof of Genetics. I have 35 years of experience in genetics research, with an emphasis on applying molecular analytical technologies to achieve a better understanding of complex genetic disorders. My team in Brest for a long time has been involved in the study of two genetic disorders particularly present in our isolated Celtic population: cystic fibrosis and haemochromatosis. We also study other disorders, such as hereditary pancreatitis and polycystic kidney disease. Focusing on cystic fibrosis (CF), we propose to illustrate what has been the road map of our research projects during the last thirty years and to show how the impact of gene discovery and genetic and genomic progresses has dramatically modified our view on predictive medicine; personalized medicine; and, not the least, patient care. 1) Mapping and cloning the gene responsible for the disorder: After the CFTR gene was cloned in the late 1990s, we immediately embarked on the CF genetic analysis consortium with the aim of identifying the molecular defects of the gene. We were the first to identify nearly all the mutants in a large population of 3 million inhabitants (Férec et al. Nat Genet 1992) and—to make a long story short—our lab has identified more than 400 mutations and set up new methods to scan the 27 exons of the gene in only one week (Audrézet et al. Hum Mol Genet 1993; Le Maréchal et al. Hum Genet 2001; Audrézet et al. J Mol Diagn 2008). We were also the first to perform a systematic screen of genomic rearrangements in the CFTR gene, leading to the identification of a large number of gross deletions (Audrézet et al. Hum Mutat 2004) and, through a worldwide collaborative study, to describe the distribution of these rearrangements in different populations of the world (Férec et al. Eur J Hum Genet 2006). We finally set up a custom CGH array assay to precisely narrow down these deletions/duplications (Quémener et al. Hum Mutat 2010).2) Study of genotype/phenotype correlations: The genotype/phenotype correlations among CF patients sharing the same mutation is complex, suggesting that the phenotype is influenced, beyond environmental factors, by factors such as modifier genes or the long-distance regulation of the gene itself (Férec et al. Hum Mol Genet 1993; Braun et al. J Cyst Fibros 2006). Knowledge of mutations in the gene has completely modified the spectrum of phenotypes associated with CFTR dysfunction. As, for example, CFTR-related disorders such as sterility in men with absence of vas deferens are associated with specific mutated alleles (Chillon et al. N Engl J Med 1995). 3) Development of genetic epidemiology: The high incidence of CF in our geographic area (Brittany) combined with our long experience in newborn screening for this disease have led us to develop, in the last twenty years, a research program devoted to the genetic epidemiology of CF. This program aims to measure the changes observed in the incidence, survival, and clinical outcomes of CF. The pilot newborn screening project implemented in our area thirty years ago was an excellent example of a successful program combining a biochemical marker test with, for the first time, a mutation screening test (Scotet et al. Lancet 2000). 4) The development of regulation and functional study of the CFTR protein: In this field, our aim is to identify new proteins interacting with the wild-type CFTR protein. We have shown for the first time that AnxA5 interacts directly with CFTR and regulates its normal function (Trouvé et al. Biochim Biophys Acta 2007). Indeed, we have shown that AnxA5 is involved in the cell surface localization of the F508del CFTR and that the Cl channel function of the mutated CFTR is increased, indicating that the mechanisms regulating AnxA5 are potential therapeutic targets in CF (Le Drevo et al. Biochim Biophys Acta 2008). We also showed, for the first time, that the altered apoptosis observed in CF under stress conditions (inflammation, infection) is due to altered Cal-1, Csp12, and mostly Csp-3 activation (Kerbiriou et al. PLoS One 2009). 5) Impact of gene discovery on health policies: The discovery of the CFTR gene, the identification of its mutations, and the development of newborn screening and the prenatal molecular diagnosis test have dramatically changed the epidemiology of CF. As a model in Brittany, a region of 3 million inhabitants where all the mutated alleles are identified, we set up a newborn screening pilot program as early as 1989, proposed a prenatal test to accurately identify at-risk families, and systematically proposed in affected families a cascade screening for mutation carrier detection. We were able to assess the impact of those public health policies (Scotet et al. Lancet 2000; Scotet et al. Prenat Diagn 2008, Duguépéroux et al. J Cyst Fibros 2016). In our area, around 37,000 births occur each year and a mean of 11 newborns are screened positive for CF. This leads to a CF incidence of 1/3300, which is decreasing (Scotet et al. Orphanet J Rare Dis. 2012). The results of those different policies have decreased the incidence of CF by one third (Scotet et al. Hum Genet 2003). I am well prepared to serve as Principal Investigator on this project, entitled "Origin of F508del-CF and Heterozygote Selective Advantage: Role of Arsenic". In fact, our INSERM team is uniquely well prepared for this project because of expertise in genetic analysis of both the genes responsible for CF (CFTR) and haemochromatosis (HFE) as well as our large number of stored DNA specimens. During 20 years of collaboration with Prof Farrell, we have explored explanations for the relatively high frequency of the F508del allele with studies of ancient DNA and modern DNA from trios to identify when and where F508del arose and its pattern of dissemination (Farrell et al. Nature Precedings 2007; Farrell et al. Eur J Hum Genet 2018). Now, we are ready to determine its origin more specifically and why there must have been a selective advantage for the F508del/wt carrier.

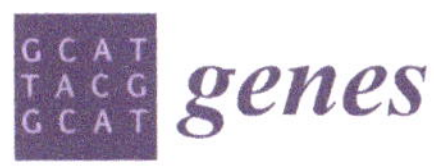 *genes* 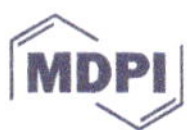

Article

Detargeting Lentiviral-Mediated CFTR Expression in Airway Basal Cells Using miR-106b

Soon H. Choi [1], Rosie E. Reeves [1], Guillermo S. Romano Ibarra [2], Thomas J. Lynch [1],
Weam S. Shahin [1], Zehua Feng [1], Grace N. Gasser [1], Michael C. Winter [1], T. Idil Apak Evans [1],
Xiaoming Liu [1], Meihui Luo [1], Yulong Zhang [1], David A. Stoltz [3], Eric J. Devor [4], Ziying Yan [1] and
John F. Engelhardt [1,*]

[1] Department of Anatomy and Cell Biology, University of Iowa, Carver College of Medicine,
Iowa City, IA 52242, USA; soon-choi@uiowa.edu (S.H.C.); rosiereeves10@gmail.com (R.E.R.);
tom-lynch@outlook.com (T.J.L.); weam-shahin@uiowa.edu (W.S.S.); zehua-feng@uiowa.edu (Z.F.);
grace-gasser@uiowa.edu (G.N.G.); michael-winter@uiowa.edu (M.C.W.); idil-apak@uiowa.edu (T.I.A.E.);
xiaoming-liu@uiowa.edu (X.L.); meihui-luo@uiowa.edu (M.L.); yulong-zhang@uiowa.edu (Y.Z.);
ziying-yan@uiowa.edu (Z.Y.)
[2] Molecular Medicine Program, University of Iowa, Carver College of Medicine, Iowa City, IA 52246, USA;
guillermo-romanoibarra@uiowa.edu
[3] Department of Internal Medicine, University of Iowa, Carver College of Medicine, Iowa City, IA 52246, USA;
david-stoltz@uiowa.edu
[4] Department of Obstetrics and Gynecology, University of Iowa, Carver College of Medicine,
Iowa City, IA 52246, USA; eric-devor@uiowa.edu
* Correspondence: john-engelhardt@uiowa.edu

Received: 12 September 2020; Accepted: 2 October 2020; Published: 6 October 2020

Abstract: Lentiviral-mediated integration of a *CFTR* transgene cassette into airway basal cells is
a strategy being considered for cystic fibrosis (CF) cell-based therapies. However, *CFTR* expression is
highly regulated in differentiated airway cell types and a subset of intermediate basal cells destined to
differentiate. Since basal stem cells typically do not express CFTR, suppressing the *CFTR* expression
from the lentiviral vector in airway basal cells may be beneficial for maintaining their proliferative
capacity and multipotency. We identified miR-106b as highly expressed in proliferating airway basal
cells and extinguished in differentiated columnar cells. Herein, we developed lentiviral vectors
with the miR-106b-target sequence (miRT) to both study miR-106b regulation during basal cell
differentiation and detarget CFTR expression in basal cells. Given that miR-106b is expressed in the
293T cells used for viral production, obstacles of viral genome integrity and titers were overcome by
creating a 293T-B2 cell line that inducibly expresses the RNAi suppressor B2 protein from flock house
virus. While miR-106b vectors effectively detargeted reporter gene expression in proliferating basal
cells and following differentiation in the air–liquid interface and organoid cultures, the CFTR-miRT
vector produced significantly less CFTR-mediated current than the non-miR-targeted CFTR vector
following transduction and differentiation of CF basal cells. These findings suggest that miR-106b
is expressed in certain airway cell types that contribute to the majority of CFTR anion transport in
airway epithelium.

Keywords: miRNA; airway basal cell; CFTR; gene therapy; lentivirus

---

1. Introduction

Cystic fibrosis (CF) is an inherited disease caused by mutations in the cystic fibrosis transmembrane
conductance regulator (*CFTR*) gene [1]. *CFTR* is expressed primarily in epithelial cells of multiple
organs. CFTR plays an important role in transepithelial anion transport important for regulating

airway surface fluid volume, viscosity, and pH [2]. Lung disease with CF involves thick viscous mucus and chronic bacterial infections and is the primary cause of mortality. Gene and cell-based therapies for CF lung disease are gaining momentum, but knowledge gaps do remain regarding the target airway cell types that can prevent or reverse lung disease once a functional *CFTR* gene is expressed [3].

Both the proximal and distal airways express CFTR, but the landscape of cell types and CFTR expression patterns differ in these two levels of the airway. In the proximal airways, basal cells are considered the major stem cell precursor for ciliated cells, goblet cells, ionocytes, and other specialized cell types [3,4]. *CFTR* is expressed at widely divergent levels in a subset of proximal airway basal cells, secretory (goblet) cells, and ionocytes [5,6]. In the distal airway, basal and club cells are generally considered multipotent or bipotent stem cells, respectively, and can both give rise to ciliated cells. CFTR is most abundantly expressed in club secretory cells of bronchioles and alveolar type II cells [3,7,8].

Delivery of the *CFTR* gene to the CF airway basal cell is of particular interest in CF cell-based therapies, as this stem cell target has the ability to self-renew and differentiate into secretory cells (goblet or club), ciliated cells, and ionocytes. Lentiviral vectors have advantages over other widely used gene delivery vectors, such as adeno-associated vector (AAV), because lentiviruses integrate into the host genome and persist following cell division. However, CFTR is not typically expressed in multipotent airway basal cells but is rather expressed in transitional (intermediate) basal cells fated to become secretory cells [3,6,7]. Given that the functional role of CFTR expression in basal cell differentiation is unknown, methods to regulate transgene-derived CFTR expression in multipotent and transitional basal cell states and mimic endogenous patterns of expression could provide greater efficacy in CF cell therapy approaches.

We hypothesized that this pattern of expression could be achieved by suppressing *CFTR* expression in multipotent basal cells via miRNA-mediated silencing. This approach of suppressing transgene expression in a specific cell type is most often referred to as "detargeting". To this end, we sought to identify a miRNA that was selectively expressed in multipotent basal cells and identified miR-106b. The target sequence of miR-106b was then incorporated into the 3′-untranslated region (UTR) of reporter and *CFTR* transgene cassettes encoded within bicistronic and bidirectional lentiviral vectors. Here, we describe the challenges and solutions for vector production using this approach, the analysis of dual reporter gene vectors that demonstrate the efficiency of basal cell detargeting of transgene expression, and the functional consequences of downregulating *CFTR* expression in CF human basal cells by assessing their capacities for generating CFTR currents following differentiation. We believe these vectors created will provide new opportunities for studying pathways that control lineage-commitment of airway basal cells, understanding cell type-specific functions of CFTR function, and ultimately aid in developing more effective gene therapy approaches for CF.

2. Materials and Methods

2.1. Proviral Vector Plasmid Construction

pLV-dt/EGFP is a proviral lentiviral transfer plasmid. It is derived from pLent6/V5-GW/lacZ (Invitrogen) by inserting a phosphoglycerate kinase 1 promoter (PGK) driven dTomato expression cassettes (PGK-dTomato or dt) in the same direction as the lentiviral genomic transcript and a human cytomegalovirus enhancer beta-actin promoter (CBA) driven nuclear EGFP expression cassettes (CBA-EGFP) in opposite orientations. The EGFP reporter has the SV40 large T antigen nuclear localization signal sequence attached to its C-terminus.

pLV-dt/ΔEGFP is derived from pLV-dt/EGFP following deletion of the CBA promoter. This vector was used to confirm that enhanced titers generated in the presence of B2 was due to antisense transcripts derived from the CBA-EGFP expression cassette.

pLV-dt/EGFP-miRT and pLV-dt/EGFP-RmiRT are derivates of pLV-dt/EGFP. pLV-dt/EGFP-miRT has four tandem 21-nt long sequences complementary to miR-106b (4× miR-target or miRT) within the 3′ UTR of the CBA-EGFP cassette. pLV-dt/EGFP-RmiRT is the control vector with the miRT sequences placed in the reverse orientation (reverse-4× miRT or RmiRT) within the 3′ UTR of the CBA-EGFP cassette.

pLV-dt/CFTR-miRT was constructed by deleting the CBA-EGFP cassette from pLV-dt/EGFP-miRT but leaving the miRT within the vector. pLV-dt/CFTR-Ø was constructed by deleting both the CBA-EGFP and cassette from pLV-dt/EGFP-miRT. Subsequently, the PGK-CFTR fragment was cloned in the opposite orientation to the Tomato cassette and the CBA promoter placed in front of the Tomato transgene cassette.

TripZ-B2 was constructed using a binary plant vector pCassRZ containing FHV RNA1 cDNA (a generous gift from Jang-Kyun Seo and ALN Rao) as template for amplifying B2 by PCR using a 5′ forward primer encoding an AgeI site (underlined) (5′-AAAAAA ACCGGTGCCGCCACCATGCCAAGCAAACTCGCGCTAATCC-3′) and a 3′ reverse primer encoding a MluI site (underlined) (5′-AAAAAAACGCGTTTTCGGGCTAGAACGGGTGTGGGTG-3′). The resulting B2 gene PCR product was digested with AgeI and MluI, and subcloned into TripZ vector (Thermo Scientific) under the control of tetracycline response element.

All lentiviral vector plasmids were amplified by transforming Stbl3 competent *Escherichia coli* (*E. coli.*) (ThermoFisher Scientific, #C7373, Waltham, MA, USA). DNA purification was carried out using QIAprep Miniprep kits (QIAGEN, #27104, Hilden, Germany) and Nucleobond Xtra Maxi EF kits (Takara, #740414, Kusatsu, Japan). All vector plasmids were Sanger sequenced to confirm integrity.

2.2. Cell Culture and Human Basal Expansion

The human embryonic kidney cell line HEK293T was used for vector production and cultured in Dulbecco's modified Eagle's medium (DMEM) with 10% fetal bovine serum (FBS) and 1% Penicillin/Streptomycin (P/S). Primary human airway epithelial cells were isolated from the dissected tracheobronchial airway of CF (ΔF508/G551D) and non-CF lungs obtained at the time of lung transplantation and were obtained from the Cells and Tissue Core at the University of Iowa Carver College of Medicine. When lentivirus transduced basal cell cultures were expanded for FACS isolation, they were cultured under dual SMAD signaling inhibition using Small Airway Epithelial Growth Medium (SAGM; Lonza, #CC-3118, Basel, Switzerland) supplemented with extra additives (SAGM-EA) on tissue culture plates precoated with Collagen IV (Sigma, #C7521, St. Louis, MO, USA), as previously described [9]. For experiments that used unsorted populations of lentivirus transduced human basal cells passaged only 2–3 times, cells were cultured in Bronchial Epithelial Cell Growth Medium BulletKit (BEGM; Lonza, #CC-3170, Basel, Switzerland) and directly seeded onto a transwell filter culture at an air–liquid interface.

2.3. Generation of Differentiated Air–Liquid Interface Cultures

Polarized human airway epithelial cultures were generated at an air–liquid interface by seeding 2×10^5 basal cells onto transwell inserts with polyester membrane (Corning, #3450, Corning, NY, USA) that was precoated with collagen IV (Sigma #C7521, St. Louis, MO, USA). Seeding occurred in SAGM-EA or BEGM, depending on the experimental design, and at 24 h post-seeding the basal cell culture medium was replaced with PneumaCult ALI medium (StemCell Technologies, Vancouver, Canada) in both the apical and basal chambers. The next day, the apical chamber media was aspirated, and the basal chamber media was replaced every other day for a minimum of 21 days before analysis.

2.4. microRNA Inhibitor Transfection

Anti-miR miRNA inhibitor for has-miR-106b (ThermoFisher Scientific, Assay ID AM10067, #AM17000, Waltham, MA, USA) and anti-miR miRNA inhibitor negative Control #1 (ThermoFisher Scientific, #AM17010, Waltham, MA, USA) were used to transfect the 293T cells transduced with LV-dt/EGFP-miRT. The transfection procedure followed the RNAi transfection protocol provided with Lipofectamine RNAiMAX Transfection Reagent (ThermoFisher Scientific, #13778100, Waltham, MA, USA).

2.5. Lentiviral Vector Production

Lentiviral vector production was performed using a previously published protocol [10] with slight modifications in 293T and 293T-B2 cells. When the 293T-B2 cells were used, doxycycline was added at the time of Ca_2PO_4 transfection (500 ng/mL) with viral production vector: pMD2.G (VSV-G envelope expressing vector), psPAX2 (packaging vector) and the proviral vector plasmid (pLV-dt/EGFP-miRT, pLV-dt/EGFP-RmiRT, pLV-dt/CFTR-miRT, or pLV-dt/CFTR-Ø). At ~12–16 h post-transfection, the medium was changed to DMEM with 2% FBS. At 24 h and 48 h after the first medium change, the medium containing lentivirus is harvested and filtered (0.4 μm pore size). The virus was concentrated ~100-fold using a Lenti-X Concentrator (Takara, #631232, Kusatsu, Japan) and then resuspended in a medium of choice. Lentiviral vector titers were calculated by serial dilution on 293T cells followed by flow cytometry for Tomato expression at 3 days post-infection, as previously described [10].

2.6. Creation of the Doxycycline-Inducible 293T-B2 Cell Line

The TripZ-B2 plasmid described above was used to produce a lentiviral vector for transduction of 293T cells. The virally transduced cells were selected with puromycin treatment (3 μg/mL) for 5 days. After that, 0.25 μg/mL of puromycin was used for 293T-B2 maintenance and expansion. B2 was induced by addition of doxycycline to the culture medium (Sigma, #D9891), as described above.

2.7. qPCR miRNA Arrays

Total RNA was extracted using the miRVana miRNA isolation kit (Ambion, #AM1560, Austin, TX, USA). RNA quality and concentrations were analyzed on a NanoDrop M-1000 spectrophotometer and an Agilent 2100 Bioanalyzer. RNAs with quality scores >7.00 were used for expression assays. RNA concentrations were standardized to 200 ng/μL. TaqMan low-density miRNA arrays (TLDAs) (Applied Biosystems, #4444913, Foster City, CA, USA) were used to assess miRNA expression levels in proliferating basal cells grown in SAGM-EA. Reverse transcription of 600 ng total RNA was carried out using a TaqMan miRNA reverse transcriptase kit (Applied Biosystems, #4366596) with Megaplex RT primers, Human Pool (Applied Biosystems, #4399966). Samples were loaded onto the TLDA, which utilizes 384 wells preloaded with specific miRNA probes and primers in each well. The TLDA data were processed on an Applied Biosystems Model 7900 Genetic Analyzer, and the data were analyzed using the Applied Biosystems StatMiner software. Each sample was analyzed in triplicate, and each Ct value was normalized to the Ct value of RNU48 endogenous RNA control. Relative quantification of each miRNA was performed using the $\Delta\Delta$Ct method. Statistical significance of the fold change was assessed using two-tailed t-tests. *p*-values of <0.05 were taken as statistically significant.

2.8. Quantitative Real-Time PCR of miRNAs

TaqMan miRNA assays for homo sapiens (has) miR-106b, miR-25, miR-93, and RNU-48 are from ThermoFisher's MicroRNA Analysis products (#4427975), and their Assay IDs are 000442, 000403, 000432, and 001006, respectively. The qPCR was performed according to their protocol (thermofisher.com/taqmanfiles, Waltham, MA, USA).

2.9. Transduction of Human Primary Airway Basal Cells

Primary human basal cells were plated on 6-well plates at 25–30% confluence for lentivirus infection in the presence of DEAE-Dextran (6 μg/mL) [11]. On the day following plating, the lentiviral vector solution was mixed with culture medium (2 mL total volume with ~5×10^6 transduction units (TU)) and added to each well and incubated overnight before the medium was changed. Typically, the level of transduction based on Tomato expression was 30–50% of cells.

2.10. Organoid Culture

The membranes of 24-well transwells (Corning) were coated with 20 μL of a 1:1 PneumaCult-ALI:cold Matrigel (Corning, #354277) mixture and then incubated at 37 °C for 30 min. The airway basal cells (~11,000 cells/well) in the medium and cold Matrigel are mixed at a 1:1 (*v/v*) ratio and 50 μL of the Matrigel/cell mixture was applied onto the transwell. After incubation at 37 °C for 30 min, PneumaCult-ALI (StemCell Technologies, #05001) was added on top of the Matrigel in the apical chamber and basal chamber. The medium was then changed every other day and the organoids were analyzed after ~3 weeks by staining with Hoescht 33342 (10 μg/mL) for one hour and imaged live on a confocal microscope (LSM 880, Zeiss, Oberkochen, Germany).

2.11. Immunohistochemistry and Microscopy

ALI membranes were fixed in 4% paraformaldehyde (PFA) overnight prior to washing with phosphate-buffered saline (PBS) and embedding in Tissue-Tek® O.C.T. Compound (OCT) frozen blocks. Frozen sections were cut at 10 μm and post-fixed in 4% PFA for 20 min, rinsed three times with PBS, and then incubated in blocking buffer containing 20% donkey serum, 0.5% triton X-100, 1 mM $CaCl_2$ in PBS for 1 h. Samples were then blocked with 1% donkey serum and then incubated with primary antibody in diluent buffer containing 1% donkey serum, 0.5% triton X-100 and 1 mM $CaCl_2$ in PBS overnight at 4 °C. Slides were then washed twice with PBS and then incubated with secondary antibody in diluent buffer at room temperature for 1 h. Nuclei were stained with Hoescht 33342 (10 μg/mL). The primary antibodies were chicken anti-GFP (1:1000, Aves Lab, #GFP-1020) and rabbit anti-keratin 5 (1:500, BioLegend, #PRB160P). The secondary antibodies used were Alexa Fluor 488 labeled donkey anti-chicken IgG (1:250, Jackson ImmunoResearch, #703-546-155, West Grove, PA, USA) and Alexa Fluor 647 labeled donkey anti-rabbit IgG (1:250, Jackson ImmunoResearch, #711-606-152, West Grove, PA, USA). Slides were washed three times with PBS and then mounted with Aquamount (Thermo Scientific, VWR #41799-008, Waltham, MA, USA). Images of stained slides were obtained using an LSM 880 confocal microscope (Zeiss, Oberkochen, Germany).

2.12. Flow Cytometry

We used fluorescence-activated cell sorting (FACS) to isolate pure populations of Tomato-positive basal cells from LV-dt/EGFP-RmiRT and LV-dt/EGFP-miRT transduced cultures. These cells were then seeded into ALI cultures and differentiated for 21 days. Cells were then dissociated with Accutase (StemCell Technologies, #07920), centrifuged at 200 RCM for 5 min, and resuspended in 1mL PBS without calcium or magnesium chloride. To evaluate EGFP expression in various cell types, cells were fixed and permeabilized using the Foxp3 Fixation/Permeabilization kit following the manufacturer's protocol (eBiosciences/ThermoFisher #005523-00, Waltham, MA, USA). Cells were stained with the following antibodies: BSND (Abcam clone EPR14270, Cambridge, UK), MUC5AC (Novus clone 45M1, Littleton, CO, USA), acetylated alpha tubulin (Cell Signaling clone D20G3 conjugated to Alexa 647), p63 (Abcam clone EPR5701 conjugated to Alexa647). BSND and MUC5AC were stained with goat anti-rabbit and goat anti-mouse polyclonal antibodies conjugated to Alexa 647 (Invitrogen/ThermoFisher; #A-21244 and #A21235, Waltham, MA, USA). Stained cells were then run on an Attune NxT Flow Cytometer (ThermoFisher, Waltham, MA, USA) and analyzed using FlowJo version 10.7 (Ashland, OR, USA).

2.13. Short-Circuit Current Measurements

Short-circuit currents were measured in CF ALI cultures generated from LV-dt/EGFP-RmiRT and LV-dt/EGFP-miRT transduced basal cells following differentiation for at least 3 weeks. Transwells were placed under VCC MC8 voltage clamps and P2300 Ussing chambers (Physiologic Instruments, San Diego, CA, USA) with low chloride buffer in the apical chamber and high chloride buffer in the basal chamber, as previously described [12,13]. The change in current was assessed after the sequential addition of the following antagonists and agonists: 100 µM amiloride (ENaC inhibitor), 100 µM 4,4'-Diisothiocyano-2,2'-stilbenedisulfonic acid (DIDS) (a general chloride channel blocker that does not affect CFTR), 100 µM 3-Isobutyl-1-methylxanthine (IBMX) and 10 µM forskolin (to increase intracellular cAMP levels which activate CFTR), and 50 µM GlyH101 (a CFTR channel blocker).

2.14. Statistical Analysis

Statistical analysis and graphical presentation were performed using Microsoft Excel (version 16.41, Redmond, WA, USA), GraphPad Prism (version 8, San Diego, CA, USA), and RStudio (version 1.3.959, Boston, MA, USA). Statistical significance in the TLDA data was analyzed using Student's *t*-test without assuming a consistent standard deviation between genes and adjusted for multiple comparisons using a false discovery rate approach using a two-stage linear step-up procedure of Benjamini, Krieger and Yekutieli, with Q = 5%. Correlation of miRNA expression between passage 3 and 18 was tested using linear regression analysis in RStudio (version 1.3.959, Boston, MA, USA). One-way ANOVA and Bonferroni's multiple comparisons test were used for lentiviral vector titration. One-way ANOVA and Tukey's multiple comparisons test were used for Isc analysis and qPCR. One-way ANOVA and Dunnett's multiple comparisons test were used for cell type analysis flow cytometry.

3. Results

3.1. Basal Cells Stably Express miR-106b in Conditional Reprogramming Proliferative Cultures for Long-Term Culture

To select a miRNA for detargeting experiments, we accessed publicly available data through NCBI Gene Expression Omnibus (GEO) under serial number GSE22145 that compared basal cells vs. columnar cells in nasal airway [14] and found seven miRNAs that were consistently expressed in basal cells but not columnar cells from the nasal epithelia of three donors (Figure 1A). To evaluate the expression of miRNA expression in our cultured human tracheobronchial basal cells expanded in SAGM-EA [9], we used a TaqMan low-density array (TLDA; Applied Biosystems) to quantify relative expression of 377 miRNAs (Supplemental Table S1). Expression of 252 miRNAs was consistently detected in basal cells at passage 3 and at passage 18 (Figure 1B). Of these miRNAs, only nine changed significantly between passage 3 and 18 (FDR test with Q = 5%) and 171 miRNAs did not exceed a ±2-fold change in expression in the passage (Figure 1C). Using a less stringent test, expression of 15 miRNAs changed significantly between passage 3 and 18 (unadjusted *t*-test $p \leq 0.05$ and absolute fold change ≥ 2) (Figure 1D).

Comparison of our array data with the nasal miRNA sequencing study demonstrated that miR-106b was one of the few miRNAs that was not expressed in columnar cells. Other miRNAs that were basal cell-specific in the nasal study included miR-184 and miR-500. miR-500 was detected at lower levels than miR-106b in our array study and miR-184 was undetectable. In this regard, miR-106b appeared to be the ideal miRNA to use in basal cell detargeting. We decided that our candidate miRNA should have a higher expression level than that of miR-455-3p, which has been reported to effectively inhibit MUC1 in human epithelial basal cells [15]. To more quantitively evaluate the expression of miR-106 in reference to low (miR-500) and very low (miR-184) basal cell expressing miRNAs, we performed single-plex qPCR for these miRNAs in comparison to that of miR-455-3p (Figure 1E). As expected, the expression levels of miR-184 expression was very low and miR-500a was absent, while miR-106b was more than 11-fold higher than the level of miR-455-3p. Moreover, miR-106b was stable on passage, decreasing by only 30% during the 15 passages. These findings confirmed the validity of the array data and suggested miR-106b was a top candidate for basal cell detargeting.

miR-106b, miR-25 and miR-93 belong to the miR-106b-25 cluster that is located in the 13th intron of mini-chromosome maintenance complex component 7 gene (*MCM7*) [16,17]. We prepared miRNA samples from six donors and analyzed the relative expression of these miRNAs (Figure 1F). The expression levels were fairly consistent between the six random donor samples. Notably, although these miRNAs are in the same cistron, their expression varied over a 10-fold range in airway basal cells (Figure 1F), and the pattern of expression of each of the three miRNAs was also different than that reported for the miR-106b-25 cluster in other tissues [18–22]. Although miR-93 was expressed at ~4.5-fold higher levels than miR-106b, we chose to move forward with miR-106b since miR-93 was observed to be expressed in differentiated human nasal columnar cells [14] (GEO dataset: GSE22145).

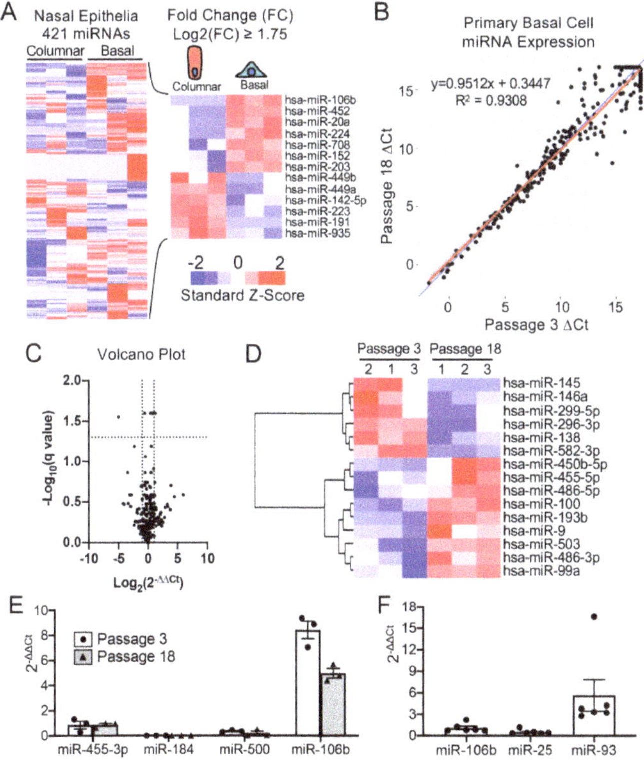

Figure 1. mMiR-106b is stably expressed at high levels in proliferating human basal cells. (**A**) Published data of miRNAs detected by high throughput sequence profiling of nasal basal cells and columnar cells (Accession: GSE22145) were used to generate a heatmap of 421 expressed miRNAs (left) and 13 miRNAs with a Log2 fold difference greater than 1.75 or less than −1.75 (right). (**B**) Correlation of miRNA expression in basal cells at Passage 3 and Passage 18 detected by qPCR array with the blue line represents a theoretical perfect correlation (x = y), and the red line represents linear regression model. (**C**) Volcano plot of miRNA array data indicating genes that were differentially expressed between passages 3 and 18. (**D**) Heatmap of miRNA array data with unsupervised hierarchical clustering of 15 miRNAs (of 252 detected) with an absolute fold change ≥ 2 and an unadjusted *p* value of ≤0.05. (**E**) Relative quantification of candidate basal cell-specific miRNAs, miR-184, miR-500, and miR-106b compared to a known basal cell-specific miR-455-3p. Freshly isolated primary human tracheobronchial cells were passaged 3 (P3) and 18 (P18) times in SAGM-EA media (*N* = 3). (**F**) Relative quantification of miRNAs belonging to miR-106b-25 cluster in passage 3 basal cells (*N* = 6). Each dot represents one donor.

3.2. Increasing the Production Yield of a Lentiviral Vector Harboring Bidirectional Expression Cassettes

In order to evaluate detargeting using a basal cell-specific miR-target (miRT) site, we sought to have two reporter genes (one detargeted and one constitutively expressed) within the lentiviral vector. Since the miRT must reside in the 3′ UTR of the targeted gene cassette, creating this vector required two transgene cassettes (each with unique promoters and 3′ UTRs) oriented in the opposite direction (Figure 2A). We chose a nuclear-targeted EGFP (EGFP-nls) and Tomato as the two transgenes, with the miRT harbored in the 3′ UTR of the EGFP-nls cassette in the reverse orientation. The Tomato transgene in the direct orientation utilized the 3′-LTR polyA site and could not accommodate a miRT without compromising the viral packaging. This vector platform, we call LV-dt/EGFP, was constructed to allow the flexible insertion of any miRT sequence for specific cell type detargeting of transgene expression.

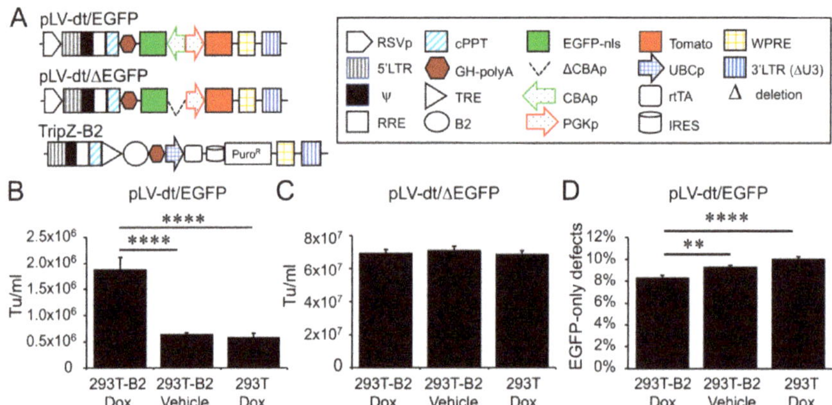

Figure 2. Suppressor of RNAi B2 protein increases titer and viral genome integrity of lentiviral vectors harboring bidirectional gene expression cassettes. (**A**) pLV-dt/ΔEGFP and pLV-dt/EGFP are the proviral vector plasmids used in production of these lentiviral vectors. TripZ-B2 is a lentiviral vector used to make the 293T-B2 cell line that expresses B2 following doxycycline treatment. The box legend to the right highlights the components of these proviral plasmids. Definitions are as follows: 5′LTR, 5′ long terminal repeat; ψ, psi, viral packaging signal sequence; RRE, rev response element, where Rev protein binds; cPPT, central polypurine tract, recognition site for proviral DNA synthesis; STOP, translation stop sequence; EGFP-nls, *EGFP* with nuclear localization signal; ΔCBAp, deletion of chicken beta-actin promoter (CBA); CBAp, CBA promoter in reverse orientation to the viral genomic transcript; PGKp, mouse phosphoglycerate kinase 1 promoter; TRE, tetracycline response element; UBCp, ubiquitin C promoter; rtTA, reverse tetracycline trans-activator; IRES, internal ribosomal entry site; WPRE, Woodchuck hepatitis virus post-transcriptional regulatory element for increasing nuclear export; 3′LTR (ΔU3), 3′ long terminal repeat with deletion in unique 3′ sequence that is necessary for activating viral genome transcription. (**B**) Comparison of LV-dt/EGFP titers produced by 293T-B2 with doxycycline treatment, 293T-B2 with vehicle treatment, and 293T with doxycycline treatment. Data show the mean+/-SEM for $N = 6$ viral preparations. (**C**) Comparison of lentiviral vector LV-dt/ΔEGFP transduction unit per milliliter (Tu/mL) produced by 293T-B2 with doxycycline treatment, 293T-B2 with vehicle (water) treatment, and 293T with doxycycline treatment. Data show the mean+/-SEM for $N = 6$ viral preparations. (**D**) Comparison of the percentage of cells positive for EGFP only among LV-dt/EGFP infected cells produced by 293T-B2 with doxycycline treatment, 293T-B2 with vehicle treatment, and 293T with doxycycline treatment. Data show the mean+/-SEM for $N = 6$ viral preparations. (**B,C**) Statistical comparisons were made by one-way ANOVA, Bonferroni's multiple comparison test. ****, $p < 0.0001$. **, $p < 0.01$.

Initial attempts to generate the LV-dt/EGFP virus gave rise to low titers, despite lacking miRT sequences. We hypothesized complementarity of antisense EGFP mRNA, expressed from the proviral plasmid following transfection, with the full-length sense-strand viral RNA genome might activate RNAi and degrade viral genomes prior to packaging. To approach this problem, we sought to suppress RNAi during packaging with the flock house virus protein B2, which is a known RNAi suppressor [23–25]. When a B2-expression plasmid was co-transfected when making LV-dt/EGFP, the resulting virus titer was ~3 times higher than that without B2 (data not shown). We then used a lentivector to stably integrate a *B2* gene expression cassette into 293T cells, however, persistent *B2* expression in 293T cells was toxic. Thus, we generated a 293T cell line that expresses a doxycycline inducible (Tet-on) B2 protein using a TRIPZ vector (Figure 2A). We first tested different concentrations of doxycycline and two time points of doxycycline addition, at the time of proviral vector transfection or at the first media change after transfection. We observed that addition of 500 ng/mL doxycycline at the time of transfection produced highest virus titer while maintaining health of the producer cells. *B2* mRNA induction by doxycycline was verified by qPCR (data not shown). Indeed, the lentiviral vector LV-dt/EGFP titer was significantly increased by doxycycline induced B2 expression during the virus production (Figure 2B). To confirm that the mechanism of reduced titers of LV-dt/EGFP was due to antisense EGFP transcripts, we created a second control vector (LV-dt/ΔEGFP) which lacked the CBA-promoter controlling EGFP expression. Titers of LV-dt/ΔEGFP, which lacked expression of EGFP transcripts with complementary to the viral genome, were not affected by the induction of B2 (Figure 2C).

To calculate viral titers in the above experiments, we used titration transduction assays on 293 cells followed by flow cytometry. We noticed that there were LV-dt/EGFP transduced cells that were positive for only EGFP or Tomato. This suggested that mutations or deletions within the proviral genomes likely occurred prior to packaging. During reverse transcription, a reverse transcriptase may change its templates 8 to 10 times [26] contributing to diversity of the lentivirus in the wild. This is a drawback to lentiviral vectors. We sought to evaluate whether inhibiting RNAi pathways with B2 would improve integrity of the packaged LV-dt/EGFP genomes. To this end, we compared the percentage of LV-dt/EGFP transduced 293T cells that only expressed EGFP (defective particles) from three types of viral preparation conditions: 1) 293T-B2 cells induced with doxycycline, 2) 293T-B2 cell not induced with doxycycline, and 3) 293T cells induced with doxycycline. Results from these flow cytometry comparisons demonstrated that group-1 and group-2 had ~20% and ~10% fewer defective particles than group-3, respectively (Figure 2D). We hypothesize that low level expression of B2 in the uninduced group-2 viral preparations improved integrity of the viral genomes when compared to 293T preparations lacking B2 (group-3).

3.3. Detargeting EGFP Expression in Proliferating Basal Cells.

To test whether the miR-106b target sequence (miRT) could be used to effectively detarget gene expression in basal cells, we generated a lentivirus vector that contained a nuclear targeted EGFP with the 3'-UTR miR-106b target sequence (pLV-dt/EGFP-miRT) and a control lentivirus vector with the miR-106bT sequence in reverse orientation (pLV-dt/EGFP-RmiRT; Figure 3A). We infected human epithelial basal cells grown in SAGM-EA with LV-dt/EGFP-miRT or LV-dt/EGFP-RmiRT and analyzed EGFP and Tomato expression by flow cytometry and fluorescent imaging. As hypothesized, the nuclei of the LV-dt/EGFP-RmiRT transduced basal cells were EGFP-positive, whereas basal cells transduced with the LV-dt/EGFP-miRT vector were EGFP-negative (Figure 3B). Thus, the miR-106b target sequence in the 3'-UTR appeared to successfully detarget EGFP expression in basal cells. To verify that miR-106b was indeed responsible for *EGFP* knock-down, we transfected FACS isolated Tomato-positive LV-dt/EGFP-miRT transduced cells with a miR-106b inhibitor. As expected, the LV-dt/EGFP-miRT transduced cells transfected with the miR-106b inhibitor recovered nuclear EGFP expression, while the mock transfected negative control cells did not (Figure 3C). The quantification of EGFP-positive only (Q4), Tomato-positive only (Q1), EGFP/Tomato-double-positive (Q2) and double-negative (Q3) cells are shown in the quadrants generated by flow cytometry (Figure 3D).

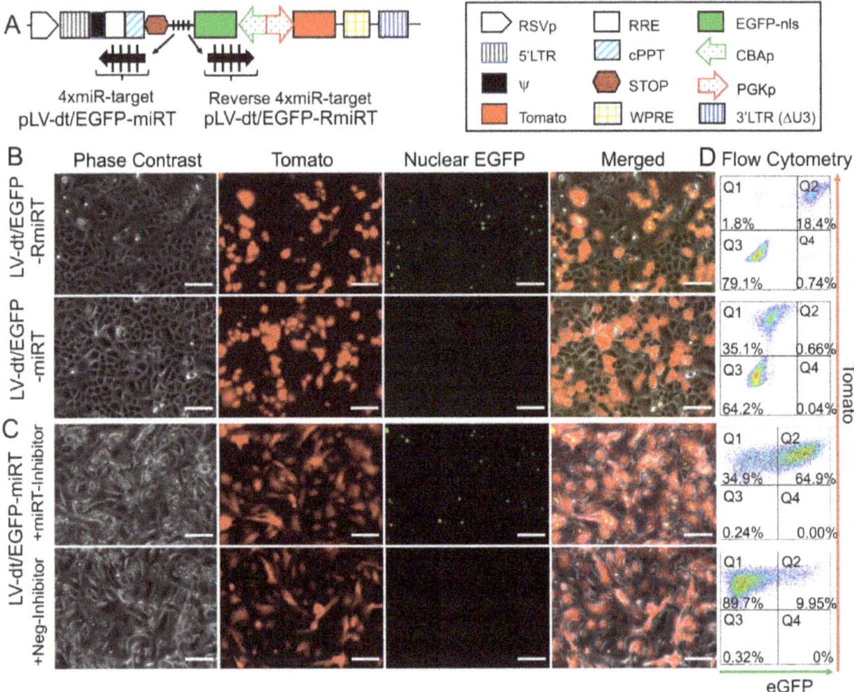

Figure 3. Incorporation of miR-106b target sequence (miRT) into the 3′-UTR of EGFP effectively detargets lentiviral-mediated expression in proliferating basal cells. (**A**) Diagram of the bidirectional promoter proviral lentiviral plasmids (pLV-dt/EGFP-miRT and pLV-dt/EGFP-RmiRT) used to generate lentivirus and test detargeting in basal cells. The box legend to the right highlights the components of these proviral plasmids as described in detail within the Figure 2A legend. LV-dt/EGFP-miRT is the experimental vector harboring a CBA promoter driven nuclear targeted EGFP (EGFP-nls) with miR-106b target sequence (4× miR target or mirT) in the reverse orientation. In the forward direction, the PGK promoter drives expression of the Tomato reporter, which is unaffected by miR-106b. LV-dt/EGFP-RmiRT is a control vector with the miRNA target sequence in the reverse orientation. (**B**) LV-dt/EGFP-miRT and LV-dt/EGFP-RmiRT viruses were used to transduce primary human airway basal cell in SAGM-EA cultures. The Tomato-positive (red) cells indicate the virally transduced cells. EGFP expression is seen in dt/EGFP-RmiRT control transduced cells but not in cells transduced with the detargeted LV-dt/EGFP-miRT vector. Scale bar, 100 μm. (**C**) Basal cells transduced with LV-dt/EGFP-miRT vector, and FACS isolated for Tomato-positive cells, were transfected with miRT-106b inhibitor sequences to block detargeting or mock transfected. Scale bar, 100 μm. (**D**) The cells in (B and C) were analyzed by flow cytometer and are shown in dot plots to the right of the corresponding images for each condition. The percentage of cells are indicated in each quadrant: Q1 (Tomato-positive only cells), Q2 (Tomato and EGFP double-positive cells), Q3 (EGFP-positive only cells), and Q4 (non-fluorescent cells).

3.4. Basal Cell miRT-106b Detargeting is Partially Maintained in Differentiated ALI Cultures and Organoids

miR-106 is highly expressed in proliferating basal cells grown in SAGM-EA media and basal cell detargeting with miRT-106b is highly effective (Figure 3). To determine if miR-106 expression in basal cells of differentiated cultures was sufficient for detargeting, we studied the EGFP expression profiles of ALI and organoid cultures generated from LV-dt/EGFP-miRT and LV-dt/EGFP-RmiRT transduced basal cells. Approximately 40% of the basal cell population was transduced and the cells were not subjected to FACS prior to making ALI cultures or airway organoids. ALI cultures generated from these two groups were sectioned and evaluated for EGFP, Tomato, and KRT5 (basal cell marker) expression. Both LV-dt/EGFP-miRT and LV-dt/EGFP-RmiRT transduced basal cells formed a pseudostratified epithelium with Tomato expression marking transduced cells and KRT5 marking the basal cell layer (Figure 4). As expected, LV-dt/EGFP-miRT transduced cultures lacked nuclear EGFP expression in the majority of KRT5-positive basal cells, confirming detargeting, but contained EGFP-positive nuclei in differentiated columnar cells (Figure 4A). Conversely, LV-dt/EGFP-RmiRT transduced control cultures contained nuclear EGFP-positive cells throughout the basal layer as well as the columnar cell differentiated layer (Figure 4B). Notably, LV-dt/EGFP-miRT transduced ALI culture lacked EGFP in ~50% of columnar cells, whereas the vast majority of columnar cells expressed EGFP in LV-dt/EGFP-RmiRT cultures. These findings suggest that miR106b may also be expressed or retained in a subset of columnar cells in ALI cultures.

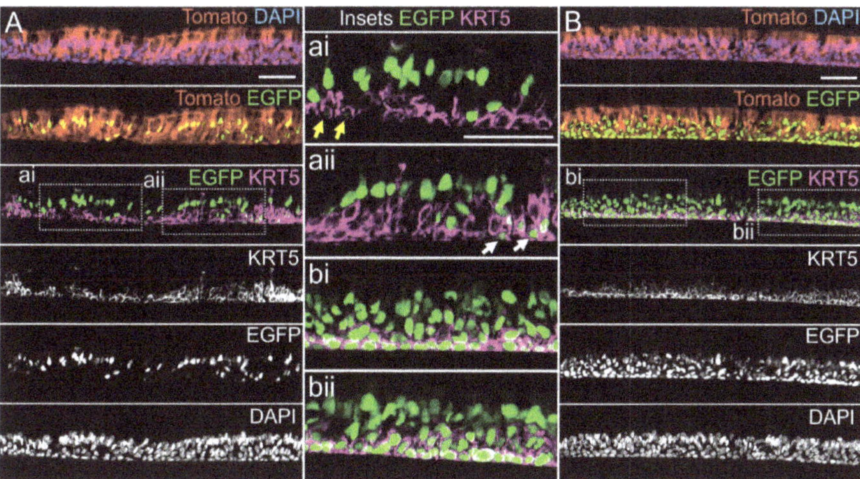

Figure 4. Lentiviral-mediated basal cell detargeting of EGFP following differentiation at an air–liquid interface. Primary human basal cells were transduced with LV-dt/EGFP-miRT or LV-dt/EGFP-RmiRT vectors and expanded for 1–2 days before seeding for differentiation in air–liquid interface (ALI) cultures. (**A,B**) Confocal microscopic images of (**A**) LV-dt/EGFP-miRT and (**B**) LV-dt/EGFP-RmiRT transduced ALI culture using sections immunostained for KRT5 (keratin-5) and imaged for KRT5, EGFP, and Tomato expression with DAPI to mark nuclei. Dual and single channel images are shown. Enlarged boxed regions in (**A,B**) are shown in the middle column. Scale bar, 50 μm.

We next performed similar studies in airway organoid cultures generated from LV-dt/EGFP-miRT and LV-dt/EGFP-RmiRT transduced basal cells (Figure 5A). These airway organoids mature with time to form an external basal cell layer and internal luminal cell layer composed of differentiated columnar cells. Similar to ALI cultures, confocal imaging of intact organoids demonstrated that LV-dt/EGFP-RmiRT transduced organoids contained EGFP expressing cells that spanned the outer basal cell layer as well as the differentiated luminal cell layer. By contrast, Tomato-positive LV-dt/EGFP-miRT transduced cells of the organoid lacked EGFP expression in the outer basal cell layer, but EGFP-positive luminal cells were observed. Tomato expression was dimmer than in the outer layer of basal cells in both groups, similar to ALI cultures, suggesting that the PGK promoter may be less active in the basal cells.

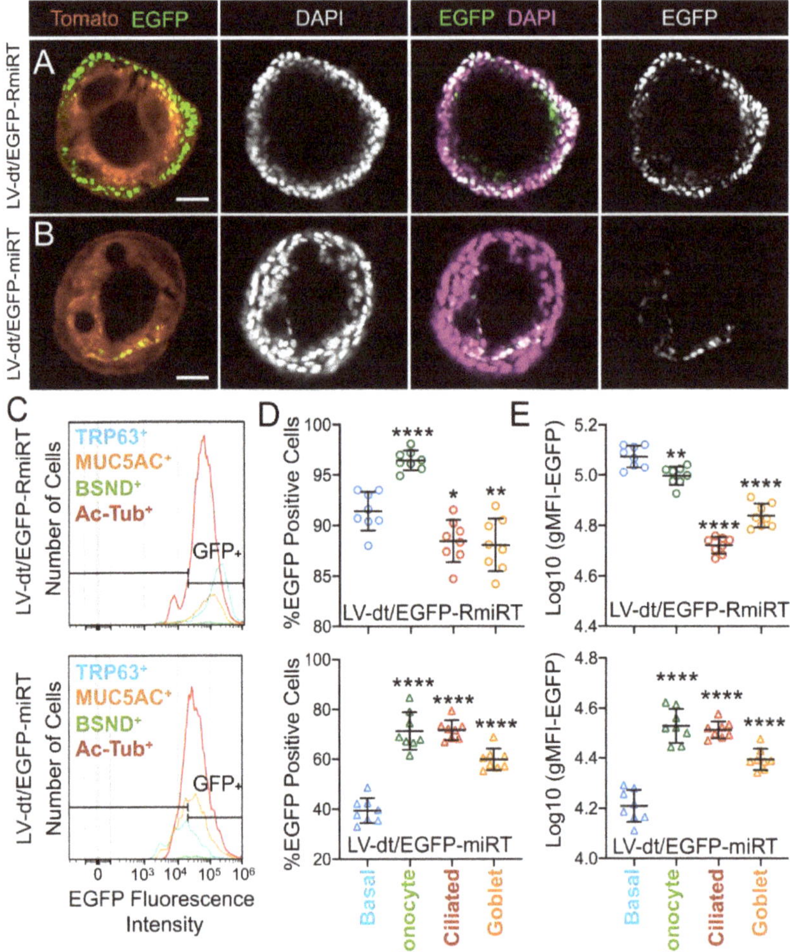

Figure 5. Basal cell detargeting of a reporter transgene in differentiated cell types of ALI cultures. (**A**,**B**) Human basal cells were transduced with (**A**) LV-dt/EGFP-RmiRT or (**B**) LV-dt/EGFP-miRT and expanded for 1–2 days prior to seeding in organoid culture. Confocal microscopic images of live organoids stained with the Hoescht 33342 nuclei marker. Single and dual channel images are pseudocolored to better project nuclear EGFP expression. Scale bar, 50μm. (**C–E**) Primary basal cells were transduced with LV-dt/EGFP-RmiRT or LV-dt/EGFP-miRT viruses and then FACS was used to isolated pure Tomato-positive basal cells. These cells were expanded in culture and then seeded into ALI cultures for differentiation and then detached and immunostained for quantification of EGFP expression in various cells types by flow cytometer. (**C**) Epithelial lineages were stained for TRP63/p63 (basal cells; blue), BSND (ionocytes; green), alpha-tubulin (ciliated), and MUC5AC (goblet cells; orange). Representative histogram distributions of lineage-labeled cell populations treated transduced with LV-dt/EGFP-RmiRT (top) or LV-dt/EGFP-miRT (bottom). (**D**) Percentage of EGFP-positive cells for each lineage using the gate shown in (**C**) which captures 90% of EGFP-positive basal cells in the control LV-dt/EGFP-RmiRT vector group. (**E**) Mean fluorescent intensity (MFI) of lineage-labeled populations. Statistics represent a one-way ANOVA with Dunnett's multiple comparison test against the basal cell population: * $p < 0.01$, ** $p < 0.05$, **** $p < 0.0001$. Data show the mean +/-SD for $N = 8$ transwells for each condition.

To quantify the extent of detargeting in basal cells, we transduced primary human basal cells with LV-dt/EGFP-miRT or LV-dt/EGFP-RmiRT vector systems and FACS isolated Tomato-positive cells for expansion in SAGM-EA prior to seeding into ALI cultures. Well-differentiated ALI cultures were then dissociated, and the single cell suspension of epithelial cells was fixed and stained for markers of basal cells (TRP63), ciliated cells (acetylated tubulin), goblet cells (MUC5AC), and ionocytes (BSND). These populations were then subjected to flow cytometer and the percentages of EGFP-positive cells for each cell phenotype quantified (Figure 5C–E). As expected from confocal imaging of ALI cultures (Figure 4), the fluorescent intensity of all cell types in the LV-dt/EGFP-miRT group was lower than that of LV-dt/EGFP-RmiRT, suggesting that inclusion of the miRT-106b target sequences generally reduces expression of the EGFP transgene. However, quantification of the percentage of EGFP-positive cells demonstrated the largest drop for miRT vs. RmiRT expression in TRP63-positive basal cells (2.3-fold) (Figure 5D). Furthermore, in LV-dt/EGFP-RmiRT transduced cells, the percentage of EGFP-positive basal cells was significantly lower than ciliated and goblet cells, whereas the opposite was observed in LV-dt/EGFP-miRT transduced cells (Figure 5D). Additionally, the mean fluorescent intensity (MFI, calculated as the geometric mean) of EGFP was the highest in basal cells of the LV-dt/EGFP-RmiRT control group, supporting confocal imaging of ALI demonstrating the strongest EGFP expression in KRT5-positive basal cells with this vector (Figure 4B, bi, bii). By contrast, the MFI was the lowest in the LV-dt/EGFP-miRT transduced basal cells as compared to ionocytes, ciliated cells and goblet cells (Figure 5E), similar to those observed histologic studies (Figure 4A, ai, aii). Overall, these findings suggest that the miRT-106b sequences effectively reduce expression of EGFP in basal cells.

An unexpected finding from these cellular phenotyping studies of LV-dt/EGFP-miRT- and LV-dt/EGFP-RmiRT-transduced epithelia was a significant shift in the number of goblet cells and ionocytes (Table 1). The largest shift occurred in the percentage of MUC5AC-positive goblet cells, rising 2-fold ($p < 0.0001$) in LV-dt/EGFP-miRT transduced epithelia as compared to the RmiRT control vector. By contrast, the percentage of ionocytes marginally declined in the LV-dt/EGFP-miRT group ($p < 0.0388$), while the percentage of basal cells and ciliated cells was not significantly different between the two groups. These findings raise the interesting possibility that high-level expression of mRNA containing the miRT sequence could potentially sequester miR-106b and impact processes involved in goblet cell and ionocyte specification.

Table 1. Distribution of cell types in differentiated ALI cultures.

Vector	% Basal Cells (TRP63+)	% Ionocytes (BSND+)	% Ciliated Cells (Ac-Tubulin+)	% Goblet Cells (MUC5AC+)
LV-dt/EGFP-RmiRT	21.8+/−3.8 *	0.82+/−0.02	44.3+/−1.6	11.2+/−0.8
LV-dt/EGFP-miRT	22.4+/−1.5	0.72+/−0.04	41.5+/−0.9	21.9+/−1.2
p-value **	0.7768	0.0388	0.1567	<0.0001

The percentage of viable cells positive for each of the phenotypic cellular markers is shown (TRP63-basal cells; BSND-ionocytes; acetylated tubulin-ciliated cells; MUC5AC-goblet cells). Cells not positive for any of the four antibodies were 21.9% and 12.5% for LV-dt/EGFP-RmiRT- and LV-dt/EGFP-miRT-transduced epithelia, respectively. * Mean +/-SEM. ** Statistical comparisons by Welch's *t* test.

3.5. Basal Cell-Detargeting of CFTR Expression Alters Functional Complementation in CF Airway Epithelia

To test our primary hypothesis that detargeting of CFTR in basal cells would improve complementation in CF airway epithelia, we replaced EGFP in LV-dt/EGFP-miRT with CFTR to generate the pLV-dt/CFTR-miRT lentiviral vector. Our control vector (pLV-dt/CFTR-Ø) was identical to pLV-dt/CFTR-miRT but lacked the miR-106b target sequences (Figure 6A). Freshly isolated CF human tracheobronchial basal cells were transduced with each vector and expanded 4 days before seeding into transwells for ALI culture. Contrary to our initial hypothesis, ALI cultures transduced with LV-dt/CFTR-Ø gave rise to ~3.5-fold greater CFTR-mediated Cl⁻ currents than that of LV-dt/CFTR-miRT transduced ALI cultures (Figure 6B), even though both cultures expressed similar levels of *CFTR* mRNA, which were 3.2-fold (LV-dt/CFTR-Ø) and 2.7-fold (LV-dt/CFTR-miRT) higher levels than the mock-infected group. Characteristic of CFTR, these currents were induced by cAMP agonists (IBMX/Forskolin) and inhibited by the CFTR channel blocker GlyH101. The slightly lower expression of CFTR mRNA in the LV-dt/CFTR-miRT transduced cultures was expected, consistent with detargeted expression in basal cells.

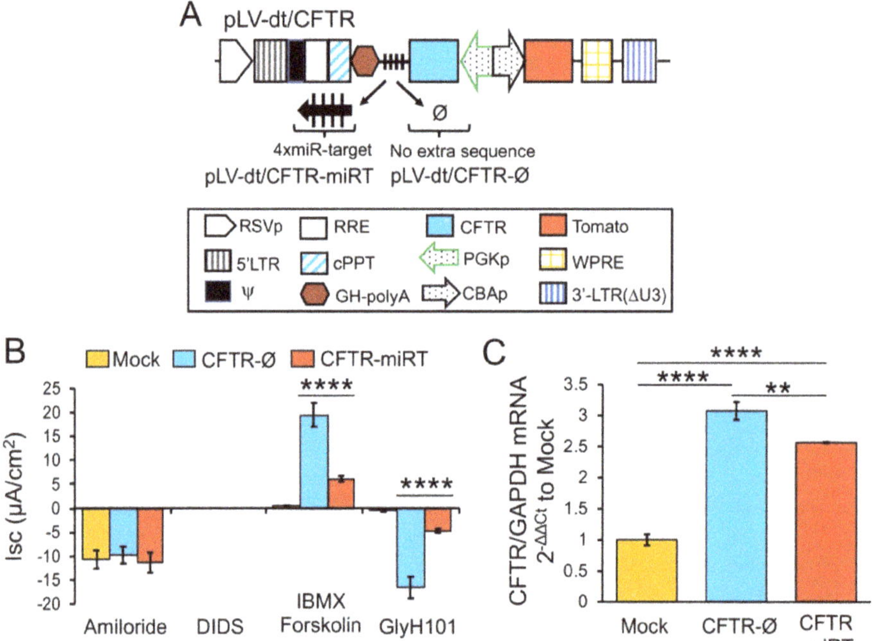

Figure 6. Detargeting CFTR expression in basal cells impacts the level of complementation in CF airway epithelia. (**A**) Diagram of lenti-vector containing CFTR expression cassette in reverse orientation. The PGK promoter (PGKp) drives expression of CFTR with the miR-106b target sequence (4× miR target or mirT) in the 3′UTR. CBA promoter drives expression of Tomato as a reporter gene for viral transduction. pLV-dt/CFTR-Ø is a control vector with no miRT sequence. Box (below) is a legend for each shape in the diagram that highlights the components of these proviral plasmids as described in detail within the Figure 2A legend. (**B**) Short-circuit current (Isc) measurements of differentiated air-liquid interface cultures seeded with transduced at basal cells. Mock, mock-infected cells. PGK-CFTR-Ø, cells transduced by LV-dt/CFTR-Ø; PGK-CFTR-miRT, cells transduced by LV-dt/CFTR-miRT. Amiloride was used to block ENaC-mediated Na$^+$ currents. 4,4′-Diisothiocyanatostilbene-2,2′-disulfonic acid (DIDS) was use to inhibit most non-CFTR chloride channel. 3-isobutyl-2-methylxanthine (IBMX) and Forskolin was used for activate CFTR channels. N-(2-naphtalenyl)-(3.5-dibromo-2.4-dihydroxyphenyl)methylene glycine hydrazide (GlyH101) was used to block CFTR. Data show the mean +/-SEM for N = 6 transwells for each condition. (**C**) Relative quantification of CFTR mRNA normalized to GAPDH mRNA from each sample used in B. For B and C, the statistics used is one-way ANOVA, Tukey's multiple comparisons test. ****, $p < 0.0001$. **, $p = 0.0025$. Data show the mean +/-SEM for N = 3 independent samples for each condition.

4. Discussion

Multipotent basal cells are generally considered the primary stem cell of the large conducting airways [27] and thus are a primary target for stem cell-based genetic therapies for CF. CFTR is expressed in a subpopulation of transitional basal cells (i.e., intermediate basal cells) that are fated to become secretory cells (i.e., goblet cells and club cells) [6,28]. CFTR is also expressed at low levels in a subpopulation of secretory cells and at high levels in pulmonary ionocytes [5,6]. The function of CFTR expression in transitional basal cells remains unclear, but it stands to reason that this expression could be a precursor state to CFTR-expressing daughter cells [3]. The contribution of CFTR expression in secretory cells and ionocytes to the overall level of transepithelial ion transport in airway epithelium is also a source of controversy [3]. Given that CFTR is not expressed in proliferating airway basal cells and the potential that basal cell CFTR expression may impact fate decisions, we reasoned that developing a lentiviral vector that could more closely reproduce endogenous multipotent and transitional basal cell CFTR expression patterns would have utility for CF cell-based therapies. Thus, we sought to develop a lentiviral vector that would repress CFTR expression in proliferating multipotent basal cells and activate CFTR expression in transitional basal cells as they commit to differentiate.

Gene replacement cell-based therapies for CF will require the expansion of basal cells in conditionally reprogrammed culture and the introduction of a corrected *CFTR* gene using an integrating approach (e.g., lentivirus) [29,30]. It was on this rationale that we designed a lentiviral vector with bi-directional promoters capable of carrying miRT sequences within a heterologous 3′-UTR of the reverse oriented target gene. Through bioinformatics and experimentation, we identified miR-106b as being highly expressed in both proliferating human tracheobronchial and nasal basal cells (Figure 1), but absent in differentiated columnar cells. Thus, the miRT for miR-106b appeared to be suitable for approaching our studies. Notably, the regulated miRT gene must be placed in the reverse orientation since a heterologous UTR in the direct orientation would prematurely terminate the viral genomic RNA during virus production [31]. Lentiviruses with reverse-oriented expression cassettes produce low viral titers due to a double-stranded RNA response and cleavage of the vector RNA genome by cellular Dicer [31,32]. However, previous attempts have successfully produced high titer virus when an inducible promoter is used to drive the reverse-oriented gene of interest [31].

Our studies required the use of a strong promoter for both expression cassettes and, like others, we found titers to be low within our bidirectional pLV-dt/EGFP vector. We improved the inherently low titer using a suppressor of RNA silencing (SRS), B2 protein from flock house virus. Although most viral infections activate RNAi responses in the cell against the virus [33,34], only a few have looked into using RNAi suppressors in animal viral vector production [35,36]. In lentiviruses, potential SRSs include Nef and Tat [37,38]; Tat is included with psPAX2 packaging plasmid and may help protect the lentiviral genome during virus production. By utilizing the B2 protein, pLV-dt/EGFP vector production was further increased 3-fold (Figure 2). In this study, we only used B2, but other SRSs of some well-known plant and animal virus SRSs [33,39,40] are worth investigating and may further improve virus production with a bi-directional vector. One downside of using the 293T-B2 cell line is that the cells seem to be even less tightly attached to the surface of the culture dish than the wild-type 293T, so when adding transfection reagents or media it should be carried out very carefully. To mitigate this problem, poly-lysine coating the culture dish may help the cells to attach more tightly and help improve the virus titer.

Our studies evaluating miR-106b-mediating detargeting using the pLV-dt/EGFP-miRT vector system demonstrated robust shut-off of the EGFP-miRT reporter in proliferating basal cells (Figure 3). Adjusting for differences in functional titer, the miRT-106b reduced EGFP expression 54-fold in proliferating human basal cells as compared to the RmiRT-106b control vector. However, when the pLV-dt/EGFP-miRT basal cells were differentiated at an ALI, there was a subset of basal cells that were not detargeted and a subset of columnar cells that were detargeted (Figure 4). We do not know whether quiescent G0 and intermediate basal cells express miR-106b and this could impact detargeting of pLV-dt/EGFP-miRT in KRT5-positive basal cells. The finding of miRT-106b detargeted columnar cells also suggests that at least in differentiated ALI culture systems, miR-106b expression is expressed or retained in a larger subset of columnar cells than previously observed in human nasal epithelia [14]. Culture conditions likely impacted miR-106b expression and the level of detargeting since organoid cultures demonstrated robust basal cell detargeting with the pLV-dt/EGFP-miRT as compared to the

RmiRT-106b control vector. It is also worth noting that in ALI cultures the CBA promoter used to drive EGFP expression in the pLV-dt/EGFP is robustly expressed in basal cells, while the PGK promoter used to drive Tomato expression is more active in columnar cells and less active in basal cells (Figure 4). These differences were even more greatly accentuated in organoid cultures (Figure 5A,B) where very weak EGFP expression was observed in the luminal cell layer for both vector systems.

Due to the relative activity of the CBA and PGK promoters in basal vs. columnar cells of ALI cultures and organoids, we altered the sequence of the promoters in our pLV-dt/CFTR-miRT and pLV-dt/CFTR-Ø vector systems. Since the PGK promoter was weaker in basal cells and stronger in columnar cells, it was used to drive CFTR expression, thus accentuating the detargeting by miRT-106b in basal cells and facilitating CFTR expression in differentiated cells that participate in ion transport (Figure 6A). Similarly, the CBA promoter had greater expression in basal cells and thus was used to drive Tomato expression. Contrary to our original hypothesis, CF ALI cultures transduced with LV-dt/CFTR-miRT had significantly less functional correction of CFTR currents as compared to LV-dt/CFTR-Ø (Figure 6B).

While the reason for the observed difference in CFTR complementation is currently unknown, there are three potential explanations that warrant further investigation. First, LV-dt/EGFP-miRT transduced ALI cultures had a subpopulation of columnar cells that were Tomato-positive and EGFP-negative. This phenotype was rarely observed in control ALI transduced with the pLV-dt/EGFP-RmiRT vector. Thus, these results would be consistent with expression of miR-106b in a subset of columnar cells that contribute to CFTR-mediated current.

Second, expression of the EGFP-miRT-106b transcript in basal cells led to significant changes in two cell populations when differentiated at ALI (i.e., ionocytes and goblet cells) (Table 1). The decrease in the percentage in ionocytes was relatively small (12%), while the increase in goblet cells was large (200%). Both of these cellular compartments express CFTR in a subpopulation of each cell type. One possibility for this vector-related shift in differentiated cell types is that high-level expression of EGFP-miRT-106b transcripts may sequester miR-106b and act like a miR-inhibitor. Thus, it is possible that inhibiting miR-106b activates differentiation toward columnar cells that cannot participate in CFTR-mediated ion transport. This possibility can be supported by two interpretations of CFTR mRNA levels shown in Figure 6C, which are not mutually exclusive. The mild reduction in total CFTR mRNA levels in LV-dt/CFTR-miRT transduced epithelia is consistent with successful CFTR detargeting in basal cells, where the decrease may represent expression of CFTR in basal cells. However, we cannot rule out that inhibiting miR-106b may have led to an expansion of cell types that cannot facilitate CFTR-mediated anion transport, and that we cannot currently account for with the flow cytometry panel described. Future studies using single-cell RNAseq could help to understand the shift in cellular compartments and their *CFTR* expression patterns.

The last formal possibility for explaining these results, however unlikely, is the contribution of basal cell CFTR expression to transepithelial anion transport. Current wisdom suggests that only channels that reside in the apical and basolateral membranes of polarized epithelia contribute to transepithelial ion movement. However, very little is known about why CFTR is expressed in basal cells, so we cannot rule this out as a formal possibility.

miR-106b is one of the three miRNAs in the polycistronic miR-106b ~25 cluster within an intron of the *MCM7* gene. MCM7 is part of the DNA replication initiation complex, but its expression is not necessarily coupled to that of miR-106b [19,20]. miR-106b can also play roles in cell-cycle regulation of both stem cells and cancer cells [16,41]. For example, expression of this miRNA enhances cell growth [42], promotes migration of certain cancer cells [43], and promotes cell cycle progression [44]. In SAGM-EA conditionally reprogramming media, basal cells are locked into a self-renewing state. However, it remains unclear if miR-106b plays a role in cell cycle progression of basal cells cultured under these conditions. We did not observe a major difference in morphology or growth of cells expressing the miRT-106b target in either EGFP or CFTR transcripts, and this might suggest that sequestration of miR-106b from its native targets does not occur if these biologic functions of miR-106b are relevant to airway basal cells.

5. Conclusions

This study has strengths and limitations. One limitation includes a clearer understanding of cellular expression patterns of miR-106b in ALI cultures. While we had initial chosen miR-106b as a candidate based on its lack of expression in nasal columnar cells, our reporter gene expression studies suggest that it may be expressed in a subset of columnar cells. Future studies evaluating miR-106b expression in FACS-isolated cell types would allow for a clearer interpretation of how the miRT-106b sequence alters CFTR complementation. A second limitation is the fact the promoters used in the bicistronic vectors studied have slightly different activities in basal vs. columnar cells. The use of a bidirectional promoter might be a better approach for future studies, however, the most commonly used major immediate-early cytomegaloviruses enhancer/promoter is typically inactivated in lentiviral vectors by methylation. A strength of these studies includes the development of miRT-106b vectors that can clearly detarget expression in proliferating basal cells. Such a vector system can be used to study basal cell differentiation through the regulated expression of transcription factors that would otherwise terminally differentiate proliferating basal cells. A second strength includes the novel findings that miR-106b appears to be expressed in specific populations of cells that contribute to CFTR-mediated transepithelial ion transport and/or that certain cell types can express CFTR mRNA but not participate in CFTR-dependent transepithelial anion transport. Although more research is needed to understand the mechanism, the finding itself has implications for CF gene therapy as it implies unique cellular targets for CFTR complementation.

Supplementary Materials: The following are available online at http://www.mdpi.com/2073-4425/11/10/1169/s1, Table S1: PCR array table.

Author Contributions: Conceptualization, S.H.C., Z.Y., and J.F.E.; methodology, S.H.C., R.E.R., E.J.D., G.S.R.I., D.A.S., T.J.L., G.N.G., Z.F., M.C.W., T.I.A.E., W.S.S., Y.Z., Z.Y., and J.F.E.; formal analysis, S.H.C., R.E.R., G.S.R.I., D.A.S., E.J.D., T.J.L., W.S.S., Z.Y., and J.F.E.; investigation, S.H.C., R.E.R., E.J.D., G.S.R.I., X.L., M.L. Z.Y., and J.F.E.; resources, E.J.D., D.A.S., Z.Y., and J.F.E.; writing—original draft preparation, S.H.C., and R.E.R.; writing—review and editing, T.J.L., G.S.R.I., D.A.S., Z.Y., and J.F.E.; supervision, Z.Y., and J.F.E.; project administration, J.F.E..; funding acquisition, J.F.E. All authors have read and agreed to the published version of the manuscript.

Funding: This work was supported by grants from the National Institutes of Health P30 DK054759, P01 HL152960, R01 DK047967 to J.F.E., and a grant from the Cystic Fibrosis Foundation to J.F.E. G.S.R.I. was supported by two T32s HL007638 and GM007337.

Acknowledgments: University of Iowa, Carver College of Medicine, Flow Cytometry core, Genomics Core, Microscopy Core, Tissue Culture Core. ALN Rao (University of California at Riverside) and Jang-kyun Seo (Seoul National University, South Korea) for the plasmid containing FHV RNA1 gene.

Conflicts of Interest: The authors declare no conflict of interest.

Abbreviations

CF	cystic fibrosis
CFTR	cystic fibrosis transmembrane conductance regulator
miR	microRNA
3'-UTR	3'-untranslated region
PGK	mouse phosphoglycerate kinase 1 promoter
CBA	CMV early enhancer-chicken beta-actin promoter
Tomato	dTomato, dt
SAGM-EA	Small Airway Epithelial Growth Medium with extra additives

References

1. Riordan, J.R.; Rommens, J.M.; Kerem, B.; Alon, N.; Rozmahel, R.; Grzelczak, Z.; Zielenski, J.; Lok, S.; Plavsic, N.; Chou, J.L.; et al. Identification of the cystic fibrosis gene: Cloning and characterization of complementary DNA. *Science* **1989**, *245*, 1066–1073. [CrossRef] [PubMed]
2. Xie, Y.; Ostedgaard, L.; Abou Alaiwa, M.H.; Lu, L.; Fischer, A.J.; Stoltz, D.A. Mucociliary Transport in Healthy and Cystic Fibrosis Pig Airways. *Ann. Am. Thorac. Soc.* **2018**, *15*, S171–S176. [CrossRef] [PubMed]
3. Tang, Y.; Yan, Z.; Engelhardt, J.F. Viral Vectors, Animal Models, and Cellular Targets for Gene Therapy of Cystic Fibrosis Lung Disease. *Hum. Gene Ther.* **2020**, *31*, 524–537. [CrossRef] [PubMed]
4. Rock, J.R.; Randell, S.H.; Hogan, B.L. Airway basal stem cells: A perspective on their roles in epithelial homeostasis and remodeling. *Dis. Model. Mech.* **2010**, *3*, 545–556. [CrossRef] [PubMed]
5. Montoro, D.T.; Haber, A.L.; Biton, M.; Vinarsky, V.; Lin, B.; Birket, S.E.; Yuan, F.; Chen, S.; Leung, H.M.; Villoria, J.; et al. A revised airway epithelial hierarchy includes CFTR-expressing ionocytes. *Nature* **2018**, *560*, 319–324. [CrossRef] [PubMed]
6. Plasschaert, L.W.; Zilionis, R.; Choo-Wing, R.; Savova, V.; Knehr, J.; Roma, G.; Klein, A.M.; Jaffe, A.B. A single-cell atlas of the airway epithelium reveals the CFTR-rich pulmonary ionocyte. *Nature* **2018**, *560*, 377–381. [CrossRef] [PubMed]
7. Carraro, G.; Mulay, A.; Yao, C.; Mizuno, T.; Konda, B.; Petrov, M.; Lafkas, D.; Arron, J.R.; Hogaboam, C.M.; Chen, P.; et al. Single Cell Reconstruction of Human Basal Cell Diversity in Normal and IPF Lung. *Am. J. Respir. Crit. Care Med.* **2020**. [CrossRef]
8. Xu, Y.; Mizuno, T.; Sridharan, A.; Du, Y.; Guo, M.; Tang, J.; Wikenheiser-Brokamp, K.A.; Perl, A.T.; Funari, V.A.; Gokey, J.J.; et al. Single-cell RNA sequencing identifies diverse roles of epithelial cells in idiopathic pulmonary fibrosis. *JCI Insight* **2016**, *1*, e90558. [CrossRef]
9. Mou, H.; Vinarsky, V.; Tata, P.R.; Brazauskas, K.; Choi, S.H.; Crooke, A.K.; Zhang, B.; Solomon, G.M.; Turner, B.; Bihler, H.; et al. Dual SMAD Signaling Inhibition Enables Long-Term Expansion of Diverse Epithelial Basal Cells. *Cell Stem Cell* **2016**. [CrossRef]
10. Barde, I.; Salmon, P.; Trono, D. Production and titration of lentiviral vectors. *Curr. Protoc. Neurosci.* **2010**, *53*, 4–21. [CrossRef]
11. Denning, W.; Das, S.; Guo, S.; Xu, J.; Kappes, J.C.; Hel, Z. Optimization of the transductional efficiency of lentiviral vectors: Effect of sera and polycations. *Mol. Biotechnol.* **2013**, *53*, 308–314. [CrossRef]
12. Sun, X.; Olivier, A.K.; Liang, B.; Yi, Y.; Sui, H.; Evans, T.I.; Zhang, Y.; Zhou, W.; Tyler, S.R.; Fisher, J.T.; et al. Lung phenotype of juvenile and adult cystic fibrosis transmembrane conductance regulator-knockout ferrets. *Am. J. Respir. Cell Mol. Biol.* **2014**, *50*, 502–512. [CrossRef] [PubMed]
13. Yan, Z.; Sun, X.; Feng, Z.; Li, G.; Fisher, J.T.; Stewart, Z.A.; Engelhardt, J.F. Optimization of Recombinant Adeno-Associated Virus-Mediated Expression for Large Transgenes, Using a Synthetic Promoter and Tandem Array Enhancers. *Hum. Gene Ther.* **2015**, *26*, 334–346. [CrossRef] [PubMed]
14. Marcet, B.; Chevalier, B.; Luxardi, G.; Coraux, C.; Zaragosi, L.E.; Cibois, M.; Robbe-Sermesant, K.; Jolly, T.; Cardinaud, B.; Moreilhon, C.; et al. Control of vertebrate multiciliogenesis by miR-449 through direct repression of the Delta/Notch pathway. *Nat. Cell Biol.* **2011**, *13*, 693–699. [CrossRef] [PubMed]
15. Martinez-Anton, A.; Sokolowska, M.; Kern, S.; Davis, A.S.; Alsaaty, S.; Taubenberger, J.K.; Sun, J.; Cai, R.; Danner, R.L.; Eberlein, M.; et al. Changes in microRNA and mRNA expression with differentiation of human bronchial epithelial cells. *Am. J. Respir. Cell Mol. Biol.* **2013**, *49*, 384–395. [CrossRef]
16. Mehlich, D.; Garbicz, F.; Wlodarski, P.K. The emerging roles of the polycistronic miR-106b approximately 25 cluster in cancer-A comprehensive review. *Biomed Pharmacother.* **2018**, *107*, 1183–1195. [CrossRef]
17. Kim, Y.K.; Kim, V.N. Processing of intronic microRNAs. *EMBO J.* **2007**, *26*, 775–783. [CrossRef]
18. Zhou, Y.; Hu, Y.; Yang, M.; Jat, P.; Li, K.; Lombardo, Y.; Xiong, D.; Coombes, R.C.; Raguz, S.; Yague, E. The miR-106b~25 cluster promotes bypass of doxorubicin-induced senescence and increase in motility and invasion by targeting the E-cadherin transcriptional activator EP300. *Cell Death Differ.* **2014**, *21*, 462–474. [CrossRef]
19. Chuang, T.D.; Luo, X.; Panda, H.; Chegini, N. miR-93/106b and their host gene, MCM7, are differentially expressed in leiomyomas and functionally target F3 and IL-8. *Mol. Endocrinol.* **2012**, *26*, 1028–1042. [CrossRef]
20. Haldar, S.; Roy, A.; Banerjee, S. Differential regulation of MCM7 and its intronic miRNA cluster miR-106b-25 during megakaryopoiesis induced polyploidy. *RNA Biol.* **2014**, *11*, 1137–1147. [CrossRef]

21. Kan, T.; Sato, F.; Ito, T.; Matsumura, N.; David, S.; Cheng, Y.; Agarwal, R.; Paun, B.C.; Jin, Z.; Olaru, A.V.; et al. The miR-106b-25 Polycistron, Activated by Genomic Amplification, Functions as an Oncogene by Suppressing p21 and Bim. *Gastroenterology* **2009**, *136*, 1689–1700. [CrossRef]

22. Smith, A.L.; Iwanaga, R.; Drasin, D.J.; Micalizzi, D.S.; Vartuli, R.L.; Tan, A.C.; Ford, H.L. The miR-106b-25 cluster targets Smad7, activates TGF-beta signaling, and induces EMT and tumor initiating cell characteristics downstream of Six1 in human breast cancer. *Oncogene* **2012**, *31*, 5162–5171. [CrossRef] [PubMed]

23. Chao, J.A.; Lee, J.H.; Chapados, B.R.; Debler, E.W.; Schneemann, A.; Williamson, J.R. Dual modes of RNA-silencing suppression by Flock House virus protein B2. *Nat. Struct. Mol. Biol.* **2005**, *12*, 952–957. [CrossRef] [PubMed]

24. Li, H.; Li, W.X.; Ding, S.W. Induction and suppression of RNA silencing by an animal virus. *Science* **2002**, *296*, 1319–1321. [CrossRef]

25. Lingel, A.; Simon, B.; Izaurralde, E.; Sattler, M. The structure of the flock house virus B2 protein, a viral suppressor of RNA interference, shows a novel mode of double-stranded RNA recognition. *EMBO Rep.* **2005**, *6*, 1149–1155. [CrossRef] [PubMed]

26. Rawson, J.M.O.; Nikolaitchik, O.A.; Keele, B.F.; Pathak, V.K.; Hu, W.S. Recombination is required for efficient HIV-1 replication and the maintenance of viral genome integrity. *Nucleic. Acids Res.* **2018**, *46*, 10535–10545. [CrossRef] [PubMed]

27. Rock, J.R.; Onaitis, M.W.; Rawlins, E.L.; Lu, Y.; Clark, C.P.; Xue, Y.; Randell, S.H.; Hogan, B.L. Basal cells as stem cells of the mouse trachea and human airway epithelium. *Proc. Natl. Acad. Sci. USA* **2009**, *106*, 12771–12775. [CrossRef] [PubMed]

28. Engelhardt, J.F.; Yankaskas, J.R.; Ernst, S.A.; Yang, Y.; Marino, C.R.; Boucher, R.C.; Cohn, J.A.; Wilson, J.M. Submucosal glands are the predominant site of CFTR expression in the human bronchus. *Nat. Genet.* **1992**, *2*, 240–248. [CrossRef]

29. Flotte, T.R.; Ng, P.; Dylla, D.E.; McCray, P.B., Jr.; Wang, G.; Kolls, J.K.; Hu, J. Viral vector-mediated and cell-based therapies for treatment of cystic fibrosis. *Mol. Ther.* **2007**, *15*, 229–241. [CrossRef]

30. Yan, Z.; McCray, P.B., Jr.; Engelhardt, J.F. Advances in gene therapy for cystic fibrosis lung disease. *Hum. Mol. Genet.* **2019**, *28*, R88–R94. [CrossRef]

31. Poling, B.C.; Tsai, K.; Kang, D.; Ren, L.; Kennedy, E.M.; Cullen, B.R. A lentiviral vector bearing a reverse intron demonstrates superior expression of both proteins and microRNAs. *RNA Biol.* **2017**, *14*, 1570–1579. [CrossRef]

32. Liu, Y.P.; Vink, M.A.; Westerink, J.T.; Ramirez de Arellano, E.; Konstantinova, P.; Ter Brake, O.; Berkhout, B. Titers of lentiviral vectors encoding shRNAs and miRNAs are reduced by different mechanisms that require distinct repair strategies. *RNA* **2010**, *16*, 1328–1339. [CrossRef] [PubMed]

33. Ding, S.W.; Han, Q.; Wang, J.; Li, W.X. Antiviral RNA interference in mammals. *Curr. Opin. Immunol.* **2018**, *54*, 109–114. [CrossRef] [PubMed]

34. Son, K.N.; Liang, Z.; Lipton, H.L. Double-Stranded RNA Is Detected by Immunofluorescence Analysis in RNA and DNA Virus Infections, Including Those by Negative-Stranded RNA Viruses. *J. Virol.* **2015**, *89*, 9383–9392. [CrossRef] [PubMed]

35. Rauschhuber, C.; Mueck-Haeusl, M.; Zhang, W.; Nettelbeck, D.M.; Ehrhardt, A. RNAi suppressor P19 can be broadly exploited for enhanced adenovirus replication and microRNA knockdown experiments. *Sci. Rep.* **2013**, *3*, 1363. [CrossRef]

36. Liu, Y.; Zhang, L.; Zhang, Y.; Liu, D.; Du, E.; Yang, Z. Functional analysis of RNAi suppressor P19 on improving baculovirus yield and transgene expression in Sf9 cells. *Biotechnol. Lett.* **2015**, *37*, 2159–2166. [CrossRef]

37. Aqil, M.; Naqvi, A.R.; Bano, A.S.; Jameel, S. The HIV-1 Nef protein binds argonaute-2 and functions as a viral suppressor of RNA interference. *PLoS ONE* **2013**, *8*, e74472. [CrossRef]

38. Bennasser, Y.; Le, S.Y.; Benkirane, M.; Jeang, K.T. Evidence that HIV-1 encodes an siRNA and a suppressor of RNA silencing. *Immunity* **2005**, *22*, 607–619. [CrossRef]

39. de Vries, W.; Berkhout, B. RNAi suppressors encoded by pathogenic human viruses. *Int. J. Biochem. Cell Biol.* **2008**, *40*, 2007–2012. [CrossRef]

40. Maillard, P.V.; van der Veen, A.G.; Poirier, E.Z.; Reis e Sousa, C. Slicing and dicing viruses: Antiviral RNA interference in mammals. *EMBO J.* **2019**, *38*. [CrossRef]

41.	Mens, M.M.J.; Ghanbari, M. Cell Cycle Regulation of Stem Cells by MicroRNAs. *Stem Cell Rev. Rep.* **2018**, *14*, 309–322. [CrossRef]

42.	Li, Y.; Wang, Y.; Zhou, H.; Yong, Y.; Cao, Y. miR-106b promoted growth and inhibited apoptosis of nasopharyngeal carcinoma cells by suppressing the tumor suppressor PTEN. *Int. J. Clin. Exp. Pathol.* **2016**, *9*, 7078–7086.

43.	Cheng, Y.; Guo, Y.; Zhang, Y.; You, K.; Li, Z.; Geng, L. MicroRNA-106b is involved in transforming growth factor beta1-induced cell migration by targeting disabled homolog 2 in cervical carcinoma. *J. Exp. Clin. Cancer Res.* **2016**, *35*, 11. [CrossRef] [PubMed]

44.	Ivanovska, I.; Ball, A.S.; Diaz, R.L.; Magnus, J.F.; Kibukawa, M.; Schelter, J.M.; Kobayashi, S.V.; Lim, L.; Burchard, J.; Jackson, A.L.; et al. MicroRNAs in the miR-106b family regulate p21/CDKN1A and promote cell cycle progression. *Mol. Cell Biol.* **2008**, *28*, 2167–2174. [CrossRef] [PubMed]

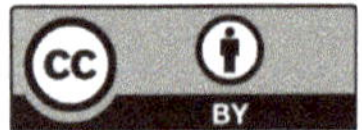

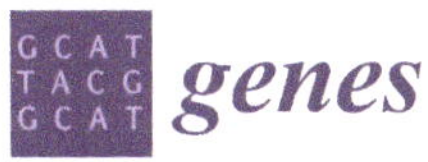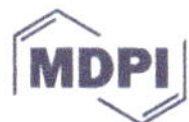

Article

Human Nasal Epithelial Organoids for Therapeutic Development in Cystic Fibrosis

Zhongyu Liu [1,2,†], Justin D. Anderson [1,2,†], Lily Deng [2], Stephen Mackay [1,2], Johnathan Bailey [2], Latona Kersh [1,3], Steven M. Rowe [1,2,3,4] and Jennifer S. Guimbellot [1,2,*]

[1] Gregory Fleming James Cystic Fibrosis Research Center, University of Alabama at Birmingham (UAB), Birmingham, AL 35294, USA; ZLiu@peds.uab.edu (Z.L.); jdanderson@peds.uab.edu (J.D.A.); MackaySS@EVMS.edu (S.M.); lkersh@peds.uab.edu (L.K.); srowe@uabmc.edu (S.M.R.)

[2] Department of Pediatrics, Division of Pulmonary and Sleep Medicine, UAB, Birmingham, AL 35233, USA; ldeng@uab.edu (L.D.); johnathb@uab.edu (J.B.)

[3] Department of Medicine, Division of Pulmonary, Allergy, and Critical Care Medicine, UAB, Birmingham, AL 35294, USA

[4] Department of Cell, Developmental and Integrative Biology, UAB, Birmingham, AL 35294, USA

[*] Correspondence: jguimbellot@peds.uab.edu; Tel.: +1-205-234-0250; Fax: +1-205-975-5983

[†] These authors contributed equally to this work.

Received: 6 April 2020; Accepted: 27 May 2020; Published: 29 May 2020

Abstract: We describe a human nasal epithelial (HNE) organoid model derived directly from patient samples that is well-differentiated and recapitulates the airway epithelium, including the expression of cilia, mucins, tight junctions, the cystic fibrosis transmembrane conductance regulator (CFTR), and ionocytes. This model requires few cells compared to airway epithelial monolayer cultures, with multiple outcome measurements depending on the application. A novel feature of the model is the predictive capacity of lumen formation, a marker of baseline CFTR function that correlates with short-circuit current activation of CFTR in monolayers and discriminates the cystic fibrosis (CF) phenotype from non-CF. Our HNE organoid model is amenable to automated measurements of forskolin-induced swelling (FIS), which distinguishes levels of CFTR activity. While the apical side is not easily accessible, RNA- and DNA-based therapies intended for systemic administration could be evaluated in vitro, or it could be used as an ex vivo biomarker of successful repair of a mutant gene. In conclusion, this highly differentiated airway epithelial model could serve as a surrogate biomarker to assess correction of the mutant gene in CF or other diseases, recapitulating the phenotypic and genotypic diversity of the population.

Keywords: cystic fibrosis; CFTR; human nasal epithelial cells; organoids; biomarker; functional assay; CFTR modulators; pre-clinical in vitro models

---

1. Introduction

Cystic fibrosis (CF) is an autosomal recessive genetic disorder caused by disease-causing variants in the CF transmembrane conductance regulator (CFTR) gene. CFTR is expressed on the epithelial cells of several organs, including the lung, intestine, pancreas, and liver. In the lung, functional CFTR regulates ion transfer in the airway lumen, balancing the salt, pH, and fluid content as well as influencing the viscosity and organization of mucus. In CF, this balance is impaired, resulting in thick secretions poorly transported out of the lung by the mucociliary apparatus, leading to a cycle of inflammation and infection that ultimately causes significant morbidity and mortality among the CF population.

Identifying an effective cure for CF is critical. While new drugs called CFTR modulators have been identified that are highly effective for the treatment of CF [1–3], they target the protein defect in CFTR but do not permanently correct the genetic mutation. Furthermore, although a recent three-drug CFTR modulator therapy was approved for ~90% of patients as defined by the genotype [4,5], no treatment for the underlying defect exists for the remaining 10%. This includes patients with rare mutations unsuccessfully rescued by modulators. Ideally, correction of the mutation using gene therapy or other nucleotide-based approaches would be permanently curative.

The availability of in vitro models to test correction of the genetic defect in CF has been somewhat limited. In this study, we describe the development of an in vitro model derived from patient samples (nasal brush biopsies), which recapitulates the highly differentiated airway epithelium. While we and others reported similar models derived from nasal tissue, some [6–9] are grown from differentiated cells already in an intact monolayer, either from excised nasal polyps or brush biopsies. In these cases, the apical membrane is to the exterior of the structure, and the basolateral side is not accessible. These spheroids are free-floating, which makes imaging difficult, are of limited quantity, and are derived from cells that are not passaged or expanded, making higher throughput applications impossible. One similar model [10] employs a labor-intensive technical approach that is not amenable to high-throughput applications, which the authors cite as a specific limitation. In contrast, our organoid assay utilizes small amounts of biopsy material that are expanded to millions of cells, which can provide sufficient replicates for moderate-to-high-throughput applications; was optimized for uniformity in organoid distribution and morphology to aid in automated imaging and analysis; and has a greater capacity to detect subtle differences. The model has several potential outcome measures, including quantitating the kinetics of CFTR rescue on fluid transport; fluorescent microscopy to qualitatively determine gene expression; and evaluating the functional activities through the use of novel imaging techniques (micro-optical coherence tomography, μOCT). These are useful to assess the impact of any curative therapy targeted to CFTR mutations [11–16]. Because this model is derived directly from patient samples, we postulate that it will reproduce the phenotypic and genotypic diversity that exists among the CF population and will be more likely to predict the effectiveness of the therapy across all patients.

2. Materials and Methods

2.1. Patient Samples

Non-CF healthy control subjects (n = 12, age 16–40 years) and subjects with CF (n = 36, age 1–51 years) were recruited to this study after written informed consent was obtained. For a subset of subjects with CF who contributed cells for functional assessment, basic descriptive data regarding their age, genotype, pancreatic sufficiency status, and baseline sweat chloride (when available) is described in the Supplementary Material S1. The study was approved by the University of Alabama Institutional Review Board under protocol number IRB-151030001. One brush biopsy from each nare was obtained using cytology brushes (Medical Packaging CYB1, Cat# CYB-1, length: 8 inches, width approximately 7 mm, Camarillo, CA, USA) under direct visualization of the inferior turbinate via an otoscope and sterile 9-mm speculum. The cell number obtained from brushing was varied between subjects, ranging from 2.5×10^5 to 2×10^6.

2.2. Cell Culture and Expansion

Expansion of primary human nasal epithelial cells (HNEs) was adapted from conditional reprogramming culture (CRC) methods that have been previously published [17,18]. In brief, after collection, cells were immediately placed in Roswell Park Memorial Institute (RPMI) 1640 media (Thermo Scientific, Waltham, MA, USA) and processed within two hours. Depending on the number of cells collected, cells were either cryopreserved and/or expanded in co-culture with irradiated 3T3 fibroblasts for up to 14 days in a T75 flask containing F-media with 10 μM Y27632 (Stemgent Stemolecule, Beltsville, MD, USA) [17]. At a seeding density of at least $2.5 \times 10^3/cm^2$, one T75 will yield 2×10^6 to 4×10^6 cells. For the initial three days of expansion culture only, Amphotericin B

2.5 µg/mL (Sigma-Aldrich Corp., St. Louis, MO, USA), Tobramycin 100 µg/mL (Alfa Aesar, Ward Hill, MA, USA), Ceftazidime 100 µg/mL (Sigma-Aldrich Corp., St. Louis, MO, USA), and Vancomycin 100 µg/mL (Alfa Aesar, Ward Hill, MA, USA) were added to the media of the CF-derived cells [10]. Cells were discarded if less than 80% confluent by day 14. HNEs were recovered after trypsinization in the expansion flask (0.05% trypsin-EDTA (ethylenediaminetetraacetic acid)). No cells greater than passage 3 were used to avoid a known reduction in CFTR expression at high passage numbers [19]. CF and non-CF cells behaved similarly during expansion, consistent with prior reports [20–22].

2.3. Differentiated HNE Culture

Organoids were cultured either in a Transwell system (polyester membrane, area 0.33 cm^2, pore size: 0.4 µm; Corning Inc., Corning, NY, USA) or 15-well angiogenesis slides (ibidi USA, Inc., Fitchburg, WI, USA). Slides were selected to enhance the optical imaging of organoids for morphology and functional assessment. For angiogenesis slides, Matrigel (Corning Inc., Corning, NY, USA) with a total protein concentration of at least 9 mg/mL was used for organoid culture. Each well of the slides was coated with 5 µL of cold 100% Matrigel on ice and slides were placed into a cell culture incubator at 37 °C for at least 30 min. HNEs were resuspended into a 20% matrigel and Ultroser-G (USG) media [23] suspension at 500 cells/µL. For each replicate well, 5 µL of the suspension (2500 cells/replicate) were seeded into imaging slide wells coated with matrigel, incubated at 37 °C for one hour, and covered with 50 µL of USG media. The media was exchanged every other day until the cells were used for experiments. For organoids grown in a Transwell system, a cold Transwell insert was coated with 100 µL of 100% Matrigel on ice, then put into a cell culture incubator at 37 °C for at least 30 min. Sixty microliters of the HNE cell suspension described above were seeded into Transwells coated with matrigel, incubated at 37 °C for one hour, then USG media was added to the lower chamber. For monolayer cultures, Transwell inserts were coated with 0.06 mg/mL in 0.2% acetic acid of human placenta collagen type IV (Sigma-Aldrich Corp., St. Louis, MO, USA). After expansion, HNEs were seeded into the Transwells with the density of 5×10^5 cells/insert in F-media for two days. USG media was exchanged every other day until the cells were well differentiated and used for the short-circuit current (Isc) experiments, around 28 days in culture [24].

2.4. Organoid Fixation and Immunoflurescence

Organoids derived from cells donated by 11 unique individals (6 with CF) were harvested after 28 days of culture by replacing media with 50 µL of cold 1X phosphate buffered saline (PBS) in each well on ice and pipetting 3–5 times. For histology and immunofluorescence of cross-sectioned organoids, all dissociated organoids from one ibidi slide (15 wells) were combined into a conical tube on ice. Total volume was adjusted to 10 mL with cold 1XPBS and centrifuged at 4 °C, at 300×g for 5 min, and supernatant was removed. Then, 60 µL of warm Histogel (Thermo Scientific, Waltham, MA, USA) was mixed with the organoid pellet, and immediately transferred to a histology mold. Once solid, the mold block was fixed with 4% paraformaldehyde overnight at 4 °C. After embedding in paraffin, the block was then cut into 5-µm cross-sections, fixed onto glass slides, and stained using hematoxylin and eosin (H&E). Some cross-sections were used for immunofluorescence with details described below. Histology was imaged by a Nikon Ts2 microscope. For whole mount immunofluorescence, organoids from one to two wells were pipetted into an eight-well glass bottom chamber slide (ibidi USA, Inc., Fitchburg, WI, USA), which was pre-treated with Cell-Tak (Corning Inc., Corning, NY, USA), removing excess liquid by pipette. The chamber slide was placed into a 37 °C incubator for 40 min to enhance organoid adherence to the glass bottom. After gently washing with 1X PBS 3 times, organoids were fixed with 4% paraformaldehyde (Electron Microscopy Sciences, Hatfield, PA, USA) for 30 min at room temperature (RT), and washed and stored in PBS until immunostaining. Immunofluorescent staining used modifications of previous methods [25–28]. Briefly, to reduce auto-fluorescence, 250 µL of 50 mM NH$_4$Cl in 1X PBS were added into each well of the slides at RT for 30 min while gently shaking. After washing with 1X PBS twice, cultures were permeabilized by 0.1% Triton X-100

(Alfa Aesar, Ward Hill, MA, USA) for 30 min at RT and then blocked with 2% BSA (Thermo Scientific, Waltham, MA, USA) plus 0.1% Triton X-100 in PBS for one hour at RT. All antibody solutions were prepared with 2% BSA plus 0.1% Triton X-100 in PBS. Cultures were incubated with primary antibodies at 4 °C for 2 days as follows: Anti-human CFTR (R&D Systems, Inc., Minneapolis, MN, R domain, MAB1660; 1:100), anti-human ZO-1 (Zona occludens 1; Thermo Scientific, Waltham, MA, USA, MA3-39100-A647; 1:1000), anti-human MUC5B (Mucin 5b; Sigma-Aldrich Corp., St. Louis, MO, USA, HPA008246; 1:100), anti-β IV tubulin (Tubulin β type IV; Abcam, Cambridge, MA, USA, ab11315; 1:100) for cilia, and anti-FOXI1 for Ionocytes (Forkhead box I1; Sigma-Aldrich Corp., St. Louis, MO, USA, HPA071469; 1:100). Cross-sections were incubated with primary antibodies at 4 °C overnight as follows: Anti-human MUC5AC (Mucin 5AC; Thermo Fisher Scientific, Waltham, MA, USA, MA512178; 1:100) for mucin and anti-acetylated tubulin (Tubulin α-4A; Sigma-Aldrich Corp., St. Louis, MO, USA, T7451; 1:100) for cilia. After thoroughly washing with PBS plus 0.3% Triton X-100 three times, 5 min for each time while shaking, all secondary antibodies from Invitrogen were diluted at 1:2000 and incubated at 4 °C for 2 days, except for cross-sections, which were incubated at RT in the dark for one hour. After incubation, the slides were washed thoroughly with PBS with 0.3% Triton X-100 and NucBlue (2 drops/mL for 30 min; 4′, 6-diamidino-2-phenylindole (DAPI); Thermo Scientific, Waltham, MA, USA) in 2% BSA plus 0.3% Triton X-100 was utilized for nuclear staining. Organoids were imaged with either a Nikon Ts2 or confocal microscope (Nikon A1R-HD25).

2.5. Imaging and Analysis of Organoids

Organoids were also imaged by either the automated image system in Biotek Lionheart FX or micro-optical coherence tomography (μOCT) [15] in an environmentally controlled chamber at 37 °C and 5% CO_2. Gen5 ImagePrime software (BioTek, Winooski, VT, USA) in the Lionheart was used for image processing and automated quantitation of the organoid size and count in each well. The forskolin-induced swelling (FIS) assay was adapted from assays described previously [9,29]. FIS assays were performed by 21 days of culture. The organoids for the FIS assay were pre-incubated with NucBlu (Thermo Scientific, Waltham, MA, USA) for 1 h prior to stimulation and imaging. All treatment conditions were diluted in Dulbecco's PBS and added to media at a 1:1 ratio. The organoids were stimulated with a cocktail of forskolin 10 μM and IBMX 100 μM (FI). Brightfield and fluorescent (DAPI) images of the organoids were then taken in each well of a slide (every 20 min, for 8 h in total) using Lionheart FX. The total surface area (TSA) from the sum of all organoids in the well was automatically determined by the software for each condition at each time point. As an additional quality control, DAPI images were compared to the brightfield to ensure accurate masking of TSA. The change in TSA relative to the baseline (time 0), or fractional change, was calculated for each well (3–5 individual wells per condition) and averaged for each time point. For calculation of the baseline luminal ratio (BLR), brightfield images of 3–5 wells per subject were masked using the polygon function of the NIS-Elements Basic Research software (Nikon Instruments Inc., Melville, NY, USA) by outlining the whole organoid and another mask outlining the lumen of the same organoid. Typically, 40 organoids were analyzed per subject between 3–5 wells, with a minimum of 10 organoids per well. Organoids with lumens that were not able to be visualized and masked accurately were excluded from the analysis. This method was chosen to avoid overestimating the severity of CFTR dysfunction for each subject by assigning these an arbitrarily chosen small area. For μOCT imaging, organoid cultures were placed in an environmentally controlled chamber, images were constructed, and the ciliary beat frequency (CBF) was determined as described previously [15,30,31].

2.6. Short-Circuit Current Measurements of Monolayers

Electrophysiological experiments to measure the transport of ions across epithelial monolayers were accomplished using established methods [32]. Reagents were introduced into bath solution in the Ussing chamber (Physiologic Instruments, San Diego, CA, USA) in the following order: Amiloride, 100 μM (apical) to inhibit the ENaC current; forskolin, 10 μM (apical and basal) to stimulate CFTR;

VX-770 10 µM (apical and basal) to further potentiate the current; and CFTRinh-172 10 µM (apical). Electrophysiological data were collected and analyzed using Acquire and Analyze 2.3 software (Physiologic Instruments, San Diego, CA, USA) [32].

2.7. Statistical Analysis

One-way ANOVA was used for baseline lumen ratio comparisons. Two-way ANOVA with Tukey's multiple comparisons test was used to evaluate differences between the average fractional change among people with a different CFTR function at 1 and at 8 h. Pearson's correlation coefficient was calculated for the correlation analysis. Fisher's exact test was used for culture success comparison between CF and non-CF. All statistical analysis was performed in GraphPad Prism 8 (GraphPad, La Jolla, CA, USA).

3. Results

3.1. HNE Organoid Morphology Reflects That of Airway Epithelial Layers In Vivo

Initial optimization of the assay included iterative testing of the Matrigel concentration, culture medium, cell seeding density, and type of culture vessel. After initial expansion of the nasal epithelial cells, we obtained organoids suitable for further testing from 88% of the successfully expanded samples. There were no significant differences in the culture success between CF and non-CF samples, similar to prior reports [20–22]. The average number of organoids formed in each well with the seeding density of 500 cells/µL was 31 (non-CF) and 37 (CF). Lumens were visible as early as day 3 of culture, and in the majority of samples by day 7 (Figure 1A–C). By 21 days of culture, the total surface area (TSA) and luminal area (LA) were significantly different between non-CF and CF patients, with two minimal function (MF) mutations or with a residual function (RF) mutation, but not between those with RF and MF (Figure 1D). Fixed cross-sections of the organoids show a robust circular culture with the apical lumen on the interior, and thick and thin epithelial walls, with evidence of cilia forming cells (Figure 2). Other than the lumen size, there were no qualitative differences observed between non-CF and CF cultures up to 42 days of weekly imaging.

Mucus expression was also assessed after 28 days of culture (Figure 3). Immunofluorescent staining of both MUC5AC and MUC5B was performed to assess the mucins produced, with similar qualitative expression regardless of the genotype. Mucus-producing cells with evidence of mucin granules were detected (Figure 3A). MUC5B shows bundles of mucins in both non-CF and CF organoids, whereas MUC5AC organizes as a diffuse web (Figure 3B,C). Although similar patterns have been seen in other published works, the differences in mucins seen may be due to the differences in the immunofluorescent techniques or CF phenotype [10,33]; while we did not observe the finding in a CF organoid, the approach did not allow for quantitative comparisons. Three-dimensional (3D) reconstruction of the confocal image demonstrates the secretion of MUC5B from mucosal cells into the lumen of the organoid (Figure 3D). Light microscopy and µOCT imaging were completed to assess luminal mucus movement (Figure 3E,F). Corresponding videos show a circular pattern of movement of the fluid and mucus within the lumen (Videos S1 and S2).

For both non-CF and CF organoids, cilia expression was assessed in histology sections (Figure 2A,C), whole-mount immunofluorescence with 3-D reconstruction (Figure 4A), immunofluorescent fixed cross-sections (Figure 4B), light microscopy (Figure 4C), and µOCT imaging (Figure 4D). Videos show cilia beating on the luminal (apical) surface of the organoid (Videos S3 and S4), and the ciliary beat frequency was readily measured (Figure S1). Cilia formation was similar across genotypes. Other markers of differentiation were also assessed with immunofluorescent staining of whole-mount fixed organoids. Apically localized tight junctions (ZO-1), CFTR, and FOXI1 (marker for ionocytes) were identified (Figure 4E–H). ZO-1 staining was similar across genotypes. The detection of CFTR was seen in both non-CF and CF cultures (MF/MF and MF/RF), similar to prior reports [34]. Apical plasma membrane localization of CFTR was presumed after co-staining with ZO-1 was visualized in a non-CF organoid (Figure S2) as previously seen in monolayers [35].

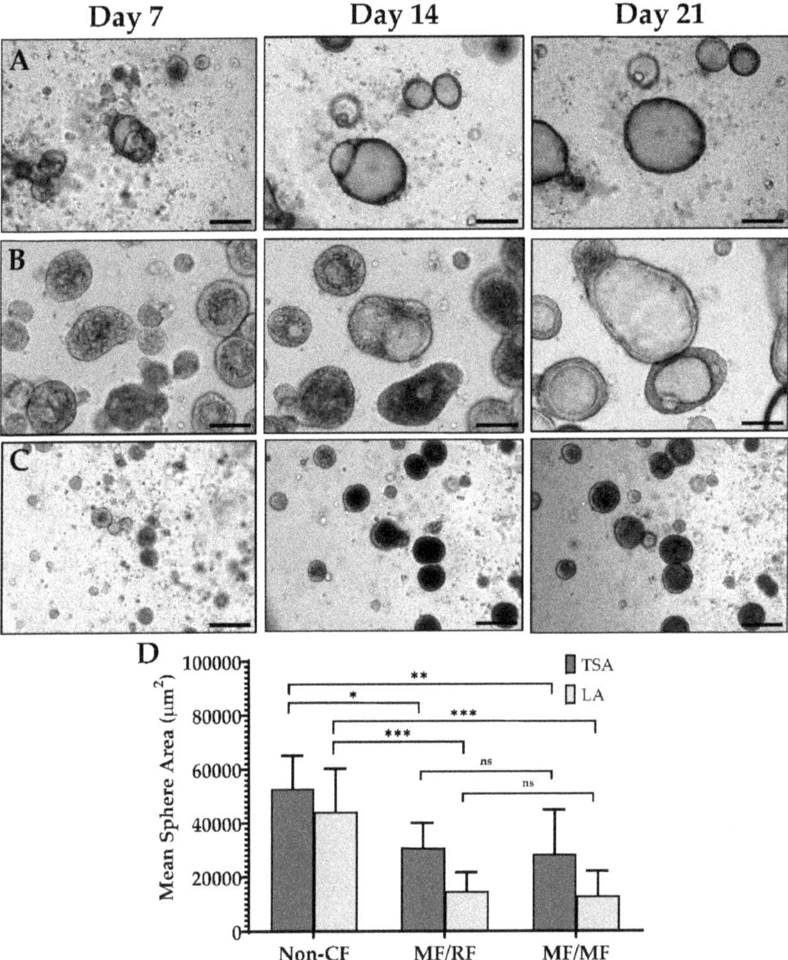

Figure 1. Nasal organoid growth characteristics. (**A–C**) Light microscopy of organoid formation over three weeks. (**A**) Non-CF (**B**) *G551D/Unknown* (MF/RF) (**C**) *F508del/F508del* (MF/MF). (**D**) The mean total surface area (TSA) and mean luminal area (LA) at 21 days of culture for non-CF (n = 6), MF/RF (n = 5), and MF/MF (n = 11) subjects' organoids. MF = Minimal Function; RF = Residual Function. Scale = 250 μm. * p = 0.02, ** p = 0.005, *** p = 0.0001, ns = not significant.

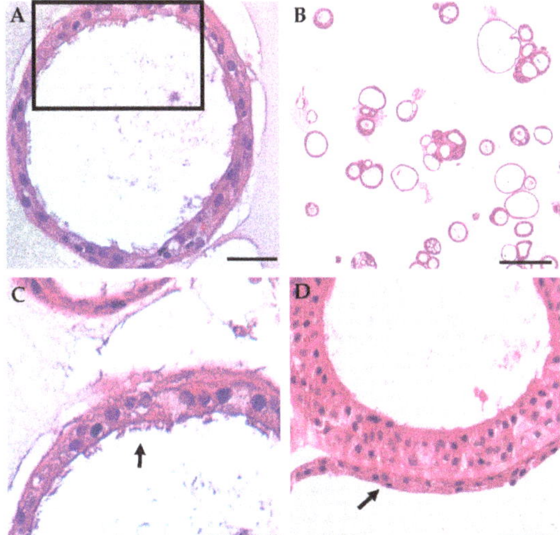

Figure 2. Representative samples of typical hematoxylin and eosin staining of HNE organoids show structural markers of differentiation. (**A**) Fully differentiated cross-section of a non-CF organoid shows a differentiated monolayer with an open lumen. Scale = 50 μm. (**B**) An example of the lower magnification of non-CF organoids demonstrates variations in the overall organoid morphology. Scale = 250 μm. (**C**) Higher magnification of the black frame in panel (**A**) showing a ciliated apical surface (arrow). Scale = 50 μm. (**D**) An example of higher magnification of G551D/unknown CF organoids showing thick and thin (arrow) epithelial walls. Scale = 50 μm.

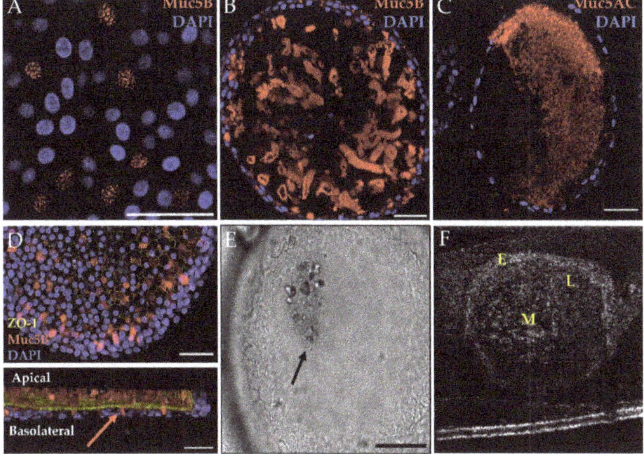

Figure 3. Mucus characteristics in HNE organoids, representative findings from CF and non-CF organoids are shown. (**A**) MUC5B granules in G551D/N1303K organoid. Scale = 50 μm. (**B**) Muc5B whole-mount IF showing a bundled mucin pattern in F508del/R117H-5T organoid. Scale = 50 μm. (**C**) MUC5AC fixed cross-section showing a diffuse mucin pattern in a non-CF organoid. Scale = 50 μm. (**D**) Top panel is the maximum projection of the 3-D hemisphere in the bottom panel. MUC5B is seen entering the lumen (arrow) through the apical surface in a non-CF organoid. Scale = 500 μm. (**E**) Brightfield microscopy showing a clump of cellular debris and/or mucus in the lumen in a non-CF organoid. Scale = 100 μm. (**F**) μOCT still of probable mucus in a non-CF organoid. (**E,F**) correspond to Videos **S1** and **S2**. E = epithelium L = lumen M = mucus.

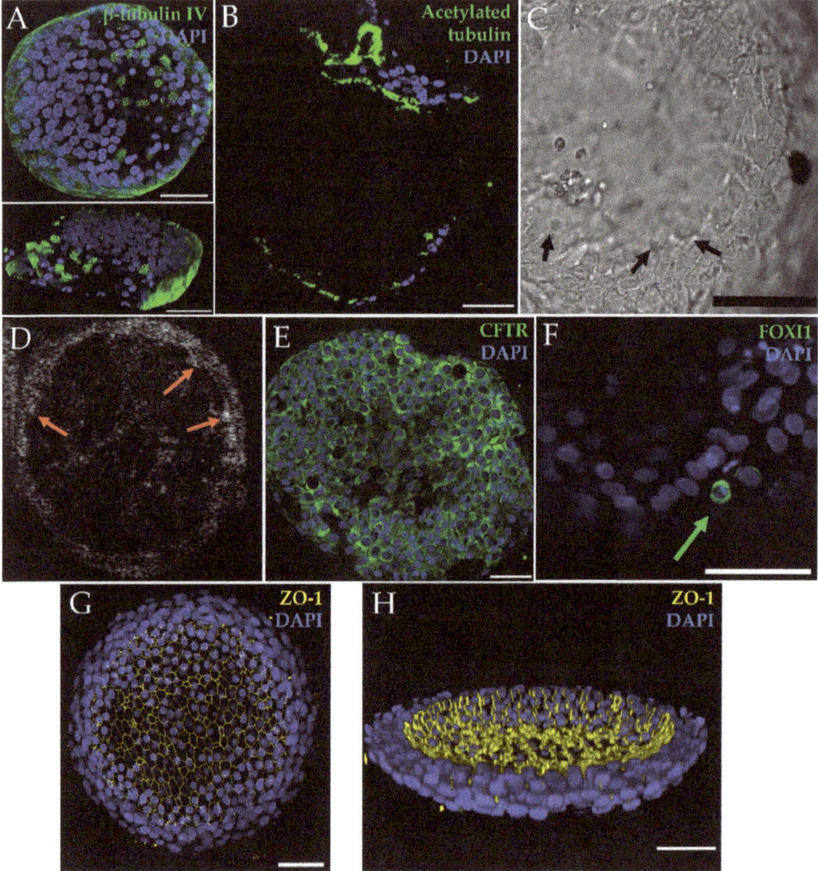

Figure 4. Other markers of airway epithelial differentiation are shown in selected images from non-CF and CF organoids. (**A**) Top panel is a confocal maximal projection of β-tubulin IV in F508del/G551D organoid with a 3-D reconstruction in the bottom panel that was sliced into to show cilia protruding. Scale = 50 μm. (**B**) Cross-section stained with acetylated tubulin in a non-CF organoid. Scale = 50 μm. (**C**) Light microscopy image of still cilia (arrows) in a non-CF organoid. Scale = 100 μm. (**D**) μOCT image of still cilia (arrows) in a non-CF organoid. (**C,D**) Stills correspond with Videos **S3** and **S4**. (**E**) Organoids also expressed CFTR, as seen in this representative example from F508del/R117H-5T organoids; co-localizion with ZO-1, seen in a non-CF organoid, is shown in Figure **S2**. Scale = 50 μm. (**F**) FOXI1-positive cell (arrow) in an F508del/F508del organoid. Scale = 50 μm. Maximal projection of tight-junction (ZO-1) staining (**G**) and a three-dimensional hemisphere demonstrating apical (luminal) localization in F508del/F508del organoids (**H**). Scale = 50 μm.

3.2. Organoid Lumen Size Differs between Different CFTR Genotypes

By day 21, organoids were determined to be sufficiently differentiated for functional evaluation. At this time point, organoids exhibited a more uniform response than younger or older cultures. Assessment of the differences between non-CF and CF organoids showed striking contrasts. In Figure 5, representative images of 21-day-old cultures of non-CF organoids are compared to cultures from patients with CF (G551D/Unknown (residual function); F508del/G551D; and F508del/F508del). While TSA and LA can broadly distinguish between non-CF and CF phenotypes (Figure 1D), the baseline luminal ratio (BLR), the fraction of LA to TSA, can distinguish between non-CF and CF and between varying levels of CFTR dysfunction (Figure 6A–C). Furthermore, BLR shows a high correlation ($r = 0.94$, $p = 0.0005$) with the baseline forskolin-stimulated Isc in HNE monolayers from the same patients (Figure 6D).

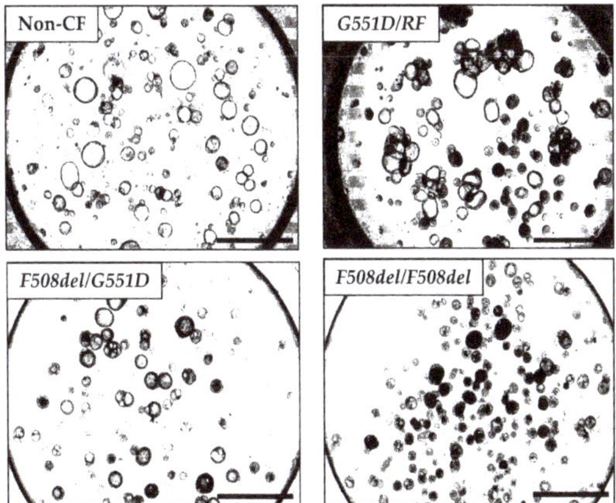

Figure 5. Light microscopy of cultures at 21 days of growth demonstrates variations in the amount of luminal fluid present within organoids of different CFTR genotypes. Scale = 1000 µm. The genotype (*G551D/unknown (MF/RF based on phenotype)*) is defined in Supplementary Material Table S1.

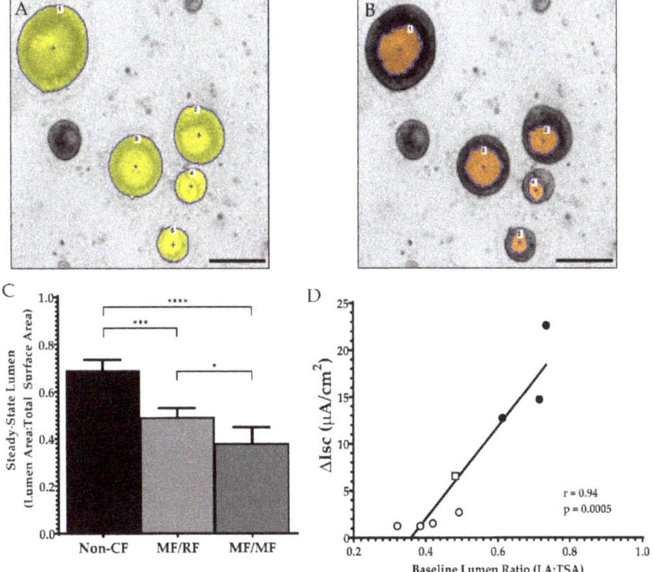

Figure 6. Baseline lumen ratio. Zoomed-in section of a well to show *F508del/G551D* organoids (**A**) masking of the organoid's total surface area and (**B**) masking of the same organoids' luminal areas. (**C**) Baseline lumen to total surface area ratio comparing non-CF (n = 6) to CF patients with residual function (n = 5) and minimal function mutations (n = 11). (**D**) Pearson correlation comparing the average organoid BLR for each person and the corresponding change in short-circuit current (ΔIsc) after forskolin stimulation in the ussing chamber. Not all subjects from (**C**) had corresponding short-circuit current measurements. Filled circle = Non-CF; Open square = MF/RF; Open circle = MF/MF. Scale = 200 µm. * $p = 0.02$, *** $p = 0.0001$, and **** $p < 0.0001$.

3.3. Optimization of Forskolin-Induced CFTR-Dependent Swelling Assay

Organoid cultures have previously been shown to be predictors of CFTR-dependent fluid transport, including to test downstream effects of gene editing [10,29,36,37]. These assays use short (1–2 h) time-lapse imaging [10,29]. We tested this organoid model for applicability for forskolin-induced swelling (FIS). We hypothesized that longer assays might show a greater dynamic range since fluid transport in epithelia is a complex process and may not be evident in a short time [11]. HNE organoids derived from cells from a healthy non-CF patient (Figure 7A), a patient with F508del/P67L (Figure 7B), and a patient with F508del/F508del (Figure 7C) CFTR are shown at 0, 1, and 8 h (Videos S5–S7). Figure 7D is the average fractional change over 8 h for three subjects with varying levels of baseline CFTR function (non-CF = normal function; F508del/P67L = residual function; and F508del/F508del=minimal function). In Figure 7E, the fractional change for each subject is shown, showing significant distinctions for the CFTR function between all three subjects at 8 h while not at 1 h.

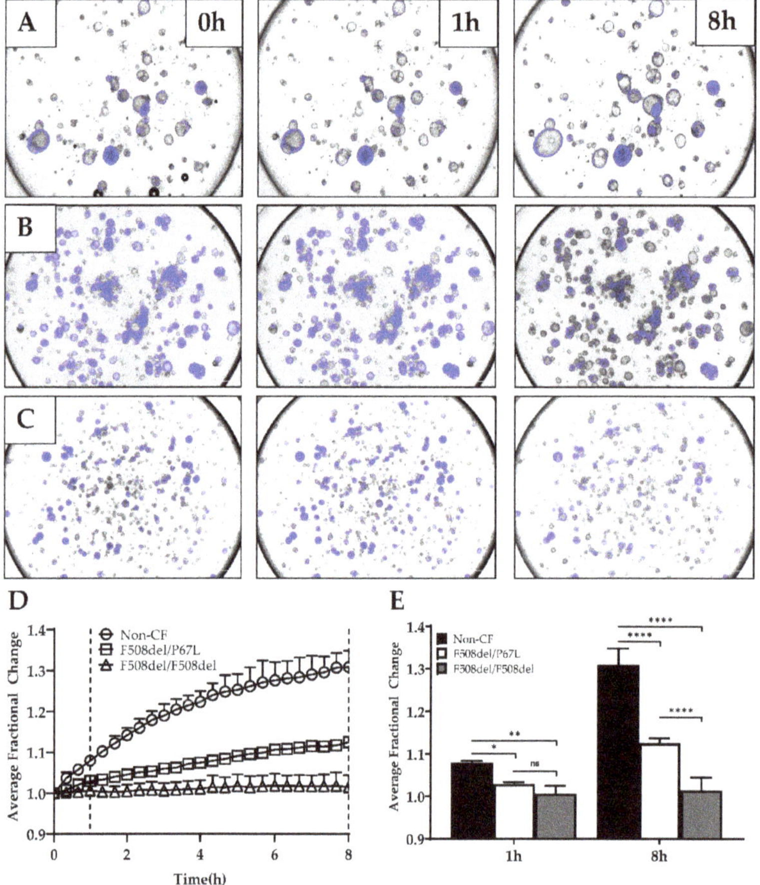

Figure 7. FIS assay. (**A–C**) Three representative brightfield and DAPI-stained images at times 0, 1, and 8 h for non-CF (**A**), F508del/P67L (**B**), and F508del/F508del (**C**) CFTR HNE organoids. (**D**) Average fractional change from baseline over 8 h for each subject, dotted lines highlighting the 1- and 8-h timepoints. (**E**) 1-h vs. 8-h time points for the average fractional change of non-CF, F508del/P67L, and F508del/F508del organoids (n = 1). (**A**) Corresponds with Video **S5**, (**B**) corresponds with Video **S6**, and (**C**) corresponds with Video **S7**. ns = not significant; * p = 0.0441, ** p = 0.0023, and **** p < 0.0001.

4. Discussion and Conclusions

In this manuscript, we provide evidence for a highly differentiated organoid culture that expresses markers consistent with human airway epithelial monolayers with reproducible cultures regardless of the genotype. The organoid culture shows distinct differences in lumen formation between non-CF and CF cultures with and without residual CFTR function, suggesting a CFTR dependence of the lumen size and fluid transport during organoid development. Along with the significant differences between the lumen formation of CF and non-CF organoids, this difference highly correlates with paralleled short-circuit measurements of baseline CFTR activity. This has not previously been evaluated in human nasal epithelial organoids, but a similar finding was seen in intestinal organoids [38]. Our swelling data suggest that this model has the potential for functional assessment of the patient phenotype, identifying both large and small differences (such as residual function, or a modest improvement of one treatment over another). Furthermore, the model has multiple applications, including FIS, assessment of mucus expression, transport, cilia activity, and fluorescence microscopy.

We present data that the full effects of CFTR restoration may not be visible over short time frames in nasal organoid studies. By lengthening the assay to eight hours, we were able to increase the distinction between differing CFTR activity levels. This result requires further testing with more subjects, but it is an interesting finding that takes into account that fluid transport may not immediately follow CFTR rescue, and the complex systems that result in fluid secretion into the lumen may take some time to show full effects. The functional assay could be useful in pre-clinical testing, where interventions designed to be delivered via systemic absorption (i.e., from the basolateral side after distribution through the blood) can be applied to an in vitro surrogate. Because it requires so little material to generate many replicates, it is amenable to higher throughput applications using novel compounds or iterative testing of different delivery mechanisms for RNA- and DNA-based therapies. Additionally, it provides a useful ex vivo marker for in vivo gene therapy trials. A nasal brush biopsy is safe, easily obtained in an outpatient clinical research setting, and can be repeatedly collected from the patient [39]. This could be tested to monitor the stability of a genetic repair, which would be helpful to confirm a corrected phenotype even if clinical measures (like lung function testing) may not be altered (for example, if a patient has a normal lung function result at the start of the study).

The differentiation of this model provides multiple readouts for CFTR functional rescue. It is highly amenable to fluorescent imaging. We used fluorescence for automated imaging of living cells as well as fixed whole organoids for immunofluorescent staining of specific markers. We observed limited evidence that the organoid can recapitulate mucin organization also seen in other models [33]. Currently, a variety of approaches to deliver gene therapy packages exist, and delivery mechanisms tagged with a fluorescent marker for measuring uptake could easily be tested across a variety of patient samples with this approach. Further, the readout for functional assessment of CFTR rescue is not limited to the measurement of the total cross-sectional area or lumen over time. Our results show that μOCT imaging can yield multiple readouts of the lumen area, mucus morphology, ciliary function, and possibly with further testing, mucus viscosity and mucociliary transport speeds.

Our study has some limitations. We present functional data (lumen size and swelling) from a limited number of subjects, while additional subject samples were used for iterative testing to optimize the culturing and assay methodology to achieve a reproducible assay. Despite the small number of subjects, the lumen measurement shows excellent distinction for differences between patient groups. The current analysis limits our baseline luminal ratio assay to manual measurements until further revisions to the automated software can be made. However, because the measurements and output for the FIS assay are automated, we will now be able to scale up the testing of many patients and correlate clinical outcome measures with the organoid data for future studies.

Our results show that a solid assay with similarities to the robust intestinal organoid forskolin-induced swelling assay can be developed with HNEs. This provides a significant advantage because not every CF center has the capacity to collect rectal biopsies on all patients, nor are all patients receptive to biopsy collection. However, many CF centers in the United States and elsewhere have experience in collecting nasal brush biopsies from infants through to adults, with risk comparable to that of a nasopharyngeal swab for virus detection. The model can assess CFTR dysfunction and rescue, both as a pre-clinical tool for systemically delivered DNA-based therapies and an ex vivo surrogate biomarker to assess the stability of DNA-based therapy in clinical trials.

Supplementary Materials: The following are available online at http://www.mdpi.com/2073-4425/11/6/603/s1, Table S1: Individual subject demographics and available clinical data for selected participants contributing functional data. Figure S1: Example measurement of μOCT ciliary beat frequencies, Figure S2: Organoid CFTR (green) co-localization with apical ZO-1 (red). (A) To illustrate the location of the ZO-1 staining within the organoid, an α-blended 3-D volume reconstruction was created with the fluorescence intensity increased to reveal the organoid's shape and orient the reader to the location of the 2D co-localization image below. (B) Magnified view of the yellow frame in (A) to better visualize the CFTR and ZO-1 overlay, Video S1: Brightfield video of luminal movement of mucus, Video S2: μOCT video of luminal movement of mucus, Video S3: Brightfield video of luminal cilia beating, Video S4: μOCT video of cilia beating, Video S5: FIS assay of non-CF organoids, Video S6: FIS assay of F508del/P67L organoids. Video S7: FIS assay of F508del/F508del organoids.

Author Contributions: Conceptualization, Z.L., J.D.A. and J.S.G.; methodology, Z.L., J.D.A., L.D., S.M. and J.S.G.; validation, Z.L., J.D.A. and J.S.G.; formal analysis, Z.L. and J.D.A.; investigation, Z.L., J.D.A., L.D. and J.B.; resources, L.K.; writing—original draft preparation, J.S.G.; writing—review and editing, Z.L., J.D.A., S.M.R. and J.S.G.; visualization, J.D.A.; supervision, J.S.G.; project administration, J.S.G.; funding acquisition, S.M.R. and J.S.G. All authors have read and agreed to the published version of the manuscript.

Funding: This work was supported by the Kaul Pediatric Research Institute Pilot Award and the Cystic Fibrosis Foundation (GUIMBE1710). J.S.G. is supported by the NIH (K23 HL143167-01A1), and the Cystic Fibrosis Foundation (GUIMBE18A0-Q). Z.L., J.D.A., L.K., and J.S.G. and S.M.R. are supported by the Gregory Fleming James Cystic Fibrosis Center (R35HL135816, NIH DK072482, CFF UAB Research and Development Program—Rowe19RO, all to S.M.R.) and the UAB Center for Clinical and Translational Science (UL1TR001417).

Acknowledgments: We gratefully acknowledge the contributions of Guillermo Tearney and Hui Min Leung, Massachusetts General Hospital and Harvard Medical School, for the invention and maintenance of the μOCT imager. We thank Susan Birket and Steven Roberts for technical assistance. We thank the UAB High Resolution Imaging Facility and the UAB Histology Core for assistance. We would also like to thank Jennifer Natt for her review and copy editing of the manuscript.

Conflicts of Interest: J.S.G. is listed as an inventor on a patent application 20170242033 from the University of North Carolina that describes a similar model. When licensed technology from UNC produces royalties, the inventors receive a share of the revenue. Otherwise, the authors declare no conflict of interest. The funders had no role in the design of the study; in the collection, analyses, or interpretation of data; in the writing of the manuscript, or in the decision to publish the results.

Abbreviations

CF   cystic fibrosis
CFTR   Cystic Fibrosis Transmembrane conductance regulator

References

1. Bell, S.C.; De Boeck, K.; Amaral, M.D. New pharmacological approaches for cystic fibrosis: Promises, progress, pitfalls. *Pharmacol. Ther.* **2015**, *145*, 19–34. [CrossRef] [PubMed]

2. Bertoncini, E.; Colomb-Lippa, D. Pulmonology: CFTR modulators for cystic fibrosis. *J. Am. Acad. Physician Assist.* **2013**, *26*, 59–60. [CrossRef] [PubMed]

3. Derichs, N. Targeting a genetic defect: Cystic fibrosis transmembrane conductance regulator modulators in cystic fibrosis. *Eur. Respir. Rev.* **2013**, *22*, 58–65. [CrossRef]

4. Middleton, P.G.; Mall, M.A.; Drevinek, P.; Lands, L.C.; McKone, E.F.; Polineni, D.; Ramsey, B.W.; Taylor-Cousar, J.L.; Tullis, E.; Vermeulen, F.; et al. Elexacaftor-Tezacaftor-Ivacaftor for Cystic Fibrosis with a Single Phe508del Allele. *N. Engl. J. Med.* **2019**, *381*, 1809–1819. [CrossRef] [PubMed]

5. Heijerman, H.G.M.; McKone, E.F.; Downey, D.G.; Van Braeckel, E.; Rowe, S.M.; Tullis, E.; Mall, M.A.; Welter, J.J.; Ramsey, B.W.; McKee, C.M.; et al. Efficacy and safety of the elexacaftor plus tezacaftor plus ivacaftor combination regimen in people with cystic fibrosis homozygous for the F508del mutation: A double-blind, randomised, phase 3 trial. *Lancet* **2019**. [CrossRef]

6. Pedersen, P.S.; Braunstein, T.H.; Jorgensen, A.; Larsen, P.L.; Holstein-Rathlou, N.H.; Frederiksen, O. Stimulation of aquaporin-5 and transepithelial water permeability in human airway epithelium by hyperosmotic stress. *Pflug. Arch.* **2007**, *453*, 777–785. [CrossRef]

7. Pedersen, P.S.; Frederiksen, O.; Holstein-Rathlou, N.H.; Larsen, P.L.; Qvortrup, K. Ion transport in epithelial spheroids derived from human airway cells. *Am. J. Physiol.* **1999**, *276*, L75–L80. [CrossRef]

8. Pedersen, P.S.; Holstein-Rathlou, N.H.; Larsen, P.L.; Qvortrup, K.; Frederiksen, O. Fluid absorption related to ion transport in human airway epithelial spheroids. *Am. J. Physiol.* **1999**, *277*, L1096–L1103. [CrossRef]

9. Guimbellot, J.S.; Leach, J.M.; Chaudhry, I.G.; Quinney, N.L.; Boyles, S.E.; Chua, M.; Aban, I.; Jaspers, I.; Gentzsch, M. Nasospheroids permit measurements of CFTR-dependent fluid transport. *JCI Insight* **2017**, *2*. [CrossRef]

10. Brewington, J.J.; Filbrandt, E.T.; LaRosa, F.J., 3rd; Ostmann, A.J.; Strecker, L.M.; Szczesniak, R.D.; Clancy, J.P. Detection of CFTR function and modulation in primary human nasal cell spheroids. *J. Cyst. Fibros* **2017**. [CrossRef]

11. Birket, S.E.; Chu, K.K.; Houser, G.H.; Liu, L.; Fernandez, C.M.; Solomon, G.M.; Lin, V.; Shastry, S.; Mazur, M.; Sloane, P.A.; et al. Combination therapy with cystic fibrosis transmembrane conductance regulator modulators augment the airway functional microanatomy. *Am. J. Physiol. Lung Cell. Mol. Physiol.* **2016**, *310*, L928–L939. [CrossRef]

12. Birket, S.E.; Chu, K.K.; Liu, L.; Houser, G.H.; Diephuis, B.J.; Wilsterman, E.J.; Dierksen, G.; Mazur, M.; Shastry, S.; Li, Y.; et al. A functional anatomic defect of the cystic fibrosis airway. *Am. J. Respir. Crit. Care Med.* **2014**, *190*, 421–432. [CrossRef] [PubMed]

13. Chu, K.K.; Mojahed, D.; Fernandez, C.M.; Li, Y.; Liu, L.; Wilsterman, E.J.; Diephuis, B.; Birket, S.E.; Bowers, H.; Martin Solomon, G.; et al. Particle-Tracking Microrheology Using Micro-Optical Coherence Tomography. *Biophys. J.* **2016**, *111*, 1053–1063. [CrossRef] [PubMed]

14. Chu, K.K.; Unglert, C.; Ford, T.N.; Cui, D.; Carruth, R.W.; Singh, K.; Liu, L.; Birket, S.E.; Solomon, G.M.; Rowe, S.M.; et al. In vivo imaging of airway cilia and mucus clearance with micro-optical coherence tomography. *Biomed. Opt. Express* **2016**, *7*, 2494–2505. [CrossRef] [PubMed]

15. Liu, L.; Chu, K.K.; Houser, G.H.; Diephuis, B.J.; Li, Y.; Wilsterman, E.J.; Shastry, S.; Dierksen, G.; Birket, S.E.; Mazur, M.; et al. Method for quantitative study of airway functional microanatomy using micro-optical coherence tomography. *PLoS ONE* **2013**, *8*, e54473. [CrossRef]

16. Tuggle, K.L.; Birket, S.E.; Cui, X.; Hong, J.; Warren, J.; Reid, L.; Chambers, A.; Ji, D.; Gamber, K.; Chu, K.K.; et al. Characterization of defects in ion transport and tissue development in cystic fibrosis transmembrane conductance regulator (CFTR)-knockout rats. *PLoS ONE* **2014**, *9*, e91253. [CrossRef]

17. Chapman, S.; Liu, X.; Meyers, C.; Schlegel, R.; McBride, A.A. Human keratinocytes are efficiently immortalized by a Rho kinase inhibitor. *J. Clin. Investig.* **2010**, *120*, 2619–2626. [CrossRef]

18. Liu, X.; Ory, V.; Chapman, S.; Yuan, H.; Albanese, C.; Kallakury, B.; Timofeeva, O.A.; Nealon, C.; Dakic, A.; Simic, V.; et al. ROCK inhibitor and feeder cells induce the conditional reprogramming of epithelial cells. *Am. J. Pathol.* **2012**, *180*, 599–607. [CrossRef]

19. Avramescu, R.G.; Kai, Y.; Xu, H.; Bidaud-Meynard, A.; Schnur, A.; Frenkiel, S.; Matouk, E.; Veit, G.; Lukacs, G.L. Mutation-specific downregulation of CFTR2 variants by gating potentiators. *Hum. Mol. Genet.* **2017**, *26*, 4873–4885. [CrossRef]

20. De Courcey, F.; Zholos, A.V.; Atherton-Watson, H.; Williams, M.T.; Canning, P.; Danahay, H.L.; Elborn, J.S.; Ennis, M. Development of primary human nasal epithelial cell cultures for the study of cystic fibrosis pathophysiology. *Am. J. Physiol. Cell Physiol.* **2012**, *303*, C1173–C1179. [CrossRef]

21. Mosler, K.; Coraux, C.; Fragaki, K.; Zahm, J.M.; Bajolet, O.; Bessaci-Kabouya, K.; Puchelle, E.; Abely, M.; Mauran, P. Feasibility of nasal epithelial brushing for the study of airway epithelial functions in CF infants. *J. Cyst. Fibros* **2008**, *7*, 44–53. [CrossRef] [PubMed]

22. Martinovich, K.M.; Iosifidis, T.; Buckley, A.G.; Looi, K.; Ling, K.M.; Sutanto, E.N.; Kicic-Starcevich, E.; Garratt, L.W.; Shaw, N.C.; Montgomery, S.; et al. Conditionally reprogrammed primary airway epithelial cells maintain morphology, lineage and disease specific functional characteristics. *Sci. Rep.* **2017**, *7*, 17971. [CrossRef]

23. Neuberger, T.; Burton, B.; Clark, H.; Van Goor, F. Use of primary cultures of human bronchial epithelial cells isolated from cystic fibrosis patients for the pre-clinical testing of CFTR modulators. In *Cystic Fibrosis*; Springer: Berlin/Heidelberg, Germany, 2011; pp. 39–54.

24. Brewington, J.J.; Filbrandt, E.T.; LaRosa, F.J., 3rd; Moncivaiz, J.D.; Ostmann, A.J.; Strecker, L.M.; Clancy, J.P. Brushed nasal epithelial cells are a surrogate for bronchial epithelial CFTR studies. *JCI Insight* **2018**, *3*. [CrossRef] [PubMed]

25. Huang, W.; Zhao, H.; Dong, H.; Wu, Y.; Yao, L.; Zou, F.; Cai, S. High-mobility group box 1 impairs airway epithelial barrier function through the activation of the RAGE/ERK pathway. *Int. J. Mol. Med.* **2016**, *37*, 1189–1198. [CrossRef] [PubMed]

26. McCray, T.; Richards, Z.; Marsili, J.; Prins, G.S.; Nonn, L. Handling and Assessment of Human Primary Prostate Organoid Culture. *J. Vis. Exp.* **2019**. [CrossRef] [PubMed]

27. Moonwiriyakit, A.; Koval, M.; Muanprasat, C. Pharmacological stimulation of G-protein coupled receptor 40 alleviates cytokine-induced epithelial barrier disruption in airway epithelial Calu-3 cells. *Int. Immunopharmacol.* **2019**, *73*, 353–361. [CrossRef]

28. Park, H.R.; O'Sullivan, M.; Vallarino, J.; Shumyatcher, M.; Himes, B.E.; Park, J.A.; Christiani, D.C.; Allen, J.; Lu, Q. Transcriptomic response of primary human airway epithelial cells to flavoring chemicals in electronic cigarettes. *Sci. Rep.* **2019**, *9*, 1400. [CrossRef] [PubMed]

29. Dekkers, J.F.; Wiegerinck, C.L.; de Jonge, H.R.; Bronsveld, I.; Janssens, H.M.; de Winter-de Groot, K.M.; Brandsma, A.M.; de Jong, N.W.; Bijvelds, M.J.; Scholte, B.J.; et al. A functional CFTR assay using primary cystic fibrosis intestinal organoids. *Nat. Med.* **2013**, *19*, 939–945. [CrossRef]

30. Wojtkowski, M.; Srinivasan, V.; Ko, T.; Fujimoto, J.; Kowalczyk, A.; Duker, J. Ultrahigh-resolution, high-speed, Fourier domain optical coherence tomography and methods for dispersion compensation. *Opt. Express* **2004**, *12*, 2404–2422. [CrossRef]

31. Liu, Z.; Mackay, S.; Gordon, D.M.; Anderson, J.D.; Haithcock, D.W.; Garson, C.J.; Tearney, G.J.; Solomon, G.M.; Pant, K.; Prabhakarpandian, B.; et al. Co-cultured microfluidic model of the airway optimized for microscopy and micro-optical coherence tomography imaging. *Biomed. Opt. Express* **2019**, *10*, 5414–5430. [CrossRef]

32. Rowe, S.M.; Pyle, L.C.; Jurkevante, A.; Varga, K.; Collawn, J.; Sloane, P.A.; Woodworth, B.; Mazur, M.; Fulton, J.; Fan, L.; et al. DeltaF508 CFTR processing correction and activity in polarized airway and non-airway cell monolayers. *Pulm. Pharmacol. Ther.* **2010**, *23*, 268–278. [CrossRef] [PubMed]

33. Ermund, A.; Meiss, L.N.; Rodriguez-Pineiro, A.M.; Bahr, A.; Nilsson, H.E.; Trillo-Muyo, S.; Ridley, C.; Thornton, D.J.; Wine, J.J.; Hebert, H.; et al. The normal trachea is cleaned by MUC5B mucin bundles from the submucosal glands coated with the MUC5AC mucin. *Biochem. Biophys. Res. Commun.* **2017**, *492*, 331–337. [CrossRef] [PubMed]

34. Schogler, A.; Blank, F.; Brugger, M.; Beyeler, S.; Tschanz, S.A.; Regamey, N.; Casaulta, C.; Geiser, T.; Alves, M.P. Characterization of pediatric cystic fibrosis airway epithelial cell cultures at the air-liquid interface obtained by non-invasive nasal cytology brush sampling. *Respir. Res.* **2017**, *18*, 215. [CrossRef] [PubMed]

35. Wong, A.P.; Bear, C.E.; Chin, S.; Pasceri, P.; Thompson, T.O.; Huan, L.J.; Ratjen, F.; Ellis, J.; Rossant, J. Directed differentiation of human pluripotent stem cells into mature airway epithelia expressing functional CFTR protein. *Nat. Biotechnol.* **2012**, *30*, 876–882. [CrossRef]

36. de Winter-de Groot, K.M.; Janssens, H.M.; van Uum, R.T.; Dekkers, J.F.; Berkers, G.; Vonk, A.; Kruisselbrink, E.; Oppelaar, H.; Vries, R.; Clevers, H.; et al. Stratifying infants with cystic fibrosis for disease severity using intestinal organoid swelling as a biomarker of CFTR function. *Eur. Respir. J.* **2018**, *52*. [CrossRef] [PubMed]

37. Schwank, G.; Koo, B.K.; Sasselli, V.; Dekkers, J.F.; Heo, I.; Demircan, T.; Sasaki, N.; Boymans, S.; Cuppen, E.; van der Ent, C.K.; et al. Functional repair of CFTR by CRISPR/Cas9 in intestinal stem cell organoids of cystic fibrosis patients. *Cell Stem Cell* **2013**, *13*, 653–658. [CrossRef]

38. Dekkers, J.F.; Berkers, G.; Kruisselbrink, E.; Vonk, A.; de Jonge, H.R.; Janssens, H.M.; Bronsveld, I.; van de Graaf, E.A.; Nieuwenhuis, E.E.; Houwen, R.H.; et al. Characterizing responses to CFTR-modulating drugs using rectal organoids derived from subjects with cystic fibrosis. *Sci. Transl. Med.* **2016**, *8*, 344ra84. [CrossRef]

39. Muller, L.; Brighton, L.E.; Carson, J.L.; Fischer, W.A., 2nd; Jaspers, I. Culturing of human nasal epithelial cells at the air liquid interface. *J. Vis. Exp.* **2013**. [CrossRef]

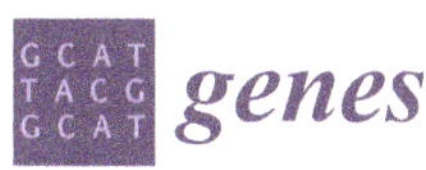 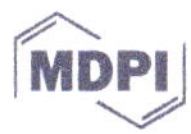

Article

Overcoming Immunological Challenges to Helper-Dependent Adenoviral Vector-Mediated Long-Term *CFTR* Expression in Mouse Airways

Huibi Cao [1], Rongqi Duan [1] and Jim Hu [1,2,*]

[1] Program of Translational Medicine, The Hospital for Sick Children, Research Institute, 686 Bay Street, Toronto, ON M5G 0A4, Canada; huibi.cao@sickkids.ca (H.C.); cathleen.duan@sickkids.ca (R.D.)

[2] Departments of Paediatrics and Laboratory Medicine and Pathobiology, University of Toronto, 1 King's College Circle, Toronto, ON M5S 1A8, Canada

* Correspondence: jim.hu@utoronto.ca; Tel.: +1-416-813-6412

Received: 10 April 2020; Accepted: 13 May 2020; Published: 18 May 2020

Abstract: Cystic Fibrosis (CF) is caused by mutations in the cystic fibrosis transmembrane conductance regulator (*CFTR*) gene, and CF patients require life-long treatment. Although *CFTR* modulators show a great potential for treating most CF patients, some individuals may not tolerate the treatment. In addition, there is no effective therapy for patients with some rare *CFTR* mutations, such as class I CF mutations, which lead to a lack of *CFTR* protein production. Therefore, other therapeutic strategies, such as gene therapy, have to be investigated. Currently, immune responses to gene therapy vectors and transgene products are a major obstacle to applying CF gene therapy to clinical applications. In this study, we examined the effects of cyclophosphamide on the modulation of host immune responses and for the improvement of the *CFTR* transgene expression in the repeated delivery of helper-dependent adenoviral (HD-Ad) vectors to mouse lungs. We have found that cyclophosphamide significantly decreased the expression of T cell genes, such as CD3 (cluster of differentiation 3) and CD4, and reduced their infiltration into mouse lung tissues. We have also found that the levels of the anti-adenoviral antibody and neutralizing activity as well as B-cell infiltration into the mouse lung tissues were significantly reduced with this treatment. Correspondingly, the expression of the human *CFTR* transgene has been significantly improved with cyclophosphamide administration compared to the group with no treatment. These data suggest that the sustained expression of the human *CFTR* transgene in mouse lungs through repeated vector delivery can be achieved by transient immunosuppression.

Keywords: cystic fibrosis; gene therapy; cyclophosphamide; transient immunosuppression

1. Introduction

Cystic fibrosis (CF) is a life-long inherited disease that affects >70,000 patients globally; it is caused by underlying genetic mutations in the cystic fibrosis transmembrane conductance regulator (*CFTR*) gene [1]. New *CFTR*-modulator drugs show promise for up to 90% of patients, including patients with *CFTR* mutations for which early modulators are ineffective [2–5]. Although *CFTR* modulators show enormous potential for treating most CF patients, they are expensive and patients require lifetime treatments [6]. In addition, some patients may not tolerate the treatments. It is understandable that pharmaceutical approaches may not always effectively fix every malfunctioning human body caused by the same genetic defect [7]. Currently, there is no remedy for some patients with rare *CFTR* mutations, such as class I mutations, which lead to a lack of production of the *CFTR* protein [8]. Therefore, alternative therapeutic strategies, such as gene therapy, should be explored.

To date, more than 2600 gene therapy clinical trials have either been completed, are going to be, or have been approved worldwide [9]. Gene therapies for inherited immune disorders, hemophilia, eye and neurodegenerative disorders, and lymphoid cancers, have recently progressed to a stage where drugs have been approved in the United States and Europe [10]. Efficient gene delivery systems are essential to gene therapy to treat human genetic diseases. Genes can be delivered to target organs and cells with viral and non-viral vectors. As therapeutics, adenoviral (Ad) vectors represent one of the promising candidates among current available advance-therapy medical products [11]. Ad vector is still one of the most commonly utilized gene transfer vectors in a variety of potential applications for lung diseases (including inherited disease and cancer gene therapy). Ad-based vector can efficiently transduce dividing and non-dividing cells. They can be easily produced and purified in high titers.

The helper-dependent adenoviral (HD-Ad) vector has been developed based on adenovirus by deleting all viral genes. This makes the HD-Ad vector less immunogenic and allows it to have a large DNA-carrying capacity [12–14]. This unique feature of large capacity makes it ideal for the delivery of large genes, such as *CFTR*, together with gene regulating components. With more than 36 kb DNA payload capacity, HD-Ad vectors can easily carry gene editing components, such as guide RNA, CRISPR-Cas9, and therapeutic donor genes with gene-regulatory elements in the same vector [15–17]. Our previous studies have demonstrated that HD-Ad vectors are efficient for transducing airway surface epithelial cells and submucosal glands [18,19]. We have shown that abundant therapeutic *CFTR* protein expression at the apical membrane of airway epithelial cells as well as the submucosal glands of the conduct airways can be achieved by HD-Ad vector delivery to the lungs of mice and pigs. More importantly, HD-Ad vectors have been shown to transduce pig airway basal cells, which are considered as stem/progenitor cells [20,21].

However, the transduction of self-renewal tissues, such as airway epithelium with episomal vectors, requires repeated administration to achieve long-term gene correction [22]. Even considering stem/progenitor cell targeting with gene editing, repeated delivery may be still needed due to the current low in vivo gene-targeting efficiency. HD-Ad vectors, as other viral vectors, evoke host innate and adaptive immune responses against capsid proteins. Studies in experimental animals and clinical trials have shown that antibody and T cell responses can limit transgene expression duration and hinder the repeated administration of gene transfer [23]. Several approaches, including vector modification and host immune system modulations, have been investigated for minimizing immune responses [24–26]. All of these approaches have shown effects on the partial reduction in inflammation and immune reactions, but they are not fruitful in improving the duration of transgene expression. The aim of this study is to investigate how pharmacological agents can modulate the host immune system to allow the sustained expression of the *CFTR* gene from HD-Ad vectors in repeated delivery to mouse airways.

2. Materials and Methods

2.1. HD-Ad Vector Preparation and Delivery to Mice Lungs

HD-Ad-*CFTR* (helper-dependent adenoviral vector expressing the human *CFTR* gene) was prepared as described previously [27]. The purity of the HD-Ad vector preparations was determined by real-time q-PCR (quantitative polymerase chain reaction). For vector delivery, adult female C57Bl/6 mice (Charles River Laboratories, Wilmington, MA, USA) were anesthetized by isoflurane inhalation, and 20 μL of 1.5×10^{10} of HD-Ad-CFTR vector in PBS (phosphate buffered saline) with 40 μg/mL of DEAE-dextran (diethylaminoethyl-dextran) and 0.1% L-α-lysophosphatidylcholine (LPC) (Sigma-Aldrich, Oakville, ON, Canada) were placed in small drops onto one nostril from which they were aspirated into the lungs. All the mice, including the experiment and control groups, were given three rounds of HD-Ad-*CFTR* vector with the same dose at day 0 (d0), day 60 (d60), and day 120 (d120). Only the experiment group was injected intraperitoneally (ip) with cyclophosphamide (50 mg/kg) at 6 h before and 4 and 8 days after the vector delivery. At 3 and 33 days following the final round of vector delivery, the mice were sacrificed and blood samples were collected by cardiac puncture. A bronchoalveolar lavage was performed three times, each with 0.9 mL of phosphate-buffered saline. The lungs were collected for RNA isolation and histological analyses. Another group of mice received a single dose of 1.5×10^{10} HD-Ad-*CFTR* vectors with the same formula and procedure, and were sacrificed 3 days following the vector delivery. The animal studies were conducted following the Animal Use Protocol (#48813) approved by the Animal Care Committee of The Hospital for Sick Children, Toronto, Canada.

2.2. RNA Isolation and Real-Time RT-qPCR

Total RNA from mouse lungs was isolated using an RNeasy kit (a simplified technology for total RNA isolation) (Qiagen, Mississauga, ON, Canada) according to the manufacturer's instructions (Invitrogen, Carlsbad, CA, USA), followed by DNase digestion. For SYBR Green real-time RT-PCR, the total RNA (1 μg) was reverse-transcribed using random hexamers and SuperScript II reverse transcriptase following the manufacturer's protocol. The resulting templates (10 ng cDNA) were used for real-time PCR (ABI Prism 7500, Applied Biosystems, Foster City, CA, USA). For relative quantification, the PCR signals were compared between groups after normalization using 18S (TaqMan, Ribosomal RNA Control Reagents, Applied Biosystems, Foster City, CA, USA) as an internal reference. The following are primer sequences for the PCR analysis of vector *CFTR* and T cell marker genes: K18CFTR-F: CCTGAGTCCTGTCCTTTCTC, K18CFTR-RCGCTGTCTGTATCCTTTCCTC; mCD3e-F: GGACGATGCCGAGAACATTGA, mCD3e-R: CCAGGTGCTTATCATGCTTCTG; mCD4-F: GCCCTCATATACACACACCTGT, mCD4-R: GCAGCAGCAGCAGCAGCAA; mCD8a-F: GCTCAGTCATCAGCAACTCG, mCD8a-R: GTGAGGGAGTTCGCAGCACT.

2.3. Anti-Ad Antibody Titer Assay

A pan-specific (IgA, IgE, IgGs, IgM) ELISA for mouse anti-human Ad5 antibodies was performed, as previously described [19,28]. A 96-well ELISA plate (Corning Costar, Acton, MA, USA) was coated with 5×10^9 viral particles of human Ad5 per well overnight at 4 °C in a 100 mM bicarbonate buffer at pH 9.6. The plate was then washed with TBS (Tris-buffered saline) and blocked with 3% BSA (bovine serum albumin) in TBS. Mouse bronchoalveolar lavage fluid (BALF) and serum diluted in 1:200 or 1:200,000 TBS, respectively, were added to the wells for overnight incubation. After washing with TBS, the plate was incubated with anti-mouse-Ig-biotin (BD Pharmingen, San Diego, CA, USA) and diluted in 1:5000 TBS for 3 hr at room temperature. The plate was washed again and incubated with avidin-alkaline phosphatase (Sigma-Aldrich, Oakville, ON, Canada), diluted 1:50,000 in TBS for 2 hr at room temperature. The plate was subsequently washed and incubated with 1 mg/mL p-nitrophenyl phosphate (Sigma-Aldrich, Oakville, ON, Canada) in 100 mM diethanolamine buffer at pH 9.8, containing 0.5 mM $MgCl_2$, for 10 min at room temperature. The reaction was stopped by the addition of 25 μL of 0.2 M EDTA (ethylenediaminetetraacetic acid) and the optical density was read at 405 nm.

2.4. Neutralizing Abs Assay

The ability of the mouse heat-inactivated serum to block the Ad5 infection of HeLa cells was measured, as described previously [28]. The diluted BALF and serum was incubated with HD-Ad-LacZ and then infected HeLa cells. After 3 days, the cells were fixed and stained with an X-gal solution. The highest dilution that resulted in a minimum 50% reduction in blue cells was recorded. When no reduction was observed, the lowest dilution was conservatively assigned.

2.5. CDs Marker Staining

Immunohistochemistry staining was performed by the Pathology Core at The Toronto Centre for Phenogenomics. Tissue sections were submitted to heat-induced epitope retrieval with citrate buffer (pH 6.0) or with Tris-EDTA buffer (pH 9.0) for 7 min, followed by the quenching of endogenous peroxidase with 0.3% hydrogen peroxide in methanol. Non-specific antibody binding was blocked with 2.5% normal horse or goat serum (Vector, Laboratories, Burlingame, CA, USA), followed by incubation for 1 h in rat anti-CD3 at a 1:150 dilution (ab11089, Abcam, Toronto, ON, Canada), rabbit anti-CD4 at a 1:500 dilution (ab183685, Abcam, Toronto, ON, Canada), rabbit anti-CD8 at a 1:1000 dilution (ab209775, Abcam, Toronto, ON Canada), or rat anti-B220 at a 1:200 dilution (14-0452-82, Invitrogen, Mississauga, ON Canada). After washes, the tissue sections were incubated for 30 min with an ImmPRESS HRP (horseradish Peroxidase) reagent anti-rabbit or anti-rat IgG polymer (Vector, Laboratories, Burlingame, CA, USA), followed by a DAB (3′,3′-Diaminobenzidine) reagent.

2.6. Statistical Analysis

Five mice were used for each group. All the data on *CFTR* mRNA, cytokine gene expression, and antibody assays were tested with Prism one-way ANOVA multiple comparisons. The data were presented as mean ± SD (standard deviation). A $p < 0.05$ was considered significant. For the *CFTR* mRNA expression, the fold change was calculated according to Livak and Schmittgen [29].

3. Results

3.1. Scheme of Experiment Design for HD-Ad-CFTR Vector Delivery and Immunosuppressant Administration

Our previous studies have shown that the HD-Ad-*CFTR* vector can efficiently transduce epithelial cells, but it induces significant inflammation and immune responses to the vector in mouse lungs [19]. In this study, we designed the experiment to investigate whether the expression of the transgene can be sustained through host immune system modulation in a model of repeated vector delivery. Three rounds of HD-Ad-*CFTR* vector were given intranasally to mice, with an interval of 2 months for each round. The immunosuppressant cyclophosphamide was administrated 6 h before vector delivery to block the initiation of inflammation and immune reaction. To maintain transiently the immunosuppression of the innate and subsequent adaptive immune responses, cyclophosphamide was given at day 4 and day 8 after the vector transduction. The immunosuppressant was administrated with a similar schedule for each round of vector delivery. As shown in Figure 1, the transgene expression and immune responses were analyzed at two time points, day 123 and day 153 following the first round of vector delivery.

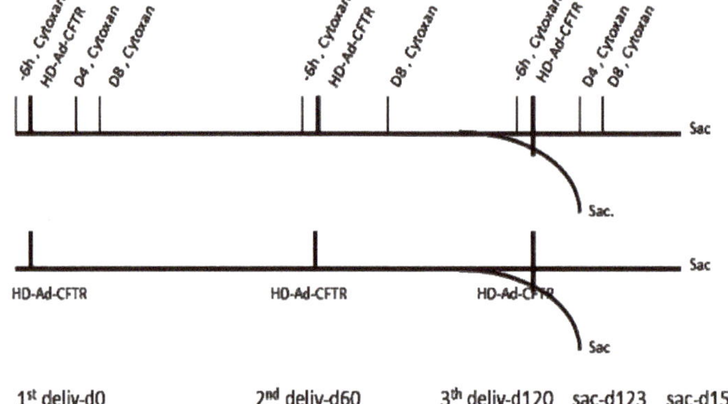

Figure 1. Time frame of the helper-dependent adenoviral (HD-Ad) vector transduction and cyclophosphamide administration. All the mice were nasally delivered HD-Ad-*CFTR* at a dose of 1.5×10^{10} viral particles in 3 rounds, each indicated by a heavy vertical line. The date of the first round of vector delivery is called d0. The second and third round was given at day 60 and day 120, respectively, following the first round. A cyclophosphamide (cytoxan) injection was administered at 6 h before (−6 h) and 4 (d4) and 8 days (d8) following the vector delivery. However, there was a glitch in the scheme where the cyclophosphamide injection at day 4 for the second round of vector delivery was missed. The samples were collected at days 3 and 33 after the last round of vector delivery, as shown in the scheme. Deliv: delivery; sac: sacrifice.

3.2. Cyclophosphamide Reduced T Cell Gene Expression

To investigate the effect of cyclophosphamide on T cells, CD3, CD4, and CD8 expression in mouse lungs was analyzed by real-time RT-qPCR. As shown in Figure 2, we observed that cyclophosphamide reduced the CD3 and CD4 gene expression by 34% and 44%, respectively, at day 3 following the last round of vector delivery compared to the mice without immunosuppression. At day 33, the CD3 and CD4 gene expression was further reduced by 38% and 47% in the cyclophosphamide-treated group. However, at this time point the difference in levels of expression between the groups with or without cyclophosphamide treatments was not statistically significant. This could be due to the small number of mice used in the experiment. Interestingly, the CD3, CD4, and CD8 gene expression decreased significantly between 3 and 33 days after the last round of vector delivery in both groups with or without cyclophosphamide administration (Figure 2). The CD3, CD4, and CD8 expression in the group with cyclophosphamide administration was reduced by 61%, 50%, and 57%, respectively, while their expression in the group without cyclophosphamide administration was reduced by 58%, 46%, and 53%, respectively. Nevertheless, these data suggested that transient immunosuppression can significantly block CD3 and CD4 gene expression. Our results were further confirmed by immunohistochemistry staining of the mouse lung tissues with antibodies against CD3, CD4, and CD8, as shown in Figure 3.

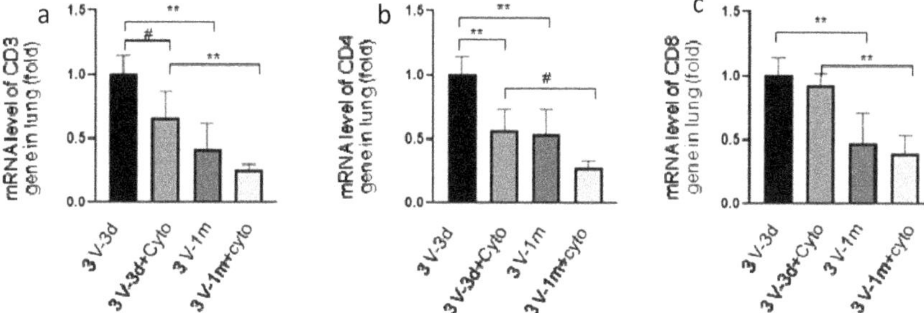

Figure 2. CD3 (cluster of differentiation 3) (**a**), CD4 (**b**), and CD8 (**c**) gene expression in mouse lungs determined by real-time RT-qPCR. RNA was isolated from mouse lung tissues, which were collected at days 3 and 33 after the last round of vector transduction from both groups of mice with or without cyclophosphamide treatments. The expression of CD3 (left panel), CD4 (middle panel), and CD8 (right panel) genes was normalized with 18S. 3V-3d: samples collected at day 3 following the third round of vector delivery; 3V-3d+cyto: samples collected from mice with the same time frame as those of 3v-3d but with cyclophosphamide treatments; 3V-1m: samples collected from mice in one month following the last round of vector delivery; 3v-1m+cyto: samples collected from mice with the same time frame as those of 3V-1m, but with cyclophosphamide treatments. Data are presented as mean ± SD (standard deviation), $n = 5$ for all groups. #: $p < 0.05$; **: $p < 0.01$.

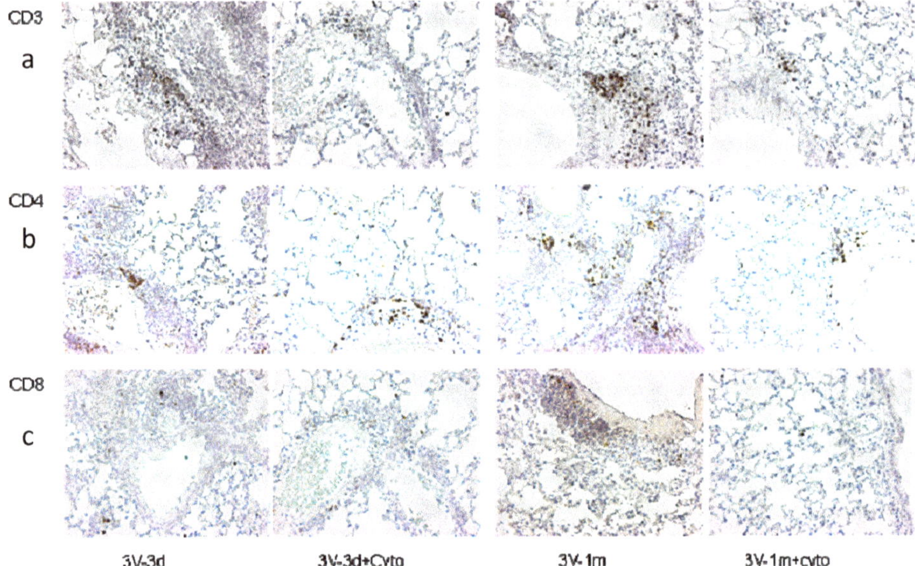

Figure 3. CD3 (**a**), CD4 (**b**), and CD8 (**c**) protein expression in mouse lungs. IHC (immunohistochemical) staining was performed in paraffin sections of mouse lungs and stained with antibodies against CD3, CD4, and CD8. The positive cells are shown in brown color. The sample labelling is the same as in Figure 2.

3.3. Cyclophosphamide Greatly Reduced B Cell Responses Induced by Repeated Vector Delivery

Our previous studies reported that cyclophosphamide can block humoral immune responses to vector delivery in mouse airways with reduced antibody production. In this study, repeated HD-Ad-*CFTR* vector delivery was expected to induce stronger immune responses to HD-Ad vector and transgene products. To test whether cyclophosphamide could still efficiently block B cell activation and functioning, we analyzed anti-adenoviral antibody and neutralizing antibodies at day 3 and day 33 after the last round of vector delivery in mouse BALF (Figure 4) and serum (Supplementary Figure S1). As shown in Figure 4a, the anti-Ad total antibodies in cyclophosphamide-treated mice were significantly lower compared to the group with no treatment at day 3. This means that cyclophosphamide administration efficiently prevented B cell function from the previous two rounds of HD-Ad-*CFTR* delivery. In contrast to CD3, CD4, and CD8 gene expression, the levels of anti-Ad antibodies were not decreased with time from day 3 to day 33 after the last round of vector delivery, when cyclophosphamide was not used.

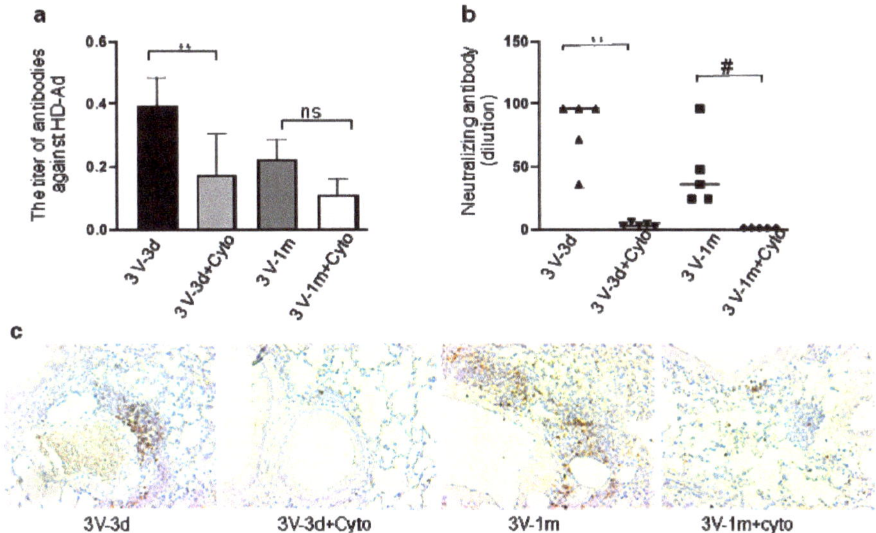

Figure 4. Host humoral immune responses to vector delivery. (**a**) The titer of anti-adenoviral antibodies in mouse bronchoalveolar lavage fluid (BALF). The total anti-Ad antibodies (IgA, IgE, IgGs, IgM) were detected with ELISA in all groups. Data were presented as mean ± SD (standard deviation). (**b**) Neutralizing antibody in mouse BALF. $n = 5$, #: $p < 0.05$; **: $p < 0.01$. (**c**) B-cell presence in mouse lungs. B-cells were detected in mouse lungs with antibodies against B220 by immunohistochemistry staining. The positive cells are shown in brown color. ns, no significant difference.

In addition, at both days 3 and 33, the BALF- and serum-neutralizing antibody was greatly reduced by the cyclophosphamide administration (Figure 4b and Supplementary Figure S1b). This indicates that cyclophosphamide reduced the neutralizing antibody production from every round of vector transduction. Congruently, IHC staining with antibodies against B220 showed less infiltration of B220-positive cells in the lungs of mice treated with cyclophosphamide compared to the group without the treatment (Figure 4c). These data suggest that cyclophosphamide treatment during vector delivery can significantly block B cell activation induced by every round of vector transduction.

3.4. Transgene Expression was Improved Significantly by Immunosuppressant

The goal of this study was to improve the long-term expression of transgene with cyclophosphamide treatment by blocking the airway inflammation and immune reaction to vector and transgene products. As shown in Figure 5a, the cyclophosphamide treatment improved the vector *CFTR* gene expression at both days 3 and 33 following the last round of vector delivery by 4.1 and 3.3 fold, respectively, compared to the vector-only group. The high level of human *CFTR* transgene expression at day 3 after the last round of transduction indicates that the cyclophosphamide treatment strongly reduced the vector-neutralizing activity in the previous rounds of vector delivery. We also observed that the *CFTR* expression level was not significantly reduced from day 3 to day 33 after the last round of delivery in the cyclophosphamide-treated group. This suggests that the cyclophosphamide treatment significantly preserved vector transduced cells. Finally, in this study of repeated vector delivery, the *CFTR* transgene expression level in cyclophosphamide-treated mice at days 123 and 153 from the first round of vector delivery remained at 83% and 63%, respectively, of that of the mice that received a single dose of vector delivery at day 3 (Figure 5b). These data clearly demonstrate that transient cyclophosphamide treatments help the targeting cells retain a relatively high level of sustained expression of the transgene in mouse lungs.

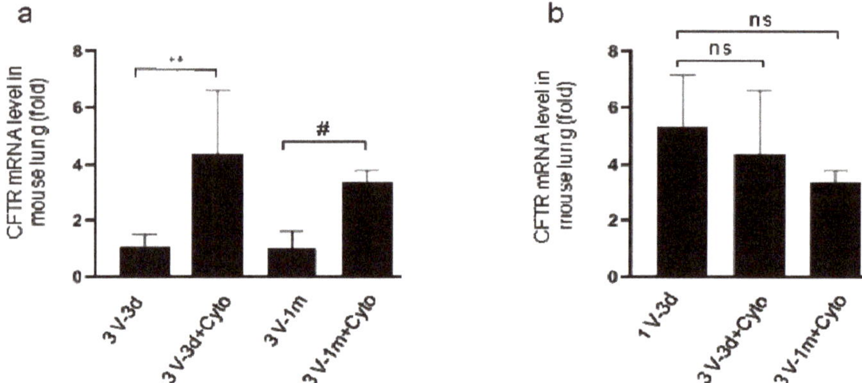

Figure 5. Expression of human cystic fibrosis transmembrane conductance regulator (*CFTR*) mRNA in mouse lungs assessed by real-time RT-qPCR. (**a**) *CFTR* mRNA levels in lung tissues of mice at days 3 and 33 following the last round of HD-Ad-*CFTR* delivery with or without cyclophosphamide treatments. The transgene expression was normalized with 18S. Data were presented as mean ± SD. $n = 5$; #: $p < 0.05$; **: $p < 0.01$. (**b**) *CFTR* mRNA levels in mouselung tissues from 3 days of single dose delivery (1V-3d), and at days 3 (3V-3d) and 33 (3V-33d) of 3 dose delivery following the last round of transduction with cyclophosphamide treatment. Data were presented as mean ± SD. Ns indicates no significant difference.

4. Discussion

In this repeated gene delivery study, we found the immunosuppressant cyclophosphamide significantly blocked the adaptive immune responses induced by the HD-Ad vector, showing a reduced T cell gene expression and T cell and B cell infiltration in mouse lungs. The transient immunosuppression resulted in a significant level of transgene expression at day 3 after three rounds of HD-Ad vector transduction and maintained a relatively high level of *CFTR* gene expression at 33 days after the last round of delivery. The slightly lower level of transgene expression in mice at day 33 may partially result from epithelial cells' turn over. These data demonstrated that the sustained expression of the transgene in mouse lungs can be achieved by the repeated delivery of HD-Ad-*CFTR* vectors with a transient cyclophosphamide administration.

The sustained expression of transgene at therapeutic levels (achieving lifelong expression) in the terminal-differentiated cells of epithelia, which are capable of self-renewal, requires the repeated administration of vectors. Immune responses against vectors and transgene products are one of the major obstacles to sustained transgene expression in repeated vector delivery. Strategies to control unwanted immune responses to transgene products and vectors are needed to achieve the sustained expression of therapeutic genes in the lung. Lungs have their own set of immune cells which function as the frontline of immunity for the airway. Adaptive immune responses can be triggered by vector antigens or vector-encoded proteins during gene delivery. We and others have shown that gene transfer with Ad or HD-Ad vectors at single doses locally or systemically resulted in the activation of T cells and humoral immune responses to transgene products and vector antigens [30]. The repeated administration of most viral vectors is hindered by the toxicity of T cells and neutralizing or opsonizing the Abs induced by the vectors.

Thus, strategies including immunosuppression, induction of immune tolerance, or modification of viral capsids have been tested in vector delivery [22]. For example, Seregin et al. reported that transient pre-treatment with glucocorticoid can significantly reduce innate and adaptive immune responses to Ad vector with systemic delivery without a transgene expression reduction in mouse liver [31]. Immune suppressant prednisone has also been shown to reduce the extent of intramuscular T-cell infiltrates in AAV-treated muscles, which may aid in achieving long-term transgene expression through promoting PD1-mediated programmed T-cell death [32]. In addition, viral vector serotype switching [33] and capsid engineering [34] have been evaluated for viral vector readministration. The repeated liver gene transfer to adult mice with mutations in the liver-specific UGT1 gene by AAV serotype switching, upon neonatal administration, resulted in the lifelong correction of total bilirubin levels in the mice [35].

Cyclophosphamide is a potent immunosuppressive agent used clinically in autoimmune disorders and the transplantation of allogeneic bone marrow or solid organs to establish peripheral allograft tolerance and suppress autoreactive T cells [36]. Our previous study found that cyclophosphamide treatment significantly improved transgene expression at day 3 following HD-Ad readministration [19]. In the repeated airway transduction mouse model, the transient use of cyclophosphamide during HD-vector administration significantly reduced the expression of the CD3 and CD4 gene and the infiltration of these cells in the targeting organ. This indicated that cyclophosphamide may cause T cell death besides its anti-mitotic and anti-replicative effects [36]. Strauss et al. have reported that the effect of cyclophosphamide on T cells is its ability to induce apoptosis, which is a fundamental difference from other immunosuppressive agents.

Cyclophosphamide up-regulated Fas (CD95) expression, triggering activation-induced cell death. Comparing the effects of other drugs such as dexamethasone and rapamycin on human peripheral blood T cells, cytotoxic cell lines, and Jurkat cells, only cyclophosphamide triggered cell death [37,38]. The induction of apoptosis is also a key mechanism to eliminate activated T cells during the termination of an immune response.

In addition to T cell effects, cyclophosphamide also affects B cell proliferation and plasma cell antibody production [39]. In this study, HD-Ad vector transduction resulted in anti-Ad antibody production. Such antibodies can bind to and prevent viral vectors from entering target cells, thereby reducing the transgene expression. Transient cyclophosphamide administration significantly prevented anti-Ad antibody production and reduced the neutralizing activity. This reduction is expected to improve the vector transduction efficiency from the next round of vector delivery and sustained transgene expression. These studies established the important concept that the transient suppression of host immune responses is efficient for the sustained expression of transgene in mouse lungs in repeated HD-Ad vector delivery.

However, one limitation of this study is that we are not sure whether our results with mice can be translated into clinical applications, because there are differences between mice and humans in the immune system. These differences include: activation of immune responses to challenge, the balance of leukocyte subsets, Toll-like receptors, and antibody subsets [40,41]. Therefore, the safety, dosage, and scheduling of cyclophosphamide administration should be further evaluated in large animal models. Cyclophosphamide has immunosuppressive and immunomodulatory properties. Considering the risk of infection for persons with CF, the immunosuppressive function of cyclophosphamide and its effect on vector transduction efficiency should be tested in proper CF animal models. In this study, we did not investigate whether cyclophosphamide affects host innate immune responses. However, our previous work has shown that there was no significant change in cytokine production to HD-Ad vector with cyclophosphamide treatment [19]. Strategies with the combination of different immunosuppressive agents to target specifically innate and adaptive immune responses at different stages may also be important. In addition, the scheduling of administration is of particular importance for the immunological effect [36]. We observed that the expression of CD3, CD4, and CD 8 genes goes down significantly with time, one month after the last round of delivery with or without cyclophosphamide treatment. This observation suggests a window for scheduling the following round of vector administration in order to avoid the peak of adaptive immune responses.

5. Conclusions

In summary, the immunosuppressant cyclophosphamide can modulate the host immune system and allow for a more sustained expression of the *CFTR* gene in repeated vector delivery to mouse airways. In combination with a gene-editing system to target airway stem cells, sustained expression with a therapeutic level of transgene may be achievable in the future.

Supplementary Materials: The following are available online at http://www.mdpi.com/2073-4425/11/5/565/s1, Figure S1: Anti-adenoviral antibodies in mouse serum. (a) The total anti-Ad antibodies (IgA, IgE, IgGs, IgM) were detected with ELISA in all groups. Data were presented as mean ± SD. (b) Neutralizing antibody in mouse sera. $n = 5$, #: $p < 0.05$; **: $p < 0.01$.

Author Contributions: Conceptualization, H.C. and J.H.; methodology, H.C. and R.D.; validation, H.C. and R.D.; formal analysis, H.C.; investigation, H.C.; resources, J.H.; data curation, H.C. and R.D.; writing—original draft preparation, H.C.; writing—review and editing, R.D. and J.H.; visualization, H.C.; supervision, J.H.; project administration, J.H.; funding acquisition, J.H. All authors have read and agreed to the published version of the manuscript.

Funding: This study was funded by the Canadian Institute for Health Research (CIHR) grants (MOP 125882), the Cystic Fibrosis Foundation Therapeutics, Inc. grant (HU15XX0), and the Cystic Fibrosis Canada grant (#3032) to JH.

Acknowledgments: The authors wish to acknowledge the contribution of Vivian Bradaschia and Milan Ganguly in the Pathology Core at The Centre for Phenogenomics for IHC staining and of Jing Wu at The Hospital for Sick Children, Research Institute for real-time RT-PCR analyses. We thank Sara Chowns for reading and commenting on the manuscript.

Conflicts of Interest: All authors have no conflict of interest to declare.

References

1. Corbyn, Z. Promising new era dawns for cystic fibrosis treatment. *Lancet* **2012**, *379*, 1475–1476. [CrossRef]
2. Davies, J.C.; Moskowitz, S.M.; Brown, C.; Horsley, A.; Mall, M.A.; McKone, E.F.; Plant, B.J.; Prais, D.; Ramsey, B.W.; Taylor-Cousar, J.L.; et al. VX-659-Tezacaftor-Ivacaftor in Patients with Cystic Fibrosis and One or Two Phe508del Alleles. *N. Engl. J. Med.* **2018**, *379*, 1599–1611. [CrossRef]
3. Heijerman, H.G.M.; McKone, E.F.; Downey, D.G.; Van Braeckel, E.; Rowe, S.M.; Tullis, E.; Mall, M.A.; Welter, J.J.; Ramsey, B.W.; McKee, C.M.; et al. Efficacy and safety of the elexacaftor plus tezacaftor plus ivacaftor combination regimen in people with cystic fibrosis homozygous for the F508del mutation: A double-blind, randomised, phase 3 trial. *Lancet* **2019**, *394*, 1940–1948. [CrossRef]
4. Keating, D.; Marigowda, G.; Burr, L.; Daines, C.; Mall, M.A.; McKone, E.F.; Ramsey, B.W.; Rowe, S.M.; Sass, L.A.; Tullis, E.; et al. VX-445-Tezacaftor-Ivacaftor in Patients with Cystic Fibrosis and One or Two Phe508del Alleles. *N. Engl. J. Med.* **2018**, *379*, 1612–1620. [CrossRef]
5. Middleton, P.G.; Mall, M.A.; Drevinek, P.; Lands, L.C.; McKone, E.F.; Polineni, D.; Ramsey, B.W.; Taylor-Cousar, J.L.; Tullis, E.; Vermeulen, F.; et al. Elexacaftor-Tezacaftor-Ivacaftor for Cystic Fibrosis with a Single Phe508del Allele. *N. Engl. J. Med.* **2019**, *381*, 1809–1819. [CrossRef]
6. Cooney, A.L.; McCray, P.B., Jr.; Sinn, P.L. Cystic Fibrosis Gene Therapy: Looking Back, Looking Forward. *Genes* **2018**, *9*, 538. [CrossRef]
7. Brody, H. Gene therapy. *Nature* **2018**, *564*, S5. [CrossRef]
8. Jennings, M.T.; Flume, P.A. Cystic Fibrosis: Translating Molecular Mechanisms into Effective Therapies. *Ann. Am. Thorac. Soc.* **2018**, *15*, 897–902. [CrossRef]
9. Ginn, S.L.; Amaya, A.K.; Alexander, I.E.; Edelstein, M.; Abedi, M.R. Gene therapy clinical trials worldwide to 2017: An update. *J. Gene Med.* **2018**, *20*, e3015. [CrossRef]
10. Dunbar, C.E.; High, K.A.; Joung, J.K.; Kohn, D.B.; Ozawa, K.; Sadelain, M. Gene therapy comes of age. *Science* **2018**, *359*. [CrossRef]
11. Gao, J.; Mese, K.; Bunz, O.; Ehrhardt, A. State-of-the-art human adenovirus vectorology for therapeutic approaches. *FEBS Lett.* **2019**, *593*, 3609–3622. [CrossRef]
12. Cao, H.; Koehler, D.R.; Hu, J. Adenoviral vectors for gene replacement therapy. *Viral Immunol.* **2004**, *17*, 327–333. [CrossRef]

13. Flotte, T.R.; Ng, P.; Dylla, D.E.; McCray, P.B., Jr.; Wang, G.; Kolls, J.K.; Hu, J. Viral vector-mediated and cell-based therapies for treatment of cystic fibrosis. *Mol. Ther.* **2007**, *15*, 229–241. [CrossRef]

14. Koehler, D.R.; Hitt, M.M.; Hu, J. Challenges and strategies for cystic fibrosis lung gene therapy. *Mol. Ther.* **2001**, *4*, 84–91. [CrossRef]

15. Zhou, Z.P.; Yang, L.L.; Cao, H.; Chen, Z.R.; Zhang, Y.; Wen, X.Y.; Hu, J. In Vitro Validation of a CRISPR-Mediated CFTR Correction Strategy for Preclinical Translation in Pigs. *Hum. Gene Ther.* **2019**, *30*, 1101–1116. [CrossRef]

16. Xia, E.; Zhang, Y.; Cao, H.; Li, J.; Duan, R.; Hu, J. TALEN-Mediated Gene Targeting for Cystic Fibrosis-Gene Therapy. *Genes* **2019**, *10*, 39. [CrossRef]

17. Xia, E.; Duan, R.; Shi, F.; Seigel, K.E.; Grasemann, H.; Hu, J. Overcoming the Undesirable CRISPR-Cas9 Expression in Gene Correction. *Mol. Ther. Nucleic Acids* **2018**, *13*, 699–709. [CrossRef]

18. Cao, H.; Machuca, T.N.; Yeung, J.C.; Wu, J.; Du, K.; Duan, C.; Hashimoto, K.; Linacre, V.; Coates, A.L.; Leung, K.; et al. Efficient gene delivery to pig airway epithelia and submucosal glands using helper-dependent adenoviral vectors. *Mol. Ther. Nucleic Acids* **2013**, *2*, e127. [CrossRef]

19. Cao, H.; Yang, T.; Li, X.F.; Wu, J.; Duan, C.; Coates, A.L.; Hu, J. Readministration of helper-dependent adenoviral vectors to mouse airway mediated via transient immunosuppression. *Gene Ther.* **2011**, *18*, 173–181. [CrossRef]

20. Cao, H.; Ouyang, H.; Grasemann, H.; Bartlett, C.; Du, K.; Duan, R.; Shi, F.; Estrada, M.; Seigel, K.; Coates, A.; et al. Transducing airway basal cells with a helper-dependent adenoviral vector for lung gene therapy. *Hum. Gene Ther.* **2018**. [CrossRef]

21. Levardon, H.; Yonker, L.M.; Hurley, B.P.; Mou, H. Expansion of Airway Basal Cells and Generation of Polarized Epithelium. *Bio. Protoc.* **2018**, *8*. [CrossRef]

22. Carlon, M.S.; Vidovic, D.; Dooley, J.; da Cunha, M.M.; Maris, M.; Lampi, Y.; Toelen, J.; Van den Haute, C.; Baekelandt, V.; Deprest, J.; et al. Immunological ignorance allows long-term gene expression after perinatal recombinant adeno-associated virus-mediated gene transfer to murine airways. *Hum. Gene Ther.* **2014**, *25*, 517–528. [CrossRef]

23. Ferrari, S.; Griesenbach, U.; Geddes, D.M.; Alton, E. Immunological hurdles to lung gene therapy. *Clin. Exp. Immunol.* **2003**, *132*, 1–8. [CrossRef]

24. Nathwani, A.C.; Tuddenham, E.G.; Rangarajan, S.; Rosales, C.; McIntosh, J.; Linch, D.C.; Chowdary, P.; Riddell, A.; Pie, A.J.; Harrington, C.; et al. Adenovirus-associated virus vector-mediated gene transfer in hemophilia B. *N. Engl. J. Med.* **2011**, *365*, 2357–2365. [CrossRef]

25. Martino, A.T.; Basner-Tschakarjan, E.; Markusic, D.M.; Finn, J.D.; Hinderer, C.; Zhou, S.; Ostrov, D.A.; Srivastava, A.; Ertl, H.C.; Terhorst, C.; et al. Engineered AAV vector minimizes in vivo targeting of transduced hepatocytes by capsid-specific CD8+ T cells. *Blood* **2013**, *121*, 2224–2233. [CrossRef]

26. Arruda, V.R.; Favaro, P.; Finn, J.D. Strategies to modulate immune responses: A new frontier for gene therapy. *Mol. Ther.* **2009**, *17*, 1492–1503. [CrossRef]

27. Palmer, D.J.; Ng, P. Methods for the production of helper-dependent adenoviral vectors. *Methods Mol. Biol.* **2008**, *433*, 33–53.

28. Koehler, D.R.; Martin, B.; Corey, M.; Palmer, D.; Ng, P.; Tanswell, A.K.; Hu, J. Readministration of helper-dependent adenovirus to mouse lung. *Gene Ther.* **2006**, *13*, 773–780. [CrossRef]

29. Livak, K.J.; Schmittgen, T.D. Analysis of relative gene expression data using real-time quantitative PCR and the 2(-Delta Delta C(T)) Method. *Methods* **2001**, *25*, 402–408. [CrossRef]

30. Schirmbeck, R.; Reimann, J.; Kochanek, S.; Kreppel, F. The immunogenicity of adenovirus vectors limits the multispecificity of CD8 T-cell responses to vector-encoded transgenic antigens. *Mol. Ther.* **2008**, *16*, 1609–1616. [CrossRef]

31. Seregin, S.S.; Appledorn, D.M.; McBride, A.J.; Schuldt, N.J.; Aldhamen, Y.A.; Voss, T.; Wei, J.; Bujold, M.; Nance, W.; Godbehere, S.; et al. Transient pretreatment with glucocorticoid ablates innate toxicity of systemically delivered adenoviral vectors without reducing efficacy. *Mol. Ther.* **2009**, *17*, 685–696. [CrossRef]

32. Cramer, M.L.; Shao, G.; Rodino-Klapac, L.R.; Chicoine, L.G.; Martin, P.T. Induction of T-Cell Infiltration and Programmed Death Ligand 2 Expression by Adeno-Associated Virus in Rhesus Macaque Skeletal Muscle and Modulation by Prednisone. *Hum. Gene Ther.* **2017**, *28*, 493–509. [CrossRef]

33. Majowicz, A.; Salas, D.; Zabaleta, N.; Rodriguez-Garcia, E.; Gonzalez-Aseguinolaza, G.; Petry, H.; Ferreira, V. Successful Repeated Hepatic Gene Delivery in Mice and Non-human Primates Achieved by Sequential Administration of AAV5(ch) and AAV1. *Mol. Ther.* **2017**, *25*, 1831–1842. [CrossRef]

34. Vandenberghe, L.H.; Wilson, J.M.; Gao, G. Tailoring the AAV vector capsid for gene therapy. *Gene Ther.* **2009**, *16*, 311–319. [CrossRef]

35. Bockor, L.; Bortolussi, G.; Iaconcig, A.; Chiaruttini, G.; Tiribelli, C.; Giacca, M.; Benvenuti, F.; Zentilin, L.; Muro, A.F. Repeated AAV-mediated gene transfer by serotype switching enables long-lasting therapeutic levels of hUgt1a1 enzyme in a mouse model of Crigler-Najjar Syndrome Type I. *Gene Ther.* **2017**, *24*, 649–660. [CrossRef]

36. Ahlmann, M.; Hempel, G. The effect of cyclophosphamide on the immune system: Implications for clinical cancer therapy. *Cancer Chemother. Pharm.* **2016**, *78*, 661–671. [CrossRef]

37. Strauss, G.; Osen, W.; Debatin, K.M. Induction of apoptosis and modulation of activation and effector function in T cells by immunosuppressive drugs. *Clin. Exp. Immunol.* **2002**, *128*, 255–266. [CrossRef]

38. Al-Homsi, A.S.; Roy, T.S.; Cole, K.; Feng, Y.; Duffner, U. Post-transplant high-dose cyclophosphamide for the prevention of graft-versus-host disease. *Biol. Blood Marrow Transplant.* **2015**, *21*, 604–611. [CrossRef]

39. Wojcik, R. Reactivity of the immunological system of rats stimulated with Biolex-Beta HP after cyclophosphamide immunosuppression. *Cent. Eur. J. Immunol.* **2014**, *39*, 51–60. [CrossRef]

40. Tao, L.; Reese, T.A. Making Mouse Models That Reflect Human Immune Responses. *Trends Immunol.* **2017**, *38*, 181–193. [CrossRef]

41. Mestas, J.; Hughes, C.C. Of mice and not men: Differences between mouse and human immunology. *J. Immunol.* **2004**, *172*, 2731–2738. [CrossRef]

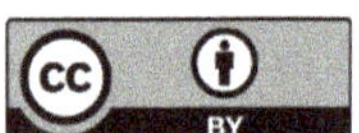

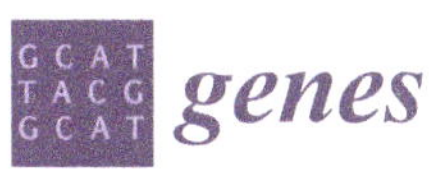
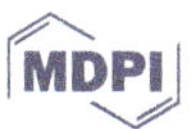

Article

Analysis of *CFTR* Mutation Spectrum in Ethnic Russian Cystic Fibrosis Patients

Nika V. Petrova *, Nataliya Y. Kashirskaya, Tatyana A. Vasilyeva, Elena I. Kondratyeva, Elena K. Zhekaite , Anna Y. Voronkova, Victoria D. Sherman , Varvara A. Galkina, Eugeny K. Ginter, Sergey I. Kutsev, Andrey V. Marakhonov and Rena A. Zinchenko

Research Centre for Medical Genetics, Moskvorechje Street, 1, 115478 Moscow, Russia; kashirskayanj@mail.ru (N.Y.K.); vasilyeva_debrie@mail.ru (T.A.V.); elenafpk@mail.ru (E.I.K.); elena_zhekayte@gmail.com (E.K.Z.); voronkova111@yandex.ru (A.Y.V.); tovika@yandex.ru (V.D.S.); vgalka06@rambler.ru (V.A.G.); ekginter@mail.ru (E.K.G.); kutsev@mail.ru (S.I.K.); marakhonov@generesearch.ru (A.V.M.); renazinchenko@mail.ru (R.A.Z.)
* Correspondence: npetrova63@mail.ru

Received: 30 March 2020; Accepted: 13 May 2020; Published: 15 May 2020

Abstract: The distribution and frequency of the *CFTR* gene mutations vary considerably between countries and ethnic groups. Russians are an East Slavic ethnic groups are native to Eastern Europe. Russians, the most numerous people of the Russian Federation (RF), make about 80% of the population. The aim is to reveal the molecular causes of CF in ethnic Russian patients as comprehensively as possible. The analysis of most common *CFTR* mutations utilized for CF diagnosis in multiethnic RF population accounts for about 83% of all CF-causing mutations in 1384 ethnic Russian patients. Variants c.1521_1523delCTT (F508del), c.54-5940_273+10250del21kb (CFTRdele2,3), c.2012delT (2143delT), c.2052_2053insA (2184insA), and c.3691delT (3821delT) are most typical for CF patients of Russian origin. DNA of 154 CF patients, Russian by origin, in whom at least one mutant allele was not previously identified (164 CF alleles), was analyzed by Sanger sequencing followed by the multiplex ligase-dependent probe amplification (MLPA) method. In addition to the 29 variants identified during the previous test for common mutations, 91 pathogenic *CFTR* variants were also revealed: 29 missense, 19 nonsense, 14 frame shift in/del, 17 splicing, 1 in frame ins, and 11 copy number variations (CNV). Each of the 61 variants was revealed once, and 17 twice. Each of the variants c.1209G>C (E403D), c.2128A>T (K710X), c.3883delA (4015delA), and c.3884_3885insT (4016insT) were detected for three, c.1766+1G>A (1898+1G>A) and c.2834C>T (S945L) for four, c.1766+1G>C (1898+1G>C) and c.(743+1_744-1)_(1584+1_1585-1)dup (CFTRdup6b-10) for five, c.2353C>T (R785X) and c.4004T>C (L1335P) for six, c.3929G>A (W1310X) for seven, c.580-1G>T (712-1G>T for eight, and c.1240_1244delCAAAA (1365del5) for 11 unrelated patients. A comprehensive analysis of *CFTR* mutant alleles with sequencing followed by MLPA, allowed not only the identification of 163 of 164 unknown alleles in our patient sample, but also expansion of the mutation spectrum with novel and additional frequent variants for ethnic Russians.

Keywords: cystic fibrosis; *CFTR* gene; common and new pathogenic variants; ethnic Russian population

1. Introduction

Cystic fibrosis (CF, OMIM#219700) is an autosomal recessive condition resulting from the pathogenic variants in the CF transmembrane regulator (*CFTR*) gene. CF is a hereditary disease caused by impaired epithelial chloride channel CFTR function. Variants are classified as disease causing, not disease causing, of variable clinical significance, or of unknown clinical significance. More than 2000 different variants of the *CFTR* gene sequence have been revealed, the pathogenicity of 20% of which is established [1,2]. In many populations the most frequent pathogenic variant of the *CFTR* gene

(*ABCC7*) is F508del, which accounts for approximately two thirds of all *CFTR* alleles, with a decreasing prevalence from Northwest to Southeast Europe. The remaining third of alleles are substantially heterogeneous, with fewer than 20 mutations occurring at a worldwide frequency of more than 0.1%. Some variants can reach a higher frequency in certain populations, due to a founder effect in religious, ethnic or geographical isolates [3]. The spectrum and frequency of *CFTR* gene sequence variants vary significantly in different countries and ethnic groups, which suggests the development of regional molecular diagnostics protocols to optimize medical and genetic care for CF patients [4].

The diagnosis of CF was proven by typical pulmonary or gastrointestinal symptoms or positive neonatal screening, or the diagnosis of CF in a sibling, as well as at least one of the following: two positive sweat chloride tests, or the identification of two *CFTR* pathologic variants in trans according to the guidelines of the European Cystic Fibrosis Society as well as the Russian National Consensus on Cystic Fibrosis [5,6].

Molecular genetic studies on CF have been conducted in the Laboratory of Genetic Epidemiology of the Research Centre for Medical Genetics for a long period of time starting from the year 1989. To date, the laboratory has analyzed the DNA of more than 3400 CF patients, the clinical diagnosis was confirmed in the Scientific-Clinical Department for Cystic Fibrosis of the Research Centre for Medical Genetics. Thereby, 87.4% of the CF patients we examined live in the European part of Russia. More than 85% are Russian or come from marriages between Russians and persons belonging to other ethnic groups. According to the Russian Registry of cystic fibrosis patients of 2017 (RF CF Registry), among at least 212 pathogenic variants of the *CFTR* gene eleven variants are the most frequent ones in the Russian Federation (their relative frequencies exceed 1% in the sample of tested patients) and they are F508del with a share of 52.81%, CFTRdele2,3—6.21%, E92K—3.00%, 2143delT—2.15%, 3849+10kbC>T—2.02%, W1282X—1.90%, 2184insA—1.85%, 1677delTA—1.81%, N1303K—1.54%, G542X—1.35%, and L138ins with 1.24% [7]. All other *CFTR* variants identified in Russian patients share 12.35%. The frequencies and spectrum of variants of the *CFTR* gene vary in different regions. This is caused by specific ethnic background of the population, as well as by different population processes occurring on different territories inhabited by the same ethnos. Thus, in the North Caucasus Federal District (NCFD), three variants are the most frequent ones: F508del (25.0%), 1677delTA (21.5%), and W1282X (17.2%) [7]. A study of *CFTR* gene variants' spectra in different NCFD ethnic groups revealed a high proportion of variant W1282X (88%) for Karachays [8], and variants 1677delTA (81.5%) and E92K (12.5%) for Chechens [9]. The most frequent variants in the Volga Federal District (VFD) are F508del (50.5%), E92K (8.7%) and CFTRdele2,3 (5.0%) [7]. A high share of E92K variant in VFD is due to the prevalence of this variant for Chuvash (55%) [10]. The second most frequent variant for Chuvash CF patients is F508del (30%) [9], although this value is lower than in the total sample of CF patients (according to the Registry of CF patients in the Russian Federation 2017, [7]).

Russian East Slavic ethnos is the most numerous people in the Russian Federation (RF) (more than 111,000,000 people), which makes 77.7% of the population of the country according to census of 2010 [11]. In the European part of RF, Russians make 85%–90% of the population.

The aim is to describe the Russian-specific spectrum of pathogenic variants of the *CFTR* gene, testing of which could increase the informativeness of DNA diagnostics in regions with a predominantly Russian population, as well to establish a basis for forming a patient base for possible targeted therapy.

2. Materials and Methods

Initially, *CFTR* genotyping of 1384 CF patients (ethnic Russians) from all-Russian sample (3457 CF patients) tested in the Laboratory of Genetic Epidemiology, Research Centre for Medical Genetics were analyzed. The diagnosis of CF was made in the Scientific-Clinical Department for Cystic Fibrosis, Research Centre for Medical Genetics or in regional CF centers according to the accepted standards [10]. Diagnosis was confirmed by analysis of clinical presentation and Gibson–Cooke sweat test, with chloride ion concentrations of 60 mmol/L or higher defining positive result. The assignment of patients' Russian ancestry was based on self- or parents' reports. The study included 154 CF Russian patients, 90% of whom came from the European part of the Russian Federation and 10% from Siberian or Far Eastern regions, for all of them at least one mutant allele was not identified.

Patients or their parents signed an informed consent to the study. The research protocol was approved by the Ethical Committee of Research Centre for Medical Genetics (Research Centre for Medical Genetics, 115522, Moscow, Moskvorechie St., 1, Russian Federation, Protocol No.17/2006 of 02.02.2006).

Molecular diagnostics consists of three consecutive stages.

First stage included analysis of 33 frequent *CFTR* variants (c.54-5940_273+10250del21kb (p.Ser18Argfs*16, CFTRdele2,3), c.254G>A (p.Gly85Glu, G85E), c.262_263delTT (p.Leu88IlefsX22, 394delTT), c.274G>A (p.Glu92Lys, E92K), c.350G>A (p.Arg117His, R117H), c.413_415dupTAC (p.Leu138dup; L138ins), c.472dupA (p.Ser158LysfsX5, 604insA), c.489+1G>T (621+1G>T), c.1000C>T (p.Arg334Trp, R334W), c.1040G>C (p.Arg347Pro, R347P), c.1397C>G (p.Ser466X, Ser466X), c.1519_1521delATC (p.Ile507del, I507del), c.1521_1523delCTT (p.Phe508del, F508del), c.1545_1546delTA (p.Tyr515X, 1677delTA), c.1585-1G>A (1717-1G>A), c.1624G>T (p.Gly542X, G542X), c.1652G>A (p.Gly551Asp, G551D), c.1657C>T (p.Arg553X, R553X), c.2012delT (p.Leu671X, 2143delT), c.2051_2052delAAinsG (p.Lys684SerfsX38, 2183AA>G), c.2052_2053insA (p.Gln685ThrfsX4, 2184insA), c.2657+5G>A (2789+5A>G), c.3140-16T>A (3272-16T>A), c.3476C>T (p.Ser1159Phe, S1159F), c.3475T>C (p.Ser1159Pro; S1159P), c.3535_3536insTCAA (p.Thr1179IlefsX17, 3667ins4), c.3587C>G (p.Ser1196X, S1196X), c.3691delT (p.Ser1231ProfsX4, 3821delT), c.3718-2477C>T (3849+10kbC-T), c.3816_3817delGT (p.Ser1273LeufsX28, 3944delGT), c.3844T>C (p.Trp1282Arg, W1282R), c.3846G>A (p.Trp1282X, W1282X), c.3909C>G (p.Asn1303Lys, N1303K), representing a routine Russian Federation panel that identifies up to 85% of mutant CF alleles as described previously [12].

Second stage included analysis of *CFTR* gene coding sequence, exon-intron junctions and 5′-UTR sequence by Sanger sequencing as described previously [12]. Variant pathogenicity status (only pathogenic or likely pathogenic variants were reported) was established using consensus recommendations of the American College of Medical Genetics and Genomics and the Association for Molecular Pathology for interpretation of sequence variants and Russian recommendations. The frequencies of identified alleles in general populations were established based on the GnomAD browser (https://gnomad.broadinstitute.org/). The predicted functional effect of missense variants was determined through SIFT, FATHMM and Radial SVM prediction algorithms as well as GERP++ and PhyloP conservation scores. Intronic and splicing variants were analyzed using Human Splicing Finder tool v. 2.4.1. Novel variants were submitted to the CFTR2 website dataset (https://cftr2.org/), CFTR1 (http://www.genet.sickkids.on.ca/cftr). Pathogenic variants of the *CFTR* gene are denoted according to the legacy nomenclature, besides novel variants named according to the HGVS nomenclature for NM_000492.4 (*CFTR*) transcript variant.

Third stage intended to search for large rearrangements in chromosome region 7q31.2 (deletions/duplications–CNV) involved the *CFTR* gene locus by the multiplex ligation-dependent probe amplification (MLPA) method in case when no pathogenic allele was detected or an allele with uncertain significance was identified at the previous stages. MLPA analysis was performed with SALSA MLPA probemix P091-D2 CFTR (MRC-Holland, Amsterdam, the Netherlands) according to the manufacturer's recommendation. The MLPA results were analyzed using Coffalyser.Net (MRC-Holland) [12].

Variants phase was checked by segregation analysis in proband and healthy parents.

The gIVS6a_415_IVS10_987Dup26817bp (CFTRdup6b-10) duplication and its boundaries were previously described by F.M. Hantash and co-authors [13]: The fragments duplicated started 415 bp downstream of exon 6a, in IVS6a, and spanned exons 6b, 7, 8, 9, and 10, breaking at 2987 bp downstream of exon 10 in IVS10. The duplicated region is 26,817 bp. Two pairs of primers have been developed to clarify the boundaries of CFTRdup6b-10 duplications identified in Russian CF patients. One flanks the junction area of rupture points of intron 11 (10 as in the legacy nomenclature) and intron 6a (6): IVS10F 5′-TCAGGAAATGGCAATGGGGT-3′ and IVS6aR 5′-GGCTCTGGTGTGATGATCCATA-3′. A 359 bp fragment from these primers is amplified only from the allele carrying the duplication. The second pair (INT10F 5′-GGGGTTGGGAAGTGATTCCA-3′ and INT10R 5′-GCCATCAGCTAGGCTTCTGTA-3′) flanks the rupture area of the intron 10, amplification occurs only from the normal sequence of the intron 10 of the *CFTR* gene leading to a product of 234 bp.

To compare variant frequencies, the Fisher test was used. The significance level was considered to be $p \leq 0.05$.

3. Results

When developing a routinely used mutation panel, the laboratory's own data [14], the results of the first collaborative study [15], and studies of other Russian laboratories (in St. Petersburg [16], Bashkortostan [17], and Tomsk [18]) were considered. The panel includes 33 pathogenic variants of the *CFTR* gene identified in patients from different regions of the Russian Federation, as well as the variants specific for certain ethnic groups [7–10], and allows identification of up to 85% of mutant alleles in all-Russian population [12].

At the first stage, the results of testing 33 pathogenic variants of the *CFTR* gene in DNA of 1384 ethnic Russians with CF (previously performed in the laboratory of genetic epidemiology) were analyzed. Thereby, 29 out of 33 tested variants were revealed (Table 1). In addition to F508del and CFTRdele2,3, eight more variants can be referred to as frequent ones for ethnic Russians (frequency of variants 2143delT, 3849+10kbC-T and 2184insA exceed 2%, variants N1303K, G542X, E92K, W1282X, and L138ins exceed 1%). The mutation detection rate of the used panel of tested variants is 83% in the sample of ethnic Russians (Table 1). In 932 patients, two mutant variants were identified, in 426 patients only one pathogenic variant was detected, both alleles were not detected in 26 patients.

Table 1. Frequencies of 33 variants of *CFTR* gene in a sample of 1384 ethnic Russians and in a nationwide sample of CF patients (RF CF Registry) [7].

No.	Variants	Number	%	% in RF CF Registry
1	c.1521_1523delCTT (p.Phe508del, F508del)	1522	54.99	52.81
2	c.54-5940_273+10250del21kb (p.Ser18Argfs*16, CFTRdele2,3)	210	7.59	6.21
3	c.2012delT (p.Leu671X, 2143delT)	75	2.71	2.15
4	c.3718-2477C>T (3849+10kbC-T)	65	2.35	2.02
5	c.2052_2053insA (p.Gln685ThrfsX4, 2184insA)	62	2.24	1.85
6	c.3909C>G (p.Asn1303Lys, N1303K)	48	1.73	1.54
7	c.1624G>T (p.Gly542X, G542X)	44	1.59	1.35
8	c.274G>A (p.Glu92Lys, E92K)	29	1.05	3.00
9	c.3846G>A (p.Trp1282X, W1282X)	32	1.16	1.90
10	c.413_415dupTAC (p.Leu138dup; L138ins)	31	1.12	1.24
11	c.3844T>C (p.Trp1282Arg, W1282R)	21	0.76	0.55
12	c.1397C>G (p.Ser466X, Ser466X)	20	0.72	0.50
13	c.3691delT (p.Ser1231ProfsX4, 3821delT)	19	0.69	0.46
14	c.1000C>T (p.Arg334Trp, R334W)	19	0.69	0.80
15	c.262_263delTT (p.Leu88IlefsX22, 394delTT)	15	0.54	0.94
16	c.3587C>G (p.Ser1196X, S1196X)	14	0.51	0.48
17	c.3816_3817delGT (p.Ser1273LeufsX28, 3944delGT)	12	0.43	0.27
18	c.2657+5G>A (2789+5A>G)	10	0.36	0.48
19	c.489+1G>T (621+1G>T)	7	0.25	0.18
20	c.3140-16T>A (3272-16T>A)	6	0.22	0.34
21	c.1657C>T (p.Arg553X, R553X)	5	0.18	0.18
22	c.1545_1546delTA (p.Tyr515X, 1677delTA)	5	0.18	1.81
23	c.3535_3536insTCAA (p.Thr1179IlefsX17, 3667ins4)	4	0.14	0.10
24	c.254G>A (p.Gly85Glu, G85E)	4	0.14	0.10
25	c.472dupA (p.Ser158LysfsX5, 604insA)	3	0.11	0.10
26	c.2051_2052delAAinsG (p.Lys684SerfsX38, 2183AA>G)	3	0.11	0.04
27	c.3475T>C (p.Ser1159Pro; S1159P)	3	0.11	0.10
28	c.1040G>C (p.Arg347Pro, R347P)	2	0.07	0.10
29	c.350G>A (p.Arg117His, R117H)	1	0.04	0.04
30	c.1519_1521delATC (p.Ile507del, I507del)	0	-	0
31	c.1585-1G>A (1717-1G>A)	0	-	0.04
32	c.1652G>A (p.Gly551Asp, G551D)	0	-	0.04
33	c.3476C>T (p.Ser1159Phe, S1159F)	0	-	0.11
	Identified	2290	82.78	
	Not identified	478	17.22	
	Total	2768		

On the second stage, 154 ethnic Russians affected by CF, for whom one or both mutant alleles were not identified when analyzing 33 mutations, were selected from the sample of 1384 CF patients for further analysis. Their genotypes were presented in Supplementary Table S2. There was a total of 164 unidentified mutant alleles of the *CFTR* gene.

As a result, in addition to 29 identified frequent mutations, 91 pathogenic (or likely pathogenic) genetic variants in the *CFTR* gene were detected (Table 2). Of these, 29 are missense mutations, 19 nonsense mutations, 14 frame-shift mutations (11 deletions and three insertions)), 17 splice-site, one in-frame insertion, 11 large rearrangements (eight deletions and three duplications).

Table 2. The *CFTR* gene variants additionally identified in 154 previously screened Russian patients.

No.	Variant According to cDNA	Protein Change	Legacy Name	Exon/Intron [1]	Number	Mutation Type
1	c.43delC	p.Leu15PhefsX1	175delC	1e	2	sd
2	c.53+1G>T		185+1G->T	1i	2	s
3	c.79G>T	p.Gly27X	G27X	2e	1	n
4	c.115C>T	p.Gln39X	Q39X	2e	1	n
5	c.223C>T	p.Arg75X	R75X	3e	1	n
6	c.252T>A	p.Tyr84X		3e	2	n
7	c.264_268delATATT	p.Leu88PhefsX21		3e	1	sd
8	c.274-6T>C		406-6T>C	3i	1	s
9	c.274G>T	p.Glu92X	E92X	4e	1	n
10	c.293A>G	p.Gln98Arg	Q98R	4e	1	m
11	c.358G>C	p.Ala120Pro		4e	1	m
12	c.422C>A	p.Ala141Asp	A141D	4e	1	m
13	c.490-1G>C			4i	1	s
14	c.580-1G>T		712-1G->T	5i	8	s
15	c.613C>A	p.Pro205Thr		6a e	1	m
16	c.650A>G	p.Glu217Gly	E217G	6a e	1	m
17	c.831G>A	p.Trp277X		6b e	1	n
18	c.940G>A	p.Gly314Arg	G314R	7e	1	m
19	c.[1075C>A;1079C>A]	p.[Gln359Lys;Thr360Lys]	Q359K/T360K	7e	1	m
20	c.1083G>A	p.Trp361X		7e	2	n
21	c.1086T>A	p.Tyr362X	Y362X	7e	1	n
22	c.1204G>T	p.Glu402X		8e	1	n
23	c.1209G>C	p.Glu403Asp	E403D	8e	3	m
24	c.[1210−12[5];1210-34TG[12]]		5T;TG12	7i	1	s
25	c.1219delG	p.Glu407AsnfsX35		9e	1	sd
26	c.1352G>T	p.Gly451Val		9e	1	m
27	c.1240_1244delCAAAA	p.Asn415X	1365del5	9e	11	sd
28	c.1364C>A	p.Ala455Glu	A455E	9e	1	m
29	c.1382G>A	p.Gly461Glu		9e	1	m
30	c.1438G>T	p.Gly480Cys	G480C	10e	1	m
31	c.1501A>G	p.Thr501Ala	T501A	10e	1	m
32	c.1513A>C	p.Asn505His		10e	1	m
33	c.1525G>C	p.Gly509Arg		10e	1	m

Table 2. *Cont.*

No.	Variant According to cDNA	Protein Change	Legacy Name	Exon/Intron [1]	Number	Mutation Type
34	c.1528delG	p.Val510PhefsX17	1660delG	10e	1	sd
35	c.1584+1G>A		1716+1G>A	10i	1	s
36	c.1589T>C	p.Ile530Thr		11e	1	m
37	c.1608delA	p.Asp537ThrfsX3		11e	2	sd
38	c.1646G>A	p.Ser549Asn	S549N	11e	1	m
39	c.1705T>C	p.Tyr569His	Y569H	12e	1	m
40	c.1735G>T	p.Asp579Tyr	D579Y	12e	2	m
41	c.1766+2T>C			12i	2	s
42	c.1766+1G>A		1898+1G>A	12i	4	s
43	c.1766+1G>C		1898+1G>C	12i	5	s
44	c.1792_1793insAAA	p.Lys598dup	K598ins	13e	1	i
45	c.1795dupA	p.Thr599AsnfsX2		13e	1	si
46	c.1911delG	p.Gln637HisfsX26	2043delG	13e	2	sd
47	c.2128A>T	p.Lys710X	K710X	13e	3	n
48	c.2195T>G	p.Leu732X	L732X	13e	1	n
49	c.2290C>T	p.Arg764X	R764X	13e	1	n
50	c.2312delA	p.Asn771ThrfsX2		13e	1	sd
51	c.2353C>T	p.Arg785X	R785X	13e	6	n
52	c.2374C>T	p.Arg792X	R792X	13e	1	n
53	c.2417A>G	p.Asp806Gly	D806G	13e	1	m
54	c.2589_2599delAATTTGGTGCT	p.Ile864SerfsX28	2721del11	14a e	2	sd
55	c.2617G>T	p.Glu873X		14a e	1	n
56	c.2658-2A>G		2790-2A->G	14b i	1	s
57	c.2780T>C	p.Leu927Pro	L927P	15e	1	m
58	c.2834C>T	p.Ser945Leu	S945L	15e	4	m
59	c.2909G>A	p.Gly970Asp	G970D	16e	1	m
60	c.2936A>T	p.Asp979Val	D979V	16e	1	m
61	c.2988+1G>A		3120+1G->A	16i	1	s
62	c.2989-2A>C			16i	1	s
63	c.2989-2A>G		3121-2A->G	16i	1	s
64	c.3107C>A	p.Thr1036Asn		17a e	1	m
65	c.3112C>T	p.Gln1038X		17a e	1	n
66	c.3189delG	p.Trp1063X		17b e	1	n

Table 2. *Cont.*

No.	Variant According to cDNA	Protein Change	Legacy Name	Exon/Intron [1]	Number	Mutation Type
67	c.3472C>T	p.Arg1158X	R1158X	19e	2	n
68	c.3484C>T	p.Arg1162X	R1162X	19e	2	n
69	c.3528delC	p.Lys1177SerfsX15	3659delC	19e	2	sd
70	c.3763T>C	p.Ser1255Pro	S1255P	20e	2	m
71	c.3775A>T	p.Arg1259X		20e	1	n
72	c.3872A>G	p.Gln1291Arg	Q1291R	20e	1	m
73	c.3874-2A>G		4006-2A->G	20i	1	s
74	c.3883delA	p.Ile1295PhefsX33	4015delA	21e	3	sd
75	c.3884_3885insT	p.Ser1297PhefsX5	4016insT	21e	3	si
76	c.3929G>A	p.Trp1310X	W1310X	21e	7	n
77	c.3963+1G>T		4095+1G->T	21i	1	s
78	c.4004T>C	p.Leu1335Pro	L1335P	22e	6	m
79	c.4242+1G>A		4374+G->A	23i	1	s
80	c.4296_4297insGA	p.Ser1435GlyfsX14	4428insGA	24e	2	si
81	c.(?-1)_(1584+1_1585-1)del		CFTRdele1-10		1	CNV
82	c.(53+2-54-1)_(273+1_274-1)del		CFTRdele2,3(non 21kb)1		1	CNV
83	c.(273+1_274-1)_(743+1_744-1)del		CFTRdele4-6a		1	CNV
84	c.(273-1_274+1)_(869+1_870-1)del(1209-1_1210+1)_(1392+1_1393+1)del		CFTRdel4-7;del9-10		2	CNV
85	c.(489+1_490-1)_(1392+1_1393-1)del		CFTRdele5-10		1	CNV
86	c.(53+1_54-1)_(164+1_165+1)del		CFTRdele21		2	CNV
87	c.(53+1_54-1)_(869+1_870+1)del		CFTRdele2-7		1	CNV
88	c.(1679+1_1680-1)_(2490+1_2491-1)del(2908+1_2909-1)del		CFTRdele12,13;del161		2	CNV
89	c.(743+1_744-1)_(1584+1_1585-1)dup		CFTRdup6b-10 (gIVS6a+415_IVS10 +2987Dup26817bp)		5	CNV
90	c.(743-1_744+1)_(869+1_870-1)dup		CFTRdup6b,7		1	CNV
91	c.(4136+1_4137-1)_(*1_?)dup		CFTRdup23,24		1	CNV

Note: ([1])–exon numbering according to legacy nomenclature, (m)-missense mutation, (n)–nonsense mutation, (sd)–frame-shift deletion, (si)-frame-shift insertion, (s)-splice-site, (i)–in-frame insertion, (CNV)–copy number variation (large rearrangement).

4. Discussion

At present, routine DNA testing of patients includes analysis for 33 pathogenic variants in the *CFTR* gene (Materials and methods section). The spectrum of variants included in the first stage of molecular genetic research was developed gradually. Therefore, 1384 ethnic Russian CF patients are included in the present study, for whom all 33 variants have been tested.

The choice of the spectrum of mutations for routine analysis is conditioned by the results obtained in the course of our own studies [14], studies conducted in different laboratories of the Russian Federation on independent samples of CF patients [6,12,16,17], and data on the prevalence of *CFTR* gene mutations in a global sample of CF patients published by the World Health Organization [18] and presented in the *CFTR* mutation database CFTR1 [19].

Mutations c.1521_1523delCTT (F508del), c.1624G>T (G542X), c.1652G>A (G551D), c.1657C>T (R553X), c.3846G>A (W1282X), c.3909C>G (N1303K), c.489+1G>T (621+1G>T), c.350G>A (R117H), and c.1585-1G>A (1717-1G>A), are among ones the most common in the world [18,20]. Therefore, first of all these mutations were included in the analysis of Russian patients. Variants c.1519_1521delATC (I507del), c.254G>A (G85E), c.3718-2477C>T (3849+10kbC-T), c.1000C>T (R334W), and c.1040G>C (R347P), although not among the most common in the world, are quite common for many populations with specific ethnic background. In 1993–1995, in order to detect pathogenic variants specific to the Russian population, a joint study of the coding sequence of the *CFTR* gene was carried out with the Institute of Biogenetics (Brest, France) by denaturing gradient gel electrophoresis with subsequent sequencing in a sample of 50 patients. It was shown that, in addition to the previously detected *CFTR* gene mutations, the mutations c.2012delT (2143delT), c.2052_2053insA (2184insA), c.262_263delTT (394delTT), and c.3691delT (3821delT) can also be considered frequent for ethnic Russian CF patients. [15]. In the collaborative study of Dörk T. with co-authors [21], in which our laboratory also participated, the predominant distribution of mutation c.54-5940_273+10250del21kb (CFTRdele2,3) was shown for the populations of Eastern Europe and the relative frequency of this mutation was determined for the studied Russian patients (7.2%); second in frequency after the mutation c.1521_1523delCTT (F508del). T.E. Ivashchenko [16] for the first time describes the variants c.1545_1546delTA (1677delTA), c.3587C>G (S1196X) and c.3844T>C (W1282R), relatively frequent for CF patients from Russia. The variant c.1545_1546delTA (1677delTA) was shown to be common for Georgian patients, whereas variants c.3587C>G (S1196X) and c.3844T>C (W1282R) were identified for Russian CF patients. In a study conducted in our laboratory, variants c.3535_3536insTCAA (3667ins4), c.3816_3817delGT (3944delGT), c.472dupA (604insA), and c.413_415dupTAC (L138ins) were identified and included in the frequent mutations' panel [14].

4.1. Similarity and Difference of Frequency Profiles of Common CF Variants in Two Samples of Russian Patients and the Data of CFTR2

A comparison of frequency profiles of 33 variants tested at the first stage shows similarity of frequency distributions for ethnic Russian patients and for patients of All-Russian sample (Table 1): the most frequent is c.1521_1523delCTT (F508del) (54.99% and 52.81%, respectively), the second in frequency is c.54-5940_273+10250del21kb (CFTRdele2,3) (7.59% and 6.21%), and frequencies of eight more variants exceed 1%. This similarity is not surprising, as ethnic Russians make up the majority (over 85%) of CF patients in the Russian Federation. However, there also are differences. Frequencies of the variants c.1521_1523delCTT (F508del) ($p = 0.059$), c.54-5940_273+10250del21kb (CFTRdele2,3) ($p = 0.018$), c.2012delT (2143delT) ($p = 0.109$), c.3718-2477C>T (3849+10kbC>T), c.2052_2053insA (2184insA), c.3909C>G (N1303K), c.1624G>T (G542X), c.3844T>C (W1282R), c.1397C>G (pSer466X), c.3691delT (3821delT), c.3816_3817delGT (3944delGT) are higher for ethnic Russian patients' sample than for the all-Russian one (Table 1, Figure 1). Perhaps, this is due to the fact that these variants are typical for ethnic Russians and may reflect this ancestry. While frequencies of other variants prevail in the all-Russian sample, which reflects the fact that these variants prevail among patients belonging to other ethnic groups. Thus, the frequency of variant c.1545_1546delTA (1677delTA) for ethnic Russians is much lower than for the all-Russian sample (0.18% and 1.81%, respectively, $p < 0.0001$). The variant c.1545_1546delTA (1677delTA) is predominantly distributed in the North Caucasus populations (Chechens, Ingush, Kumyks) [9,12]. The frequency of variant c.262_263delTT (394delTT) for ethnic Russians is lower than for the all-Russian sample (0.54% vs. 0.94%, $p = 0.074$, although difference is not significant). In the Russian Federation, it is more often found among the population associated with the past settlement of the Finno-Ugric peoples in northwestern European regions and in the Volga-Ural region [12,17]. The frequency of variant c.274G>A (E92K) for ethnic Russian patients is almost three times less than for the all-Russian sample (1.05% vs. 3.00%, $p < 0.0001$). The frequency of variant c.274G>A (p.Glu92Lys, E92K) is maximum for Chuvash (up to 55%) [10], high for Tatars (6.67%), Bashkirs (6.25%) [7], Chechens (12.5%) [9]. The frequency of c.3846G>A (p.Trp1282X, W1282X) is significant higher in the all-Russian sample (RF CF Registry) than in ethnic Russian patients (1.16% vs. 1.90%, $p = 0.012$).

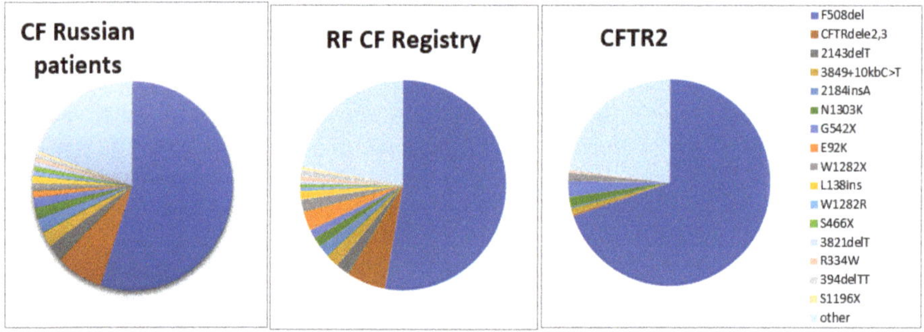

Figure 1. Frequency distribution of *CFTR* gene variants in three samples of CF patients: ethnic Russians, CF RF Registry, CFTR2 database [22].

When comparing CF-causing variant frequencies in ethnic Russian CF patients to the CFTR2 database [22], significant frequency difference was found (Fig. 1, Supplementary Table S1). So, the frequencies of c.54-5940_273+10250del21kb (p.Ser18Argfs*16, CFTRdele2,3), c.2012delT (p.Leu671X, 2143delT), c.3718-2477C>T (3849+10kbC-T), c.2052_2053insA (p.Gln685ThrfsX4, 2184insA), c.274G>A (p.Glu92Lys, E92K), c.413_415dupTAC (p.Leu138dup; L138ins) and some other variants appear higher in ethnic Russian patients while the frequencies of c.1521_1523delCTT (p.Phe508del, F508del), c.1624G>T (p.Gly542X, G542X), c.2657+5G>A (2789+5A>G), c.489+1G>T (621+1G>T), c.1657C>T (p.Arg553X, R553X), c.254G>A (p.Gly85Glu, G85E), c.1040G>C (p.Arg347Pro, R347P), c.350G>A (p.Arg117His, R117H) were lower. Variants c.3844T>C (p.Trp1282Arg, W1282R), c.3140-16T>A (3272-16T>A), and c.3816_3817delGT (p.Ser1273LeufsX28, 3944delGT) were not listed in CFTR2. Variants c.1652G>A (p.Gly551Asp, G551D), c.1585-1G>A (1717-1G>A), and c.3476C>T (p.Ser1159Phe, S1159F) were not found in tested cohort of Russian patients (Supplementary Table S1). However, the differences in frequencies in these latter series involve rare variants and their significance remains unknown.

4.2. Sanger Sequencing Detection of the CFTR Gene Variants

As a result of analysis of the coding sequence and regions of exon-intron junctions 80 variants in addition to preliminary tested common *CFTR* gene variants were identified. 61 variants identified in this work were identified on one chromosome and 17 on two chromosomes (Table 2). Each of the variants c.1209G>C (E403D), c.2128A>T (K710X), c.3883delA (4015delA) and c.3884_3885insT (4016insT) were detected for three, c.1766+1G>A (1898+1G>A) and c.2834C>T (S945L) for four, c.1766+1G>C (1898+1G>C) and c.(743+1_744-1)_(1584+1_1585-1)dup (CFTRdup6b-10) for five, c.2353C>T (R785X) and c.4004T>C (L1335P) for six, c.3929G>A (W1310X) for seven, c.580-1G>T (712-1G>T) for eight, and c.1240_1244delCAAAA (1365del5) for 11 unrelated patients (Table 2).

Some of genetic variants identified in sequencing were first discovered in this study. Description of 15 is presented in a previously published paper [23]. Nine of these variants are nonsense mutations (c.252T>A (p.Tyr84X), c.831G>A (p.Trp277X), c.1083G>A (p.Trp361X), c.3112C>T (p.Gln1038X)) or frame-shift mutations (c.264_268delATATT (p.Leu88PhefsX21), c.1219delG (p.Glu407AsnfsX35), c.1608delA (p.Asp537ThrfsX3), c.1795dupA (p.Thr599AsnfsX2), c.3189delG (p.Trp1063X), resulting in the formation of premature stop codon (Table 1). Variant c.490-1G>C breaks the acceptor site of 5 exon splicing. These variants belong to the category of PVS1 null variants (pathogenic variant sequence) according to the criteria of classification of pathogenicity of genetic variants [24]. Variant c.1792_1793insAAA (p.Lys598dup) leads to the insertion of lysine into position 598, and clinical significance of the variant is assessed as pathogenic. The clinical significance of the missense mutations (c.358G>C (p.Ala120Pro), c.1382G>A (p.Gly461Glu), c.1513A>C (p.Asn505His), c.1525G>C (p.Gly509Arg)) is assessed as probably pathogenic.

Eight more variants are presented for the first time. Two variants-nonsense mutations (c.1204G>T (p.Glu402X), c.2617G>T (p.Glu873X)) and one deletion with frame shift (c.2312delA (p.Asn771ThrfsX2)) are concluded to be PVS1 null variants according to the ACMG classification. Variant c.2989-2A>C is a violation of the 19 exon splicing site. Three missense mutations (c.613C>A (p.Pro205Thr), c.1352G>T (p.Gly451Val), c.1589T>C (p.Ile530Thr), c.3107C>A (p.Thr1036Asn)), the clinical significance of which is assessed as probably pathogenic according to the recommendations [24]. The characteristics of the phenotypes of patients who carry rare missense variants are presented in Supplementary Table S3.

4.3. CNV in Russian CF Patients Detected by MLPA

Large rearrangements of the *CFTR* gene were found for 18 unrelated patients, which is 10.8% (18/166) of the tested mutant alleles and should account for about 1% in the total sample of all mutant alleles in Russians. The MLPA method revealed 11 large rearrangements of the *CFTR* gene: three duplications and eight deletions (Table 1). Four of the large rearrangements were detected in several families. Thus, the duplication of a fragment covering 7–11 (6b–10) exons was detected for five unrelated patients. The testing system we developed allowed us to confirm that the duplication detected had the same frames as previously described in the literature [13]. In the RF CF Registry 2017, this variant was noted for six more unrelated patients. Thus, CFTRdup6b-10 was detected in eleven unrelated patients. Six of them live in the Volga-Ural region, three in the Central region. It should be noted that two patients from the Volga-Ural region belong to the other ethnic groups: one-Bashkir and one-Udmurt.

Each of the deletions, c.(53+1_54-1)_(164+1_165-1)del (CFTRdele2), c.[(1679-1_1680+1)_(2490+1 _2491-1)del[;](2908+1_2989-1)del] (CFTRdele12,13;del16) and c.(273-1_274+1)_(869+1_870-1)del(1209-1 _1210+1)_(1392+1_1393+1)del (CFTRdele4-7;del9-10) was detected twice. Complex deletion, CFTRdele12,13;del16, was detected for two patients from unrelated families living in the Moscow region; deletion CFTRdele4-7;del9-10 for two families from the Kaliningrad region and the Republic of Buryatia; deletion CFTRdele2 in families from the Transbaikal region and Irkutsk region.

4.4. Detection Rate of Three-Stage Analysis of CFTR Gene in Russian CF Patients

As a result of analysis of the coding sequence and regions of exon-intron junctions and subsequent search for large rearrangements, 163 out of 164 alleles were identified that were not detected after preliminary testing of frequent variants of the *CFTR* gene.

In one patient only variant E217G with the F508del in trans was detected after sequencing and MLPA. In NCBI-ClinVar database variant E217G is considered to be variant of conflicting interpretation of pathogenicity (benign; likely benign; uncertain significance) [25]. In the study by Lee J.H. et al. [26] it was shown that non-synonymous E217G mutation in the M470 background caused a 60%–80% reduction in *CFTR*-dependent Cl⁻ currents and HCO₃⁻ transport activities. So we might suggest that the clinical presentation in that patient is due to complex allele E217G-M470 (Supplementary Table S3).

The second mutant allele of the *CFTR* gene could not be identified in one sample. Failure to identify the second pathologic mutation in the *CFTR* gene after sequencing the coding sequence and searching for large rearrangements may be due to the location of the pathogenic variant either in inner regions of the introns, or in regulatory regions of the *CFTR* gene, or in regulatory regions outside the *CFTR* gene. Indeed, such variants have been recently identified, for example, c.1680-883A>G, c.2989-313A>T, c.3469-1304C>G, or c.3874-4522A>G, that lead to the creation of a new donor splice site and the activation of a cryptic acceptor splice site, resulting in the inclusion of an additional pseudo-exon (PE) and the loss of wild type (WT) CFTR transcripts [27].

5. Conclusions

In a representative sample of CF patients (ethnic Russians), the spectrum of 33 routinely analyzed (in Russia) variants of the *CFTR* gene was studied. It was shown that, out of 29 identified variants, frequencies of only 10 exceed 1%, and the mutation detection rate of testing did not exceed 85%. Consistent use of sequencing and MLPA methods has allowed us to identify a significant variety of *CFTR* gene mutations spectrum (91 additional genetic variants), to expand the spectrum of frequent variants (c.1766+1G>C (1898+1G>C), c.2353C>T (R785X), c.(743+1_744-1)_(1584+1_1585-1)dup (CFTRdup6b-10), c.4004T>C (L1335P), c.3929G>A (W1310X), c.580-1G>T (712-1G>T), c.1240_1244delCAAAA (1365del5), detected for five and more unrelated patients, to increase the detection rate of identified mutant alleles for Russian CF patients up to 99.4%, consistently using the strategy of Sanger sequencing and MLPA analysis. This information can be useful for the further optimization of medical genetic counseling in CF high-risk families, for improving the neonatal screening program for CF, and for making decision about the possible CFTR modulators therapy in the future. The identification of previously unknown CF-pathogenic or likely-pathogenic variants is a useful piece of information for diagnostic testing not only in Russia, but worldwide, and can be considered as a contribution to the general knowledge about the *CFTR* variant heterogeneity.

Supplementary Materials: The following are available online at http://www.mdpi.com/2073-4425/11/5/554/s1, Table S1: Frequencies of 33 variants of *CFTR* gene in the samples of 1384 ethnic Russians and in the CF patients from CFTR2 database [22], Table S2: Genotypes and *CFTR* gene variants in 154 Russian patients tested for 33 common *CFTR* variants, Table S3: Clinical and demographic characteristics of CF patients with rare missense variants.

Author Contributions: Data curation, N.V.P. and N.Y.K.; Formal analysis, N.V.P. and T.A.V.; Funding acquisition, S.I.K. and R.A.Z.; Investigation, N.V.P.; Project administration, E.K.G., S.I.K. and R.A.Z.; Resources, N.Y.K., E.I.K., E.K.Z., A.Y.V., V.D.S. and V.A.G.; Supervision, E.K.G. and R.A.Z.; Validation, T.A.V. and A.V.M.; Writing–original draft, N.V.P.; Writing–review & editing, A.V.M. All authors have read and agreed to the published version of the manuscript.

Funding: The research was partially supported by grant RFBR 20-015-0061A and within the state task of the Ministry of education and science of Russia.

Acknowledgments: The authors are grateful to Stanislav Krasovsky and Elena Amelina for their input to the collection of the clinical data of adult CF patients. Also the authors would like to thank the National CF Patient Registry for providing access to patients data and thank the individual regional CF centers representatives for allowing the use of data, https://mukoviscidoz.org/mukovistsidoz-vrossii.html.

Conflicts of Interest: The authors declare no conflict of interest. The funders had no role in the design of the study; in the collection, analyses, or interpretation of data; in the writing of the manuscript, or in the decision to publish the results.

References

1. Sosnay, P.R.; Raraigh, K.S.; Gibson, R.L. Molecular Genetics of Cystic Fibrosis Transmembrane Conductance Regulator: Genotype and Phenotype. *Pediatr. Clin. North Am.* **2016**, *63*, 585–598. [CrossRef] [PubMed]
2. Farrell, P.M.; White, T.B.; Howenstine, M.S.; Munck, A.; Parad, R.B.; Rosenfeld, M.; Sommerburg, O.; Accurso, F.J.; Davies, J.C.; Rock, M.J.; et al. Diagnosis of Cystic Fibrosis in Screened Populations. *J. Pediatr.* **2017**, *181S*, S33–S44. [CrossRef] [PubMed]

3. Castellani, C.; Cuppens, H.; Macek, M., Jr.; Cassiman, J.J.; Kerem, E.; Durie, P.; Tullis, E.; Assael, B.M.; Bombieri, C.; Brown, A.; et al. Consensus on the use and interpretation of cystic fibrosis mutation analysis in clinical practice. *J. Cyst. Fibros.* **2008**, *7*, 179–196. [CrossRef] [PubMed]

4. De Boeck, K.; Vermeulen, F.; Dupont, L. The diagnosis of cystic fibrosis. *Presse Med.* **2017**, *46*, e97–e108. [CrossRef] [PubMed]

5. Castellani, C.; Duff, A.J.A.; Bell, S.C.; Heijerman, H.G.M.; Munck, A.; Ratjen, F.; Sermet-Gaudelus, I.; Southern, K.W.; Barben, J.; Flume, P.A.; et al. ECFS best practice guidelines: The 2018 revision. *J. Cyst. Fibros.* **2018**, *17*, 153–178. [CrossRef] [PubMed]

6. National Consensus Project. *Cystic Fibrosis: Definition, Diagnostic Criteria, Treatment 2018*; Kondratyeva, E.I., Kashirskaya, N.Y., Kaprqanov, N.I., Eds.; Company BORGES Ldt.: Moscow, Russia, 2018; p. 356.

7. MEDPRAKTIKA-M. *Registry of Patients with Cystic Fibrosis in the Russian Federation. 2017*; Voronkova, A.Y., Amelina, E.A., Kashirskaya, N.Y., Kondratyeva, E.I., Krasovsky, S.A., Starinova, M.A., Kapranov, N.I., Eds.; MEDPRAKTIKA-M: Moscow, Russia, 2019; p. 68. (in Russian)

8. Petrova, N.V.; Kashirskaya, N.Y.; Vasilieva, T.A.; Timkovskaya, E.E.; Voronkova, A.Y.; Shabalova, L.A.; Kondrateva, E.I.; Sherman, V.D.; Kapranov, N.I.; Zinchenko, R.A.; et al. High proportion of W1282X mutation in CF patients from Karachai-Cherkessia. *J. Cyst. Fibros.* **2016**, *15*, e28–e32. [CrossRef] [PubMed]

9. Petrova, N.V.; Kashirskaya, N.Y.; Saydaeva, D.K.; Polyakov, A.V.; Adyan, T.A.; Simonova, O.I.; Gorinova, Y.V.; Kondratyeva, E.I.; Sherman, V.D.; Novoselova, O.G.; et al. Spectrum of CFTR mutations in Chechen cystic fibrosis patients: High frequency of c.1545_1546delTA (p.Tyr515X; 1677delTA) and c.274G>A (p.Glu92Lys, E92K) mutations in North Caucasus. *BMC Med. Genet.* **2019**, *20*, 44. [CrossRef]

10. Stepanova, A.A.; Abrukova, A.V.; Savaskina, E.N.; Poliakov, A.V. Mutation p.E92K is the primary cause of cystic fibrosis in Chuvashes. *Russ. J. Genet.* **2012**, *48*, 731–737. [CrossRef]

11. StatData.ru. Available online: http://www.statdata.ru/nacionalnyj-sostav-rossii (accessed on 8 February 2020).

12. Petrova, N.V.; Kondratyeva, E.I.; Krasovsky, S.A.; Polyakov, A.V.; Ivachshenko, T.E.; Pavlov, A.E.; Zinchenko, R.A.; Ginter, E.K.; Kutsev, S.I.; Odinokova, O.N.; et al. National Consensus Project «Cystic fibrosis: Definition, diagnostic criteria, treatment» Section «Genetics of Cystic Fibrosis. Molecular genetic diagnosis of cystic fibrosis». *Meditsinskaya Genet.* **2016**, *11*, 29–45. (in Russian).

13. Hantash, F.M.; Redman, J.B.; Goos, D.; Kammesheidt, A.; McGinniss, M.J.; Sun, W.; Strom, C.M. Characterization of a recurrent novel large duplication in the cystic fibrosis transmembrane conductance regulator gene. *J. Mol. Diagn.* **2007**, *9*, 556–560. [CrossRef]

14. Petrova, N.V.; Timkovskaya, E.E.; Zinchenko, R.A. The analysis of *CFTR* mutations frequencies in different populations of Russia. *Eur. J. Hum. Genet.* **2008**, *16*, 387.

15. Verlingue, C.; Kapranov, N.I.; Mercier, B.; Ginter, E.K.; Petrova, N.V.; Audrezet, M.P.; Ferec, C. Complete screening of mutations in the coding sequence of the CFTR gene in a sample of CF patients from Russia: Identification of three novel alleles. *Hum. Mutat.* **1995**, *5*, 205–209. [CrossRef] [PubMed]

16. Ivaschenko, T.E.; Baranov, V.S. *Biochemical and Molecular Genetic Basis of Cystic Fibrosis Pathogenesis*; Intermedika: Saint-Petersburg, Russia, 2002; p. 256. (in Russian)

17. Korytina, G.F.; Victorova, T.V.; Baykova, G.V.; Khusnutdinova, E.K. Analysis of the Spectra of Mutations and Polymorphic Loci of Cystic Fibrosis Transmembrane Conductance Regulator in the Population of Bashkortostan. *Rus. J. Genet.* **2002**, *38*, 1076–1081. [CrossRef]

18. WHO Human Genetics Programme. *The Molecular Genetic Epidemiology of Cystic Fibrosis. Report of a Joint Meeting of WHO/ECFTN/ICF(M)/ECFS/World Health Organization (WHO)*; WHO: Genoa, Italy, 2002; Available online: https://www.cfww.org/docs/who/2002/who_hgn_cf_wg_04.02.pdf (accessed on 8 February 2020).

19. Cystic Fibrosis Mutation Database. Available online: http://www.genet.sickkids.on.ca (accessed on 5 February 2020).

20. Bobadilla, J.L.; Macek, M., Jr.; Fine, J.P.; Farrell, P.M. Cystic fibrosis: A worldwide analysis of CFTR mutations—Correlation with incidence data and application to screening. *Hum. Mutat.* **2002**, *19*, 575–606. [CrossRef] [PubMed]

21. Dörk, T.; Macek, M., Jr.; Mekus, F.; Tümmler, B.; Tzountzouris, J.; Casals, T.; Krebsová, A.; Koudová, M.; Sakmaryová, I.; Macek, M.S.; et al. Characterization of a novel 21-kb deletion, CFTRdele2,3(21kb), in the CFTR gene: A cystic fibrosis mutation of Slavic origin common in Central and East Europe. *Hum. Genet.* **2000**, *106*, 259–268. [CrossRef] [PubMed]

22. CFTR2. Clinical and Functional Translation of CFTR. Available online: https://www.cftr2.org/ (accessed on 5 February 2020).

23. Petrova, N.V.; Marakhonov, A.V.; Vasilyeva, T.A.; Kashirskaya, N.Y.; Ginter, E.K.; Kutsev, S.I.; Zinchenko, R.A. Comprehensive genotyping reveals novel CFTR variants in cystic fibrosis patients from the Russian Federation. *Clin. Genet.* **2018**, *95*, 1–4. [CrossRef] [PubMed]

24. Richards, S.; Aziz, N.; Bale, S.; Bick, D.; Das, S.; Gastier-Foster, J.; Grody, W.W.; Hegde, M.; Lyon, E.; Spector, E.; et al. Standards and guidelines for the interpretation of sequence variants: A joint consensus recommendation of the American College of Medical Genetics and Genomics and the Association for Molecular Pathology. *Genet. Med.* **2015**, *17*, 405–424. [CrossRef] [PubMed]

25. National Center for Biotechnology Information (NCBI-ClinVar). Available online: https://www.ncbi.nlm.nih.gov/clinvar/ (accessed on 5 February 2020).

26. Lee, J.H.; Choi, J.H.; Namkung, W.; Hanrahan, J.W.; Chang, J.; Song, S.Y.; Park, S.W.; Kim, D.S.; Yoon, J.-H.; Suh, Y.; et al. A haplotype-based molecular analysis of CFTR mutations associated with respiratory and pancreatic diseases. *Hum. Mol. Genet.* **2003**, *12*, 2321–2332. [CrossRef] [PubMed]

27. Bergougnoux, A.; Délétang, K.; Pommier, A.; Varilh, J.; Houriez, F.; Altieri, J.P.; Koenig, M.; Férec, C.; Claustres, M.; Lalau, G.; et al. Functional characterization and phenotypic spectrum of three recurrent disease-causing deep intronic variants of the CFTR gene. *J. Cyst. Fibros.* **2019**, *18*, 468–475. [CrossRef] [PubMed]

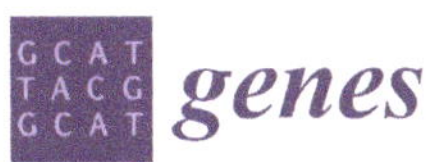 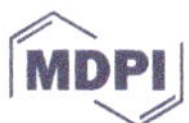

Article

Establishment of a Recombinant AAV2/HBoV1 Vector Production System in Insect Cells

Xuefeng Deng [1], Wei Zou [1], Ziying Yan [2] and Jianming Qiu [1,*]

[1] Department of Microbiology, Molecular Genetics and Immunology, University of Kansas Medical Center, Kansas City, KS 66160, USA; xuefeng2251@gmail.com (X.D.); zouw@umich.edu (W.Z.)

[2] Department of Anatomy and Cell Biology, University of Iowa, Iowa City, IA 52242, USA; ziying-yan@uiowa.edu

* Correspondence: jqiu@kumc.edu

Received: 27 March 2020; Accepted: 15 April 2020; Published: 17 April 2020

Abstract: We have previously developed an rAAV2/HBoV1 vector in which a recombinant adeno-associated virus 2 (rAAV2) genome is pseudopackaged into a human bocavirus 1 (HBoV1) capsid. Recently, the production of rAAV2/HBoV1 in human embryonic kidney (HEK) 293 cells has been greatly improved in the absence of any HBoV1 nonstructural proteins (NS). This NS-free production system yields over 16-fold more vectors than the original production system that necessitates NS expression. The production of rAAV with infection of baculovirus expression vector (BEV) in the suspension culture of Sf9 insect cells is highly efficient and scalable. Since the replication of the rAAV2 genome in the BEV system is well established, we aimed to develop a BEV system to produce the rAAV2/HBoV1 vector in Sf9 cells. We optimized the usage of translation initiation signals of the HBoV1 capsid proteins (Cap), and constructed a BEV Bac-AAV2Rep-HBoV1Cap, which expresses the AAV2 Rep78 and Rep52 as well as the HBoV1 VP1, VP2, and VP3 at the appropriate ratios. We found that it is sufficient as a trans helper to the production of rAAV2/HBoV1 in Sf9 cells that were co-infected with the transfer Bac-AAV2ITR-GFP-luc that carried a 5.4-kb oversized rAAV2 genome with dual reporters. Further study found that incorporation of an HBoV1 small NS, NP1, in the system maximized the viral DNA replication and thus the rAAV2/HBoV1 vector production at a level similar to that of the rAAV2 vector in Sf9 cells. However, the transduction potency of the rAAV2/HBoV1 vector produced from BEV-infected Sf9 cells was 5–7-fold lower in polarized human airway epithelia than that packaged in HEK293 cells. Transmission electron microscopy analysis found that the vector produced in Sf9 cells had a high percentage of empty capsids, suggesting the pseudopackage of the rAAV2 genome in HBoV1 capsid is not as efficient as in the capsids of AAV2. Nevertheless, our study demonstrated that the rAAV2/HBoV1 can be produced in insect cells with BEVs at a comparable yield to rAAV, and that the highly efficient expression of the HBoV1 capsid proteins warrants further optimization.

Keywords: rAAV2/HBoV1; baculovirus; insect cells

---

1. Introduction

Adeno-associated virus (AAV) and human bocavirus (HBoV) are members in different genera of the parvovirus family [1]. AAV is a nonpathogenic parvovirus and its productive replication needs the function of a helper virus [2,3]. In contrast, HBoV1 is a human pathogen that causes lower respiratory tract infections in young children worldwide [4–12]. In vitro, HBoV1 infects only polarized human airway epithelium cultured at an air–liquid interface (HAE-ALI), and replicates autonomously [13–16]. While both are nonenveloped, small, single-stranded (ss) DNA viruses, AAV packages both the plus- and minus-strand genome with equal efficiency, whereas HBoV1 prefers packaging the minus-strand [14]. HBoV1 has a genome of 5543 nucleotides (nts) in length, which is 18.5% (864 nts) larger than the AAV2 genome of 4679 nts [14].

The genome organizations of these two viruses are quite different. HBoV1 uses one promoter to express all viral nonstructural (NS) and structural or capsid (Cap) proteins, but AAV uses three different promoters [4,17]. The coding sequence of AAV consists of two large open reading frames (ORFs) encoding the nonstructural or replication (Rep) proteins and the Cap proteins at the left and right half of the AAV genome, respectively [18]. The large Rep78/68 and the small Rep52/40 proteins are expressed from the viral mRNAs that are transcribed by an upstream promoter at unit 5 of the genome (P5) and an internal promoter (P19), respectively. Three AAV Cap proteins, VP1, VP2 and VP3, are expressed from the mRNA transcribed by the P40 promoter [2,19]. In addition, a small NS protein, assembly-associated protein (AAP), is alternatively translated from the P40-transcribed Cap-coding mRNA [20], which plays a role in capsid assembly [21–24]. Recently, another small NS protein, membrane-associated accessory protein (MAAP), has been identified, which is also expressed from the P40-transcribed mRNA through alternative translation [25]. It exists in all AAV serotypes and was believed to play a role in the life cycle of AAV. HBoV1 expresses five NS proteins, NS1, NS2, NS3, NS4, and nuclear protein (NP1), and three Cap proteins, VP1, VP2, and VP3, as well as a bocaviral noncoding small RNA (BocaSR) [26–29]. The middle ORF, which is located at the center of the genome between the left ORF encoding NS1-4 and the right ORF encoding VP1-3, encodes NP1 [4]. NP1 plays an important role in viral DNA replication [30], as well as in regulation of HBoV1 cap expression [28,31].

The sequences at both termini of AAV and HBoV1 contain important motifs that are necessary for viral genome replication and virion assembly. In AAV, they are inverted terminal repeats (ITRs) [2,19], but in HBoV1 they are asymmetric with a non-perfectly palindromic hairpin at the left end terminus and a perfectly palindromic hairpin at the right terminus [14]. The transfection of the plasmid clone of a complete AAV genome in human embryonic kidney (HEK)293 cells leads to the production of AAV virions, but this only occurs in the presence of infection of a helper virus, such as adenovirus or co-transfection of a plasmid helper harboring all the adenoviral helper genes (*E2*, *E4Orf6*, and *VA RNA*) [32]. While HEK293 cells are not permissive to HBoV1 infection, the transfection of the cloned HBoV1 genome can produce HBoV1 infectious virions. The progeny virions infect HAE-ALI with a robustly high efficiency, even at a multiplicity of infection (MOI) of at 0.001 viral genome per cell [14,15].

Trans-complementation supports the replication and package of the gutless rAAV2 genome containing only cis elements of their termini and a gene of interest, which have been effectively developed as rAAV vectors for gene therapy of genetic diseases [2,19,33]. The safety profiles of the rAAV genome have been proven from tremendous preclinical studies and clinical trials of human gene therapy [34–41]. Up to date, two rAAV-based drugs, Luxturna and Zolgensma, have been approved by the US FDA. Similarly, a recombinant HBoV1 vector (rHBoV1) was produced in HEK293 cells via trans-complementation [42]. rHBoV1 efficiently transduced HAE-ALI from the apical membrane; however, the safety concern of being derived from a human pathogen limits its application. To overcome this disadvantage for a safe vector to transduce human airway epithelium from the airway lumen with the emphasis on gene therapy for cystic fibrosis (CF) lung disease, we successfully developed a cross-genera chimeric parvovirus vector, rAAV2/HBoV1 [42], in which the safety-proven rAAV2 genome was packaged into the airway tropic HBoV1 capsid. Importantly, the rAAV2/HBoV1 expands the package capacity of the rAAV2 genome by 20%, up to 5.8-kb [42]. Apical application of an rAAV2/HBoV1 carrying a full-length CF transmembrane conductance regulator (CFTR) cDNA of 5.4-kb to CF HAE-ALI cultures, which were made of primary airway epithelial cells of CF patients, efficiently corrected CFTR-dependent chloride transport [42]. In addition, the rAAV2/HBoV1 vector efficiently transduced ferret airways in vivo [43]. Therefore, it holds much promise for gene delivery to human airways, as well as for preclinical trials of CF gene therapy using CF ferret models [44]. Recently we have increased the production efficiency of the rAAV2/HBoV1 vector in HEK293 cells through optimization of cap expression, which approaches a similar level of rAAV2 production in HEK293 cells [45]. However, a robust vector production system is in demand for future CF gene therapy in preclinical and human trials using the rAAV2/HBoV1 vector.

Traditional rAAV vector productions utilize HEK293 cells. During the rAAV2 or the rAAV2/HBoV1 production in HEK293 cells, the rescue and replication of the rAAV2 genome require the expression of AAV *rep* in addition to the adenoviral helper genes [19,46]. rAAV2 can also be produced in insect cells by the infection of baculovirus expression vectors (BEVs). The AAV-BEV production system represents a robust and scalable bioprocess [47–52], which only requires one of the large Rep78/68 and one of the small Rep52/40 [53]. AAP is required for efficient production of certain serotypes of rAAV vectors in Sf9 cells [54,55]. Co-infection of BEVs—one carrying an rAAV2 genome and one expressing AAV2 Rep78 and Rep52 along with AAV2 VP1, VP2, and VP3—has been used to produce the rAAV vector in a large quantity at a yield of up to ~10^5 copies per Sf9 cell, compared to the yield of ~10^3 copies per HEK293 cell [47,53,54,56].

In this report, we explored the possibility of rAAV2/HBoV1 vector production in the BEV system. Our study demonstrated that the rAAV2/HBoV1 vector can be efficiently produced in a suspension Sf9 culture. In the presence of the expression of HBoV1 NP1, a vector yield similar to that of rAAV2 was achieved in Sf9 cells. To our knowledge, this is the first report that the parvoviral cross-genera pseudopackage is also effective in insect cells.

2. Materials and Methods

2.1. Cell and Cell Culture

Human embryonic kidney (HEK) 293 cells: HEK293 cells (CRL-1573), obtained from American Type Culture Collection (ATCC; Manassas, VA, USA), were cultured in Dulbecco's modified Eagle's medium (GE Healthcare Life Sciences, Piscataway, NJ, USA) with 10% fetal bovine serum (#F0926, MilliporeSigma, St. Louis, MO, USA)

Insect cells: Sf9 cells (CRL-1711, ATCC) were cultured in suspension in SFX-Insect medium (GE Healthcare, Marlborough, MA, USA) with 2% fetal bovine serum (#F0926, Millipore Sigma; St. Louis, MO, USA) at 27 °C.

HAE-ALI cultures: primary human airway cells were isolated from human lung tissues, and this procedure was carried out at the Tissue and Cell Culture Core of the Center for Gene Therapy, University of Iowa. The primary cells were cultured in the airway basal cell expansion medium (#CC-3118, Lonza, Basel, Switzerland), supplemented with 10 μM of ROCK inhibitor Y-276322, 1 μM of A8301, 1 μM of DMH-1, and 1 μM of CHIR99021 (Tocris Biosciences, Minneapolis, MN, USA) until confluency [57]. Then, the cells were collected and seeded onto collagen-coated inserts (Transwells; #3470, Corning, Tewksbury, MA, USA) with a density of 50,000 cells/well. After cell attachment for two days, the apical and basolateral medium were removed and replaced with a complete Pneumacult-ALI medium (StemCell, Vancouver, Canada) at the basolateral chamber to initiate an airway–liquid interface. The medium was changed every two days, and the ALI-cultured HAE took about four weeks to be fully differentiated. We monitored the cultures with a transepithelial electrical resistance using an epithelial Ohmvoltmeter (Millicell-ERS; EMD-Millipore, Burlington, MA, USA), and only HAE-ALI cultures with a resistance value of over 1000 $\Omega \cdot cm^2$ were used for subsequent transduction.

2.2. Construction of Baculoviral Expression Shuttle Plasmids and Other HEK293 Cell-Expressing Plasmids

pFastBacDual(m): the plasmid pFastBacDual (Invitrogen, Carlsbad, CA, USA) was modified by inserting a 0.83-kb fragment of λ DNA which contains a SbfI site at each end through SnaBI at nt 3983 and MfeI at nt 4815 to obtain the plasmid pFastBacDual (m).

pBac-AAV2ITR-GFP-Luc (5.4-kb): this BAC-AAV transfer plasmid was constructed by replacing the 0.83-kb λ DNA in pFastBacDual(m) with a 5444-nt ITR-flanked (rAAV) proviral DNA into the at two SbfI sites (Figure 1A). The intermediate rAAV proviral plasmid pAAV-CMV(P10)-GFP-SV40-Luc-bGHpA was derived from pAAV-MCS vector (Cell Biolabs, Inc., San Diego, CA, USA). Foreign

DNA flanking with a pair of SbfI sites was cloned into EcoRI and BamHI digested pAAV-MCS, including the P10 promoter, an open reading frame (ORF) of an enhanced green fluorescent protein (GFP; excised from pEGFP1, Clontech, Palo Alto, CA, USA), SV40 polyadenylation signal (polyA), SV40 early promoter, a FLAG-tagged ORF of firefly luciferase (Luc) and a stuffer from λ DNA (to make the rAAV2 genome of 5444-nt).

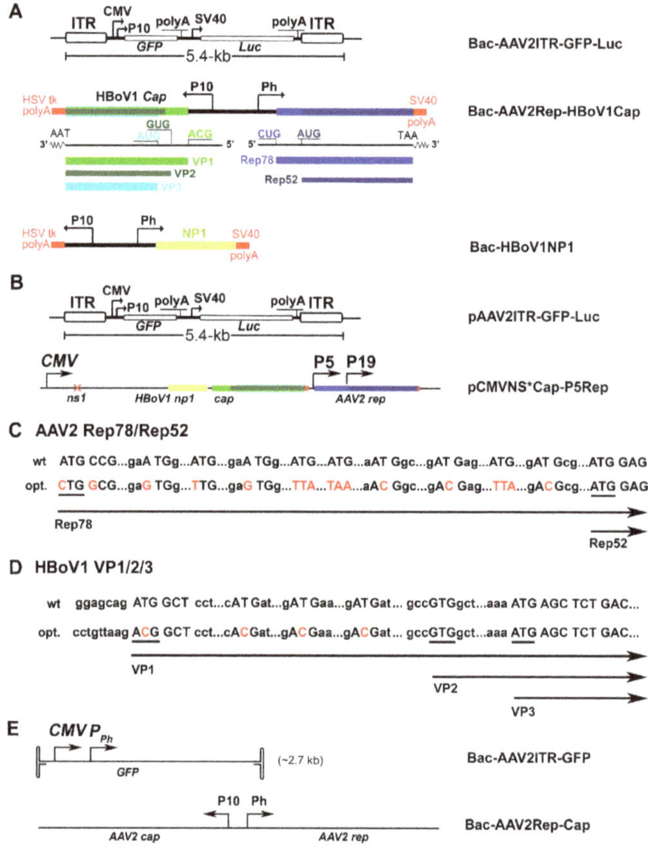

Figure 1. Construction of baculoviral transfer plasmids for vector production in Sf9 cells and the plasmids for rAAV2/HBoV1 vector production in HEK293 cells. (**A**) BEVs for rAAV2/HBoV1 production. Schematically diagrammed are structures inside the BEVs that were involved in rAAV2/HBoV1 production. Bac-AAV2ITR-GFP-Luc carries an rAAV2 genome of 5.4-kb; Bac-AAV2Rep-HBoV1Cap expresses AAV2 Rep proteins and HBoV1 capsid proteins as shown; and Bac-HBoV1NP1 expresses HBoV1 NP1. P10 and Ph are baculoviral promoters, and CMV and SV40 are cytomegaloviral immediate early and SV40 virus early promoters, respectively. PolyA: polyadenylation signal; Luc: firefly luciferase. (**B**) Plasmids used for vector production in HEK293 cells. pAAV2ITR-GFP-Luc carries the same rAAV2 genome as shown in panel A. pCMVNS*Cap-P5Cap is a two-in-one plasmid. It was derived from the plasmid pHBoV1CMVNS*Cap [28], in which the NS1/2 ORF was early terminated. An AAV2 P5 and P19 driven *rep* gene was cloned after the CMV promoter-driven HBoV1 *cap* gene expression cassette. (**C,D**) Codon optimization. Both wild type (wt) and optimized (opt.) sequences between ATGs of the AAV2 Rep78 and Rep52 ORFs (**C**) and of the HBoV1 VP1 and VP3 ORFs (**D**) are diagrammed. Nucleotides in red indicate mutations. (**E**) BEVs for rAAV2 production in Sf9 cells. Bac-AAV2ITR-GFP carries a GFP expression cassette under both the CMV and P10 promoters. Bac-AAV2Rep-Cap carries expression cassettes of AAV2 *cap* and AAV2 *rep* under the P10 and Ph promoters, respectively.

pBac-AAV2Rep-HBoV1Cap: to obtain a modified AAV2 *rep* gene expression cassette of a bifunctional Rep78- and Rep52-encoding mRNA, we synthesized a 637-bp DNA fragment containing a partially codon-optimized (opt)Rep78 ORF [56] (Figure 1C), and amplified the full-length optRep78/52 ORF using overlapped PCR, which was cloned into pFastBacDual through BglII (BamHI)-XbaI sites and resulted in pFastBacDual-AAV2Rep. We also synthesized a fragment of 390-bp containing an optimized HBoV1 sequence between VP1 AUG and VP3 AUG [28,58], as shown in Figure 1D, and amplified the full length optVP1/2/3 ORF using overlapped PCR, which was then cloned into the pFastBacDual-AAV2Rep through XhoI-NheI sites to obtain the BEV transfer plasmid pBac-AAV2Rep-HBoV1Cap (Figure 1A).

pBac-HBoV1NP1: HBoV1 NP1 ORF was cloned into pFastBacDual between the XhoI-KpnI sites to get the transfer construct pBac-HBoV1-NP1 (Figure 1A).

pAAV2ITR-GFP-Luc: to parallel compare the capability of the Sf9 cell and HEK293 cell systems, we made a plasmid, pAAV2ITR-GFP-Luc (Figure 1B), based on the backbone of pAAV-MCS promoterless (Cell Biolabs). This was achieved by cloning the fragments from the plasmid of pFastBacDual(m)-AAV2-ITR-GFP-Luc through two NotI sites.

pCMVNS*Cap-P5Rep: this was the HBoV1 *cap* and AAV2 *rep* expression two-in-one helper plasmid (Figure 1B), which was constructed by cloning the P5- and P19-driven AAV2 *rep* expression cassette from the pAV-Rep2 plasmid [42] into the pCMVNS*Cap [28], which expresses HBoV1 capsid proteins under the cytomegalovirus immediate early promoter (CMV) through a SacII site.

All the plasmids were sequenced to confirm the expressing genes and the critical elements for virus production at MCLAB (South San Francisco, CA, USA).

2.3. Recombinant Baculovirus Expression vector (BEV) Production

BEVs were generated by transfection of the BEV shuttle plasmid into DH10Bac™ *E. coli* competent cells, following the instructions of the Bac-to-Bac Baculovirus Expression System (Invitrogen, Carlsbad, CA). Bac-AAV2ITR-GFP (Bac-GFP) [47] and Bac-AAV2Rep-Cap (Bac-RepCap2) [56] (Figure 1E) were obtained from The University of Iowa Viral Vector Core Facility. BEVs were titrated in plaque forming units (pfu) by a plaque assay as described in the manual of the Bac-to-Bac Baculovirus Expression System (Invitrogen) or quantified using quantitative real-time PCR (qPCR) with an amplicon targeting to the gentamicin-resistance gene (Probe: 5′ 6FAM-ACA TTC ATC GCG CTT GCT GCC TTC-3′ ZEN /Iowa Black FQ; forward primer: 5′-CGG GAA CTT GCT CCG TAG TAA-3′, and reverse primer: 5′-CGC CAA CAA CCG CTT CTT-3′).

2.4. rAAV vector Production

For production of AAV vectors in insect cells, 200 mL of Sf9 cells in suspension culture at a density of 2×10^6 cells/mL were co-infected with BEVs at an MOI of ~10 (pfu/cell). At 72 hrs post-infection, cells were collected by centrifugation and lysed in phosphate-buffered saline, pH7.4 (PBS). After four times of freezing-thawing, the cells were sonicated at the setting of 70% power for 3 min (1 min sonicate with 1 min of interval), followed by DNase I treatment at 37 °C for 45 min and 10% deoxycholate with 0.25% Trypsin-EDTA incubation at 37 °C for another 30 min. Then, CsCl was added into cell crude lysate at a final concentration of 0.472 g/mL and incubated at 37 °C for 30 min. The mixture was centrifuged at 3,500 rpm for 30 min, the clarified virus/CsCl solution was transferred into another tube and adjusted to a final density of about 1.40 g/mL. The final clear mixture was loaded into tubes and centrifuged at 41,000 rpm for 36 hrs at 20 °C using an TH641 rotor in a Sorvall™ WX (Thermo Scientific). After two rounds of CsCl banding, an aliquot (500 μL) of gradient fractions was collected using a Gradient Station (BioComp Instruments, Fredericton, N.B., Canada), determined for values of refractive index using an Abbe Refractometer, and quantified by qPCR for vector genomes. The peak fractions were dialyzed against PBS buffer.

For the HEK293 cell system, the rAAV2/HBoV1 vector was generated by co-transfection of pAAV2ITR-GFP-Luc, pCMVNS*Cap-P5Rep, and pHelper that expresses adenoviral E2, E4Orf6 protein and VA RNA [3] into twenty 150-cm^2 plates of HEK293 cells (80% confluency) at a ratio 2:3:1, as previously described [42]. At 72 hrs post-transfection, cell pellets were collected and treated, and recombinant vector was purified as described above for infected Sf9 cells.

2.5. Western Blot and Southern Blot Analyses

Western blotting was performed as previously described [59]. For Southern blotting, low molecular weight (Hirt) DNA was extracted from BEV infected Sf9 cells, and the analysis was performed as previously described [60], using an AAV2 *cap* gene probe.

2.6. Quantitative Real Time PCR (qPCR) Analysis of rAAV2/HBoV1

The titers of rAAV2 and rAAV2/HBoV1 in DNase I digestion-resistant particles (DRP) were determined by a qPCR method that has been used previously [42]. Briefly, 50 μL aliquots of the samples were incubated with 20 units of Benzonase (MilliporeSigma) for 2 hrs at 37 °C, followed by 20 μL of proteinase K (15 mg/mL) at 56 °C for 10 min. Viral DNA was extracted using a QIAamp blood mini kit (Qiagen, Hilden, Germany), and then eluted in 50 μL of deionized water. A plasmid containing a GFP ORF was used to establish a standard curve for absolute quantification. The amplicon primers and dual-labeled probe were designed using Primer Express (Applied Biosystems, Foster City, CA, USA) and synthesized at IDT Inc. (Coralville, Iowa, USA). The sequences of the primers and probe specific to the GFP coding sequence are as follows: forward primer, 5′-CTG CTG CCC GAC AAC CA-3′; reverse primer, 5′-TGT GAT CGC GCT TCT CGT T-3′; and dual-labeled probe, 5′ 6FAM-TAC CTG AGC ACC CAG TCC GCC CT-3′ Iowa Black FQ. Probe qPCR MasterMix (Applied Biological Materials Inc., Vancouver, Canada) was used for qPCR following a standard protocol on a 7500 Fast Real-Time PCR System (Applied Biosystems, Foster City, CA, USA), and 2 μL of extracted DNA was used in a reaction volume of 20 μL.

2.7. Transmission Electron Microscopy

For each recombinant virus, aliquots of 50 μL in the peak fractions were performed for electron microscopy analysis in the Electron Microscopy Research Laboratory (EMRL) of the University of Kansas Medical Center. Briefly, two to five μL of each sample were spotted onto formvar-coated, carbon-stabilized, 200-mesh copper grids for 1 min and then washed with deionized water. Staining was achieved by adding five drops of 2% uranyl acetate. Excess staining was removed immediately by adsorption to filter paper, and the samples were then air dried. The grids were examined on a Transmission Electron Microscope (JEM-1400; JEOL, Peabody, MA, USA) at a magnification setting of 30,000 × and an accelerating voltage of 100 KV.

2.8. rAAV2/HBoV1 Transduction of HAE-ALI Cultures

We followed a previously described protocol to infect HAE-ALI cultures with rAAV2/HBoV1 [42]. Briefly, proteasome inhibitor doxorubicin and N-acetyl-l-leucyl-l-leucyl-l-norleucine (LLnL) at the final concentrations of 2.5 μM and 20 nM, respectively, were added into the culture medium of the basolateral chamber. Then, a total of 10^9 DRP of rAAV2/HBoV1 in 50 μL of medium were applied directly onto the apical surface of the airway epithelia at an MOI of ~2000 DRP/cell. At 12 hrs post-infection, the medium and virus were removed from the apical surface, and the basal medium was replaced with fresh medium without addition of proteasome inhibitors.

2.9. Measurement of Luciferase Reporter Expression

Luciferase enzyme activity was examined using a Luciferase Assay System kit (Promega, Madison, WI, USA) following the manufacturer's instructions. Briefly, HAE cells were collected after EDTA and trypsin treatments of the HAE-ALI cultures, and equal numbers of the cells from compared HAE-ALI cultures were transferred into wells of a 96-well plate. The wells were then added with 20 μL of 1× Lysis reagent, followed by mixing with 100 μL of Luciferase Assay Reagent and the light produced on a Synergy H1 microplate reader (Synergy H1, BioTek, Winooski, VT, USA) was measured.

2.10. Antibodies Used

A monoclonal antibody (clone 303.9) that reacts with AAV2 Rep78 and Rep52 and a monoclonal antibody (clone B1) that reacts with AAV2 Cap were purchased from American Research Products, Inc. (Waltham, MA, USA). Rat anti-HBoV1 Cap that reacts with VP1, VP2, and VP3 and rat anti-HBoV1 NP1 that recognizes the NP1 protein were made in house and have been described previously [26,31].

3. Results

3.1. Design of the Baculovirus Expression vector System

We used two BEVs, Bac-AAV2ITR-GFP and Bac-AAV2Rep-Cap (Figure 1E), to produce rAAV2 in Sf9 cells, which serves as a comparative control for the test of the production of the rAAV2/HBoV1 vector. In Bac-AAV2Rep-Cap, the AAV2 *rep* and *cap* genes were modified to allow expression of the Rep78 and Rep52 proteins and the VP1, VP2, and VP3 proteins from two species of mRNAs transcribed from Ph and P10 baculovirus promoters, respectively [56]. To generate the rAAV2/HBoV1 vector, we similarly made two BEVs, Bac-AAV2ITR-GFP-Luc, which harbors a 5.4-kb oversized rAAV2 genome, and Bac-AAV2Rep-HBoV1Cap (Figure 1A), which expresses AAV2 Rep78 and Rep52 under the Ph promoter and HBoV1 VP1, VP2 and VP3 under the P10 promoter. In addition, we made Bac-HBoV1NP1 that expresses the HBoV1 NP1 protein to look for a role of the NP1 in vector production.

We also compared the production and biologic properties of the rAAV2/HBoV1 vectors from insect cell and mammalian cell systems in parallel. To this end, we made the cis and trans plasmid constructs for rAAV2/HBoV1 vector production in HEK293 cells in the format similar to those used in the BEVs. The pAAV2ITR-GFP-Luc (5.4-kb) harbors the identical 5.4-kb rAAV2 genome that was in the transfer BEV Bac-AAV2ITR-GFP-Luc. The pCMVNS*Cap-P5Rep is the HBoV1 *cap* and AAV2 *rep* two-in-one expression plasmid, which expresses HBoV1 NS (NP1, NS3 and NS4) and Cap (VP1, VP2, and VP3) under the cytomegalovirus immediate early promoter (CMV) [27,28] and AAV2 Rep78 and Rep 52 under the AAV2 P5 and P19 promoters, respectively (Figure 1B).

3.2. Analyses of Protein Expression and Replication of the rAAV2 Genome in Sf9 Cells

To characterize the expression of AAV Rep and Cap, Sf9 cells grown in suspension culture were infected with Bac-AAV2Rep-Cap, Bac-AAV2Rep-HBoV1Cap, and Bac-HBoV1NP1, respectively. The infected cells were collected at 72 hrs post-infection, and the expression of viral proteins was analyzed by Western blotting. We first examined the expression of AAV2 Rep from the Sf9 cells infected with Bac-AAV2Rep-Cap (Figure 2A) and Bac-AAV2Rep-HBoV1Cap (Figure 2B), respectively. The results of Western blotting showed that the expressions of the AAV2 Rep by the P10 promoter from these two BEVs demonstrated a similar pattern, which both expressed AAV2 Rep78 and Rep52 at a ratio close to ~1:2. Of note, when we constructed the Bacmid pBac-AAV2Rep-HBoV1Cap, the codon optimization of AAV2 rep (Figure 1C) was adopted from one mRNA transcript, which was used in Bac-AAV2Rep-Cap [56]. The HBoV1 Cap expression from the Sf9 cells infected with Bac-AAV2Rep-HBoV1Cap was also analyzed with Western blotting, which confirmed that the optimization of initiation codons (Figure 1D) led to the expression levels of HBoV1 VP1, VP2, and VP3 at a ratio close to ~1:1:10 (Figure 2C), similar to that was observed from the transfection of the pCMVNS*Cap in HEK293 cells [28]. The cryptic polyadenylation signals (pA) resided inside the unique sequence in the VP1 ORF, which serve as the proximal pA preventing HBoV1 *cap* transcription in mammalian cells in the absence of NP1 expression [28], appeared to not be effective in the insect cells. These results confirmed that the expression strategy that Bac-AAV2Rep-Cap utilized to express the overlapping genes *rep* and *cap* from the baculoviral promoters P10 and Ph was applicable for the construction of Bac-AAV2Rep-HBoV1Cap. This AAV2/HBoV1 trans helper possessed the same capability to express AAV2 Rep proteins and also HBoV1 VP1, VP2 and VP3, and more importantly, they were expressed at the expected ratios. Thus, one BEV was able to express the parvoviral proteins from different genera efficiently without mutual disruption.

To determine the function of HBoV1 NP1 during the replication of the rAAV2 genome, we made a
Bac-HBoV1NP1. It expressed HBoV1 NP1 at ~25 kDa (Figure 2D). Then, Sf9 cells were co-infected with
Bac-AAV2ITR-GFP-Luc and Bac-AAV2Rep-HBoV1Cap, with or without Bac-HBoV1NP1. The infected
cells were sampled at 72 hrs post-infection and analyzed for the presence of rAAV2 replicative-form
(RF) DNA intermediates by Southern blotting (Figure 2E). Although ssDNA was not obviously detected
in both groups, clearly much more double replicative form (dRF) DNA was observed in the presence of
NP1 expression (Figure 2E, compare lanes 2 vs 3). Although NP1 is not required to modulate the HBoV1
cap expression in Sf9 cells as it does in mammalian cells, it positively enhances the replication of rAAV2
genomes. The mechanism of NP1's involvement in rAAV2 replication in Sf9 cells remains unclear.

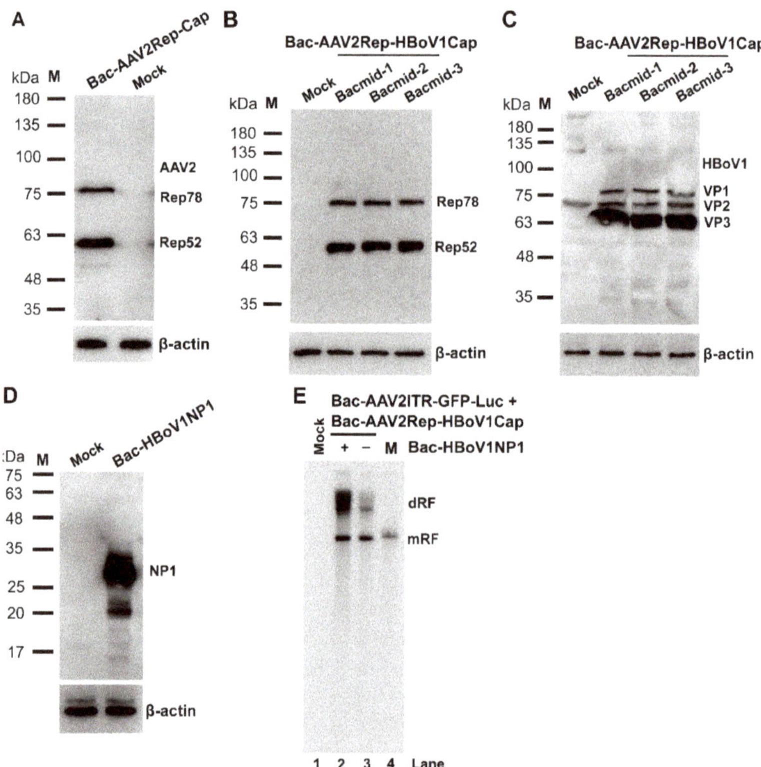

Figure 2. Expression of AAV2 Rep and Cap proteins and HBoV1 Cap and NP1 proteins in
BEV-infected Sf9 cells. (**A–D**) Western blotting. Sf9 insect cells were infected with Bac-AAV2Rep-Cap
(**A**), Bac-AAV2Rep-HBoV1Cap (**B,C**), or Bac-HBoV1NP1 (**D**). The infected cells were collected at 72 hrs
post-infection and subjected to Western blot analysis. (**A**) AAV2 Rep proteins were detected with an
anti-Rep monoclonal antibody. (**B,C**) Bac-AAV2Rep-HBoV1Cap generated from transfection of three
bacmid (Bacmid-1-3) were infected with Sf9 cells independently. (**B**) AAV2 Rep proteins were detected
with an anti-Rep monoclonal antibody, and (**C**) HBoV1 Cap protein expression was detected with
an anti-HBoV1 Cap protein antiserum. (**D**) HBoV1 NP1 was detected with a rat anti-HBoV1 NP1
antiserum. β-actin served as a loading control. Mock, uninfected cells. (**E**) Southern blotting. Sf9 cells
were infected with Bac-AAV2ITR-GFP-Luc and Bac-AAV2Rep-HBoV1Cap with (+) or without (-)
co-infection of Bac-HBoV1NP1. Cells were collected at 72 hrs post-infection and subjected to extraction
of lower molecular weight (Hirt) DNAs, which were analyzed by Southern blotting. Mock, uninfected
Sf9 cells as a control; M, a marker of a rAAV2ITR-GFP-Luc proviral replicative form (RF) genome of
5.4 kb. dRF and mRF, double and monomer RF.

3.3. rAAV2/HBoV1 vector is Successfully Produced in Sf9 Cells and NP1 Plays a Role in Increasing vector Yield

As a parallel control, we infected 200 mL of Sf9 cells with Bac-AAV2ITR-GFP and Bac-AAV2Rep-Cap for rAAV2 vector production. At 72 hrs post-infection, the infected cells were collected and lysed, and rAAV2 was purified by CsCl density gradient centrifugation. Fractions at a volume of 500 μL were collected and quantified for DRP by qPCR and demonstrated a peak at a refractive index of 1.372 (a density of ~1.40 g/mL) (Figure 3A, left). An electron micrograph of the rAAV2 produced is shown (Figure 3A, right) displaying particles of ~25 nm in diameter, a typical morphologic feature of AAV. In the peak fraction, the rAAV2 vector yield reached 7.52×10^9 DRP/μL, indicating that the Sf9 system to produce rAAV vector was successful at a yield of ~1×10^4 DRP/Sf9 cell from 200 mL Sf9 cells at a density of 2×10^6 cells/mL, a total 4×10^8 cells.

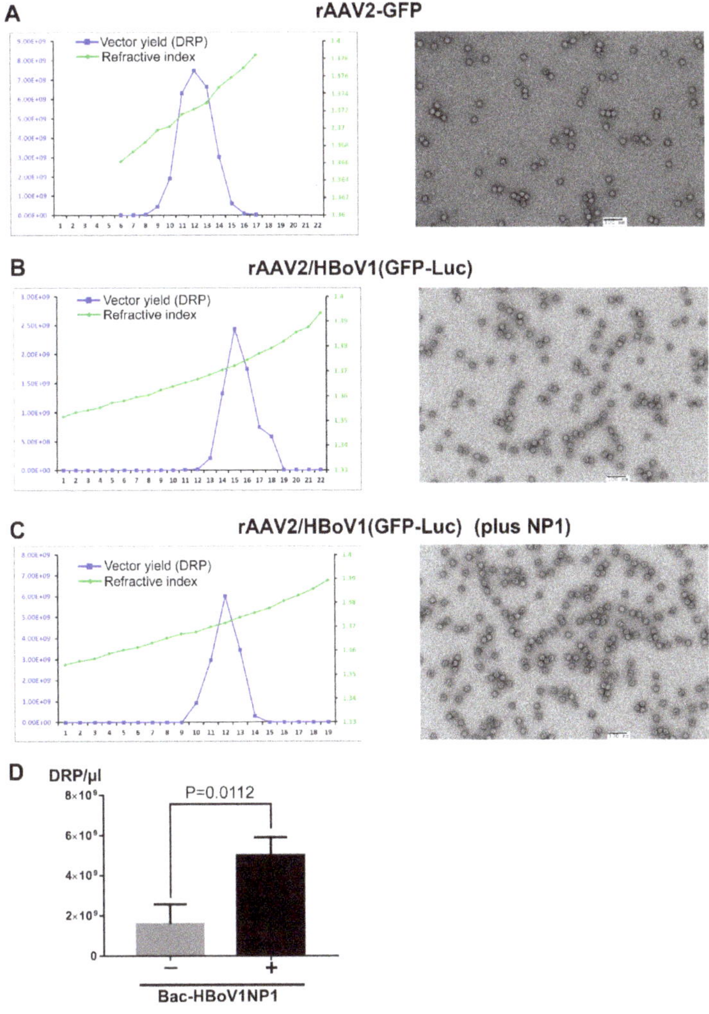

Figure 3. Purification of rAAV2 and rAAV2/HBoV1 vectors produced from BEV-infected Sf9 cells. (**A–C**) Vector production. Sf9 cells were co-infected with Bac-AAV2ITR-GFP and Bac-AAV2Rep-Cap (**A**), Bac-AAV2ITR-GFP-Luc and Bac-AAV2Rep-HBoV1Cap (**B**), or Bac-AAV2ITR-GFP-Luc, Bac-AAV2Rep-HBoV1Cap, and Bac-HBoV1NP1 (**C**). Cell lysates from infected cells were fractionated

by CsCl equilibrium ultracentrifugation. Left panel: qPCR analysis was used to determine the DRP in each fraction of 0.5 mL (blue line); the density of each fraction was determined as refractive index and is shown by the line in green. Right panel: transmission electron micrographs of rAAV2 or rAAV2/HBoV1 vectors, which were negatively stained with a 1% uranyl acetate solution. Bar = 100 nm. (**D**) Comparison of rAAV2/HBoV1 production with or without NP1 expression in Sf9 cells. The experiments in panels B&C were repeated three times in parallel. Purified vectors at the peak fraction were quantified and compared. Averages and standard deviations are shown. Statistical analysis was performed to get the P value using student "t" test.

The production of the rAAV2/HBoV1 vector was performed with BEV infection to Sf9 cells under the same conditions for rAAV2. We compared two groups of BEVs with or without expression of HBoV1 NP1 in parallel by infecting 4×10^8 cells of Sf9 cells: Group I, with Bac-AAV2ITR-GFP-Luc and Bac-AAV2Rep-HBoV1Cap; Group II, with Bac-rAAV2ITR-GFP-Luc, Bac-AAV2Rep-HBoV1Cap, and Bac-HBoV1NP1. At three days post-infection, the infected cells were collected and lysed, and vectors were purified by CsCl density gradient centrifugation. The refractive index and DRP of each fraction are shown at the left in Figure 3B,C, and the transmission electron microscopy demonstrated that the rAAV2/HBoV1 vector had a typical parvovirus icosahedral structure that was ~25 nm in diameter as shown at the right in Figure 3B,C. Without expression of HBoV1 NP1, an average vector yield was 1.6×10^9 DRP/μL in the peak fraction of 500 μL; however, there was a significant increase to 5.0×10^9 DRP/μL with the help of Bac-HBoV1NP1, confirming that expression of NP1 significantly increased vector yield by three times (Figure 3D). Notably, the expression of NP1 led to an increase in rAAV2 replicative-form (RF) DNA intermediates (Figure 2E), which could be responsible for the enhanced production.

3.4. Comparison of the Transduction Efficiencies Between rAAV2/HBoV1 vectors Produced in Sf9 Cells and in HEK293 Cells

It is encouraging that the yield of rAAV2/HBoV1 produced from the Sf9 cell system was comparable to that of rAAV2 in Sf9 cells in the presence of NP1 expression (5.0×10^9 vs 7.5×10^9 DRP/ul in the peak fraction of 500 μL). We next characterized its biological function in transducing HAE-ALI cultures. To this end and for fair comparison, we produced rAAV2/HBoV1(293) by transfection of pAAV2ITR-GFP-Luc, pCMVNS*Cap-P5Rep and pHelper into HEK293 cells of 20 × 145-mm plates and obtained a yield of 2.3×10^9 DRP/μL at the peak fraction (Figure 4A). We apically infected the well-differentiated HAE-ALI cultures, which were generated from airway epithelial cells from two different donors, with equal amounts of vectors produced from Sf9 cells or HEK293 cells. Proteasome inhibitors LLnL and doxorubicin were only applied in the basal chamber during the infection period of 12 hrs [42]. At seven days post-infection, cells were examined for the GFP expression under a fluorescence microscope, and images were taken at the same setting (Figure 4B,D). We observed more green cells from the infection of rAAV2/HBoV1(293) with relatively stronger intensity of fluorescence than its counterpart infection transduced of the rAAV2/HBoV1(Sf9). Next, the cells were lysed for quantification of the luciferase activity (Figure 4C,E), which revealed that the rAAV2/HBoV1(293) vector has a transduction efficiency 5–7 times higher than the rAAV2/HBoV1(Sf9) vector.

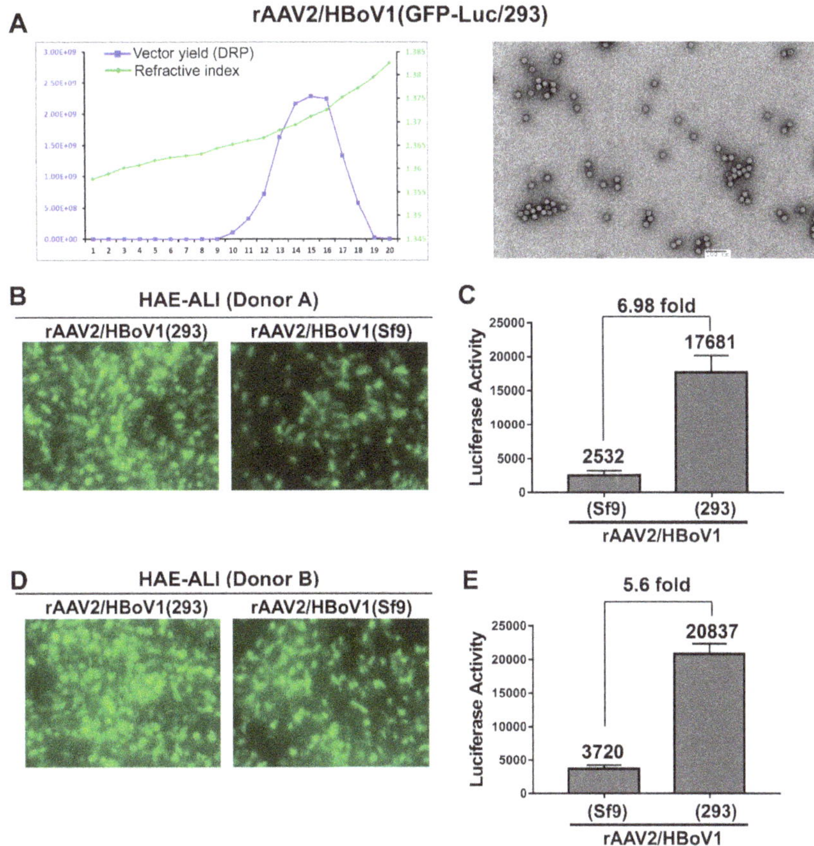

Figure 4. Comparison of the transduction efficiency between the rAAV2/HBoV1 vectors produced in Sf9 cells and HEK293 cells. (**A**) rAAV2/HBoV1 vector produced from HEK293 cells. HEK293 cells were transfected with pAAV2ITR-GFP-Luc, pCMVNS*Cap-P5Rep, and pHelper. Cell lysates from infected cells were fractionated by CsCl equilibrium ultracentrifugation. Left panel: qPCR analysis was used to determine the DRP in each fraction (blue line); the density of each fraction was determined as refractive index using an Abbe refractometer and is shown by the line in green. Right panel: a transmission electron micrograph of rAAV2/HBoV1(293) vectors. (**B–E**) rAAV2/HBoV1 transduction of HAE-ALI. HAE-ALI cultures prepared form Donor A (**B,C**) and Donor B (**D,E**) were transduced with rAAV2/HBoV1 either produced from Sf9 or HEK293 cells at an MOI of ~2000 DRP/cell from the apical surface. The rAAV2/HBoV1 vector was applied directly onto the apical surface of the airway epithelia. HAE cells were examined for GFP expression at 10 days post-transduction. Images were taken with an Eclipse Ti-S microscope (Nikon, Melville, NY, USA) at a magnification of × 20 (**B&D**). Luciferase activity was assayed at 10 days post-transduction (**C&E**). Averages and standard deviations generated from at least three independent experiments are shown. Statistical analysis was performed to get the P value using student "t" test.

4. Discussion

Cross-genera pseudopackaging between parvoviruses was first established by pseudotyping a rAAV genome into a capsid of human parvovirus B19 [61] for a chimeric AAV-B19 vector in HEK293 cells, which demonstrated high tropism to human erythroid cells. In 2013, we successfully packaged an rAAV2 genome into the capsid of HBoV1 in HEK293 cells, generating rAAV2/HBoV1 chimeric vector [42]. The rAAV2/HBoV1 vector has a high tropism for polarized human airway epithelia and is able to encapsidate an oversized rAAV2 genome of 5.8-kb, representing one of the best rAAV vectors for gene delivery to human airways and holding much promise for use in preclinical trials of CF gene therapy in ferrets and human trials of CF patients [62].

To meet the high demand of rAAV2/HBoV1 vector production at a large quantity, in this study, we took advantage of the rAAV2 vector production system in insect cells. We modified HBoV1 *cap* gene in Bac-AAV2Rep-HBoV1Cap that expressed VP1, VP2, and VP3 at a ratio of ~1:1:10 in Sf9 cells, and proved that the rAAV2/HBoV1 vector was produced in Sf9 cells. More importantly, with the co-infection of a BEV expressing HBoV1 NP1, the rAAV2/HBoV1 vector was produced at a yield of 5.0×10^9 DRP/μL, an equivalent efficiency as that of the rAAV2 vector in Sf9 cells (7.5×10^9 DRP/μL in the peak fraction) from a small suspension culture (200 mL of Sf9 cells at a density of 2 million/mL) (Table 1).

Table 1. Comparison of vector production in Sf9 vs HEK293 and with or without NP1 expression.

Vector	Helper *	Vector Yield in the Peak Fraction (500 μL)
rAAV2/HBoV1(Sf9)	None	1.6×10^9 DRP/μL
rAAV2/HBoV1(Sf9)	Bac-HBoV1NP1	5.0×10^9 DRP/ul
rAAV2(Sf9)	None	7.5×10^9 DRP/μL
rAAV2/HBoV1(293)	pHelper	2.3×10^9 DRP/μL

Note: 200 mL of Sf9 cells at a density of 2×10^6 cells/mL (a total of 4×10^8) and 20 145-mm plates of HEK293 cells (a total of 5×10^8) were infected /transfected for rAAV vector production. Vectors in the peak fraction that has the density of 1.40 g/mL in CsCl were quantified after dialyzed. * Helper: other than *rep/cap* trans complementary.

The yield of rAAV2/HBoV1 in Sf9 cells is ~10–100-fold higher than in HEK293 cells, considering a yield per cell [47,53,54,56]. The infection of the BEVs to Sf9 cell suspension is simpler than the plasmid transfection to HEK293 cells, and the process is easily scalable for large preparation, e.g., with a Bio-Reactor. It was previously reported that the biological characteristics of Sf9 cell-produced rAAV is equivalent to the HEK293 cell-produced rAAV [47,48,53,63]. However, in contrast, we observed that the transduction activity of the rAAV2/HBoV1(Sf9) vector produced from Sf9 cells is 5–7 times lower than that of the rAAV2/HBoV1(293) vector packaged in HEK293 cells (Figure 4C,E). We speculated that the rAAV2 genomes may not be as well packaged in HBoV1 capsids as that in AAV2 capsids, thus we examined these vector preps under transmission electron microscopy. We noticed that the rAAV2/HBoV1(293) vector barely had any empty particles (>95% full particles) (Figure 4A) as did the rAAV2 vector produced from Sf9 cells (Figure 3A, right panel), whereas rAAV2/HBoV1(Sf9) vectors had a high level of empty particles (only 50–60% full particles) (Figure 3B,C, right panels). Infection of BEV-Rep2Cap2, which was made following the Kotin strategy of Bac-AAV2Rep-Cap [56], expressed AAP in Sf9 cells, and knockout of the AAP decreased rAAV2 yield by 10 times [55]. This suggested that the AAP plays an important role in rAAV vector production in Sf9, which is likely through facilitation of the assembly of AAV capsids [22–24]. We currently do not know whether HBoV1 *cap* also expresses an AAP-like protein that may facilitate the assembly of the HBoV1 capsid, which warrants further investigation. Recently, glycosylation of rAAV has been reported and likely affects the potency of vector [64]. The possible variations in glycosylation between the vectors produced in HEK293 and Sf9 cells may also impact the transduction.

While the replication of the rAAV2 genome in Sf9 is not the rate limiting step for both rAAV2 and rAAV2/HBoV1 productions, it appears the trans functions for the pseudopackage of the rAAV2 genome in HBoV1 are less efficient than that for packaging it in the capsid of AAV2 or another AAV serotype. We have demonstrated an HBoV1 NS-free production system for rAAV2/HBoV1 in HEK293 cells [45]. In such a case, it appears that the expressions of AAV Rep proteins together with the helper components of adenovirus are sufficient for the cross-genera pseudopackage. It is clear that the adenovirus helper functions are not essential to the production of rAAV2 in Sf9 cells; however, it remains unknown whether they play a role in assisting the package of the rAAV2 genome into the HBoV1 capsid in HEK293 cells. Of note, the helper components from adenovirus are absent in the BEV system. Thus, the AAV2 Rep proteins, especially the AAV2 Rep52, might not be acting as efficiently in Sf9 cells as it does for pseudopackage of the rAAV2 genome in the HBoV1 capsid in HEK293 cells. For future improvement, we will tackle whether incorporation of one or more adenovirus helper components will solve this problem. Another consideration is the potent involvement of HBoV1 small NS proteins, despite the fact that the NS-free rAAV2/HBoV1 vector production system in HEK293 cells is against such action [45]. However, it is possible that they might confer necessary function in the absence of adenovirus function. Among them, the NS3 might be the first choice for the test, as it fully contains the helicase domain of the NS1, which is similar to the AAV2 Rep52 in structure [27] and executes helicase activity during viral genome packaging as the AAV2 Rep52 does [65].

In conclusion, we have established a rAAV2/HBoV1 vector production system in suspension culture of Sf9 cells for pseudopackage of the rAAV2 genome into the HBoV1 capsid. The yield of the rAAV2/HBoV1 vector is similar to that of rAAV2 produced in suspension Sf9 culture in a small volume, which is scalable in a large culture of Sf9 cells [49–51,53,66,67]. However, the current rAAV2/HBoV1-BEV system tends to produce more empty particles than the counterpart rAAV2 vector system. In the future, we will optimize the Sf9 cell production and purification system to reduce empty particles and to produce the rAAV2/HBoV1 vector in a large quantity as the suspension Sf9 cell culture can be easily scaled, which will enable the use of the vector for gene therapy of CF lung disease in large animal models.

Author Contributions: Conceptualization, Z.Y. and J.Q.; methodology, X.D.; validation, X.D.; formal analysis, X.D.; investigation, X.D.; resources, X.D. and W.Z.; data curation, X.D.; writing—original draft preparation, X.D. and J.Q.; writing—review and editing, X.D., W.Z., Z.Y., and J.Q.; visualization, X.D.; supervision, J.Q.; project administration, J.Q.; funding acquisition, Z.Y. and J.Q. All authors have read and agreed to the published version of the manuscript.

Funding: This study was supported by PHS grants AI150877 and AI139572 from the National Institute of Allergy and Infectious Diseases. This study was also supported by grant YAN19XX0 from the Cystic Fibrosis Foundation. The Electron Microscope Research Laboratory is supported, in part, by NIH/NIGMS COBRE grant P20GM104936. The JEOL JEM-1400 transmission electron microscope was purchased with funds from NIH grant 1S10RR027564. The funders had no role in study design, data collection and interpretation, or the decision to submit the work for publication.

Acknowledgments: We thank the members of the Qiu lab for technical support and valuable discussions. We acknowledge the Electron Microscope Research Laboratory, The University of Kansas Medical Center, for help with transmission of electron microscopy.

Conflicts of Interest: The authors declare no conflict of interest.

References

1. Cotmore, S.F.; Agbandje-McKenna, M.; Canuti, M.; Chiorini, J.A.; Eis-Hubinger, A.M.; Hughes, J.; Mietzsch, M.; Modha, S.; Ogliastro, M.; Penzes, J.J.; et al. Ictv Report Consortium ICTV virus taxonomy profile: Parvoviridae. *J. Gen. Virol.* **2019**, *100*, 367–368. [CrossRef]
2. Berns, K.I.; Giraud, C. Biology of adeno-associated virus. *Curr. Top. Microbiol. Immunol.* **1996**, *218*, 1–23.
3. Wang, Z.; Deng, X.; Zou, W.; Engelhardt, J.F.; Yan, Z.; Qiu, J. Human bocavirus 1 is a novel helper for adeno-associated virus replication. *J. Virol.* **2017**, *91*, e00710-17. [CrossRef]
4. Qiu, J.; Söderlund-Venermo, M.; Young, N.S. Human parvoviruses. *Clin. Microbiol. Rev.* **2017**, *30*, 43–113. [CrossRef]
5. Allander, T.; Jartti, T.; Gupta, S.; Niesters, H.G.; Lehtinen, P.; Osterback, R.; Vuorinen, T.; Waris, M.; Bjerkner, A.; Tiveljung-Lindell, A.; et al. Human bocavirus and acute wheezing in children. *Clin. Infect. Dis.* **2007**, *44*, 904–910. [CrossRef]
6. Lin, F.; Zeng, A.; Yang, N.; Lin, H.; Yang, E.; Wang, S.; Pintel, D.; Qiu, J. Quantification of human bocavirus in lower respiratory tract infections in China. *Infect. Agents Cancer* **2007**, *2*, 3. [CrossRef] [PubMed]

7. Christensen, A.; Nordbø, S.A.; Krokstad, S.; Rognlien, A.G.; Døllner, H. Human bocavirus in children: Mono-detection, high viral load and viraemia are associated with respiratory tract infection. *J. Clin. Virol.* **2010**, *49*, 158–162. [CrossRef] [PubMed]

8. Deng, Y.; Gu, X.; Zhao, X.; Luo, J.; Luo, Z.; Wang, L.; Fu, Z.; Yang, X.; Liu, E. High viral load of human bocavirus correlates with duration of wheezing in children with severe lower respiratory tract infection. *PLoS ONE* **2012**, *7*, e34353. [CrossRef] [PubMed]

9. Don, M.; Söderlund-Venermo, M.; Valent, F.; Lahtinen, A.; Hedman, L.; Canciani, M.; Hedman, K.; Korppi, M. Serologically verified human bocavirus pneumonia in children. *Pediatr. Pulmonol.* **2010**, *45*, 120–126. [CrossRef]

10. Edner, N.; Castillo-Rodas, P.; Falk, L.; Hedman, K.; Soderlund-Venermo, M.; Allander, T. Life-threatening respiratory tract disease with human bocavirus-1 infection in a four-year-old child. *J. Clin. Microbiol.* **2011**, *50*, 531–532. [CrossRef]

11. Kantola, K.; Hedman, L.; Arthur, J.; Alibeto, A.; Delwart, E.; Jartti, T.; Ruuskanen, O.; Hedman, K.; Söderlund-Venermo, M. Seroepidemiology of human bocaviruses 1–4. *J. Infect. Dis.* **2011**, *204*, 1403–1412. [CrossRef] [PubMed]

12. Martin, E.T.; Kuypers, J.; McRoberts, J.P.; Englund, J.A.; Zerr, D.M. Human Bocavirus-1 Primary Infection and Shedding in Infants. *J. Infect. Dis.* **2015**, *212*, 516–524. [CrossRef] [PubMed]

13. Dijkman, R.; Koekkoek, S.M.; Molenkamp, R.; Schildgen, O.; van der Hoek, L. Human bocavirus can be cultured in differentiated human airway epithelial cells. *J. Virol.* **2009**, *83*, 7739–7748. [CrossRef] [PubMed]

14. Huang, Q.; Deng, X.; Yan, Z.; Cheng, F.; Luo, Y.; Shen, W.; Lei-Butters, D.C.; Chen, A.Y.; Li, Y.; Tang, L.; et al. Establishment of a reverse genetics system for studying human bocavirus in human airway epithelia. *PLoS Pathog.* **2012**, *8*, e1002899. [CrossRef]

15. Deng, X.; Yan, Z.; Luo, Y.; Xu, J.; Cheng, Y.; Li, Y.; Engelhardt, J.; Qiu, J. In vitro modeling of human bocavirus 1 infection of polarized primary human airway epithelia. *J. Virol.* **2013**, *87*, 4097–4102. [CrossRef]

16. Deng, X.; Li, Y.; Qiu, J. Human bocavirus 1 infects commercially available primary human airway epithelium cultures productively. *J. Virol. Methods* **2014**, *195*, 112–119. [CrossRef]

17. Qiu, J.; Pintel, D.J. The adeno-associated virus type 2 Rep protein regulates RNA processing via interaction with the transcription template. *Mol. Cell. Biol.* **2002**, *22*, 3639–3652. [CrossRef]

18. Qiu, J.; Yoto, Y.; Tullis, G.E.; Pintel, D. Parvovirus RNA processing strategies. In *Parvoviruses*; Kerr, J.R., Cotmore, S.F., Bloom, M.E., Linden, M.E., Parish, C.R., Eds.; Hodder Arnold: London, UK, 2006; pp. 253–274.

19. Samulski, R.J.; Muzyczka, N. AAV-mediated gene therapy for research and therapeutic purposes. *Annu. Rev. Virol.* **2014**, *1*, 427–451. [CrossRef]

20. Sonntag, F.; Schmidt, K.; Kleinschmidt, J.A. A viral assembly factor promotes AAV2 capsid formation in the nucleolus. *Proc. Natl. Acad. Sci. USA* **2010**, *107*, 10220–10225. [CrossRef]

21. Sonntag, F.; Kother, K.; Schmidt, K.; Weghofer, M.; Raupp, C.; Nieto, K.; Kuck, A.; Gerlach, B.; Bottcher, B.; Muller, O.J.; et al. The assembly-activating protein promotes capsid assembly of different adeno-associated virus serotypes. *J. Virol.* **2011**, *85*, 12686–12697. [CrossRef]

22. Earley, L.F.; Kawano, Y.; Adachi, K.; Sun, X.X.; Dai, M.S.; Nakai, H. Identification and characterization of nuclear and nucleolar localization signals in the adeno-associated virus serotype 2 assembly-activating protein. *J. Virol.* **2015**, *89*, 3038–3048. [CrossRef] [PubMed]

23. Tse, L.V.; Moller-Tank, S.; Meganck, R.M.; Asokan, A. Mapping and Engineering Functional Domains of the Assembly-Activating Protein of Adeno-associated Viruses. *J. Virol.* **2018**, *92*, e00393-18. [CrossRef] [PubMed]

24. Maurer, A.C.; Cepeda Diaz, A.K.; Vandenberghe, L.H. Residues on adeno-associated virus capsid lumen dictate interactions and compatibility with the assembly-activating protein. *J. Virol.* **2019**, *93*, e02013-18. [CrossRef] [PubMed]

25. Ogden, P.J.; Kelsic, E.D.; Sinai, S.; Church, G.M. Comprehensive AAV capsid fitness landscape reveals a viral gene and enables machine-guided design. *Science* **2019**, *366*, 1139–1143. [CrossRef]

26. Chen, A.Y.; Cheng, F.; Lou, S.; Luo, Y.; Liu, Z.; Delwart, E.; Pintel, D.; Qiu, J. Characterization of the gene expression profile of human bocavirus. *Virology* **2010**, *403*, 145–154. [CrossRef]

27. Shen, W.; Deng, X.; Zou, W.; Cheng, F.; Engelhardt, J.F.; Yan, Z.; Qiu, J. Identification and Functional Analysis of Novel Non-structural Proteins of Human Bocavirus 1. *J. Virol.* **2015**, *89*, 10097–10109. [CrossRef]

28. Zou, W.; Cheng, F.; Shen, W.; Engelhardt, J.F.; Yan, Z.; Qiu, J. Nonstructural Protein NP1 of human bocavirus 1 plays a critical role in the expression of viral capsid proteins. *J. Virol.* **2016**, *90*, 4658–4669. [CrossRef]
29. Wang, Z.; Shen, W.; Cheng, F.; Deng, X.; Engelhardt, J.F.; Yan, Z.; Qiu, J. Parvovirus expresses a small noncoding RNA that plays an essential role in virus replication. *J. Virol.* **2017**, *91*, e02375-16. [CrossRef]
30. Shen, W.; Deng, X.; Zou, W.; Engelhardt, J.F.; Yan, Z.; Qiu, J. Analysis of the cis and trans requirements for DNA replication at the right end hairpin of the human bocavirus 1 genome. *J. Virol.* **2016**, *90*, 7761–7777. [CrossRef]
31. Wang, X.; Xu, P.; Cheng, F.; Li, Y.; Wang, Z.; Hao, S.; Wang, J.; Ning, K.; Ganaie, S.S.; Engelhardt, J.F.; et al. Cellular cleavage and polyadenylation specificity factor 6 (CPSF6) mediates nuclear import of human bocavirus 1 NP1 protein and modulates viral capsid protein expression. *J. Virol.* **2020**, *94*, e01444-19. [CrossRef] [PubMed]
32. Samulski, R.J.; Srivastava, A.; Berns, K.I.; Muzyczka, N. Rescue of adeno-associated virus from recombinant plasmids: Gene correction within the terminal repeats of AAV. *Cell* **1983**, *33*, 135–143. [CrossRef]
33. Kearns, W.G.; Afione, S.A.; Fulmer, S.B.; Pang, M.C.; Erikson, D.; Egan, M.; Landrum, M.J.; Flotte, T.R.; Cutting, G.R. Recombinant adeno-associated virus (AAV-CFTR) vectors do not integrate in a site-specific fashion in an immortalized epithelial cell line. *Gene Ther.* **1996**, *3*, 748–755.
34. Cideciyan, A.V.; Hauswirth, W.W.; Aleman, T.S.; Kaushal, S.; Schwartz, S.B.; Boye, S.L.; Windsor, E.A.; Conlon, T.J.; Sumaroka, A.; Roman, A.J.; et al. Vision 1 year after gene therapy for Leber's congenital amaurosis. *N. Engl. J. Med.* **2009**, *361*, 725–727. [CrossRef] [PubMed]
35. Nathwani, A.C.; Tuddenham, E.G.; Rangarajan, S.; Rosales, C.; McIntosh, J.; Linch, D.C.; Chowdary, P.; Riddell, A.; Pie, A.J.; Harrington, C.; et al. Adenovirus-associated virus vector-mediated gene transfer in hemophilia B. *N. Engl. J. Med.* **2011**, *365*, 2357–2365. [CrossRef] [PubMed]
36. Gaudet, D.; Methot, J.; Dery, S.; Brisson, D.; Essiembre, C.; Tremblay, G.; Tremblay, K.; de Wal, J.; Twisk, J.; van den Bulk, N.; et al. Efficacy and long-term safety of alipogene tiparvovec (AAV1-LPLS447X) gene therapy for lipoprotein lipase deficiency: An open-label trial. *Gene Ther.* **2013**, *20*, 361–369. [CrossRef] [PubMed]
37. Flotte, T.R.; Trapnell, B.C.; Humphries, M.; Carey, B.; Calcedo, R.; Rouhani, F.; Campbell-Thompson, M.; Yachnis, A.T.; Sandhaus, R.A.; McElvaney, N.G.; et al. Phase 2 clinical trial of a recombinant adeno-associated viral vector expressing alpha1-antitrypsin: Interim results. *Hum. Gene Ther.* **2011**, *22*, 1239–1247. [CrossRef] [PubMed]
38. Gaudet, D.; Methot, J.; Kastelein, J. Gene therapy for lipoprotein lipase deficiency. *Curr. Opin. Lipidol.* **2012**, *23*, 310–320. [CrossRef]
39. Spencer, H.T.; Riley, B.E.; Doering, C.B. State of the art: Gene therapy of haemophilia. *Haemophilia* **2016**, *22*, 66–71. [CrossRef]
40. Bennett, J.; Wellman, J.; Marshall, K.A.; McCague, S.; Ashtari, M.; DiStefano-Pappas, J.; Elci, O.U.; Chung, D.C.; Sun, J.; Wright, J.F.; et al. Safety and durability of effect of contralateral-eye administration of AAV2 gene therapy in patients with childhood-onset blindness caused by RPE65 mutations: A follow-on phase 1 trial. *Lancet* **2016**, *388*, 661–672. [CrossRef]
41. Feuer, W.J.; Schiffman, J.C.; Davis, J.L.; Porciatti, V.; Gonzalez, P.; Koilkonda, R.D.; Yuan, H.; Lalwani, A.; Lam, B.L.; Guy, J. Gene Therapy for Leber Hereditary Optic Neuropathy: Initial Results. *Ophthalmology* **2016**, *123*, 558–570. [CrossRef]
42. Yan, Z.; Keiser, N.W.; Song, Y.; Deng, X.; Cheng, F.; Qiu, J.; Engelhardt, J.F. A novel chimeric adeno-associated virus 2/human bocavirus 1 parvovirus vector efficiently transduces human airway epithelia. *Mol. Ther.* **2013**, *21*, 2181–2194. [CrossRef] [PubMed]
43. Yan, Z.; Feng, Z.; Sun, X.; Zhang, Y.; Zou, W.; Wang, Z.; Jensen-Cody, C.; Liang, B.; Park, S.Y.; Qiu, J.; et al. Human bocavirus type-1 capsid facilitates the transduction of ferret airways by adeno-associated virus genomes. *Hum. Gene Ther.* **2017**, *28*, 612–625. [CrossRef] [PubMed]
44. Yan, Z.; Stewart, Z.A.; Sinn, P.L.; Olsen, J.C.; Hu, J.; McCray, P.B., Jr.; Engelhardt, J.F. Ferret and pig models of cystic fibrosis: Prospects and promise for gene therapy. *Hum. Gene Ther. Clin. Dev.* **2015**, *26*, 38–49. [CrossRef] [PubMed]
45. Yan, Z.; Zou, W.; Feng, Z.; Shen, W.; Park, S.Y.; Deng, X.; Qiu, J.; Engelhardt, J.F. Establishment of a high-yield recombinant adeno-associated virus/human bocavirus vector production system independent of bocavirus nonstructural proteins. *Hum. Gene Ther.* **2019**, *30*, 556–570. [CrossRef] [PubMed]

46. Samulski, R.J.; Sally, M.; Muzyczka, N. Adeno-associated virus vector. In *The Development of Human Gene Therapy*; Friedmann, T., Ed.; Cold Spring Harbor: New York, NY, USA, 1999.

47. Urabe, M.; Ding, C.; Kotin, R.M. Insect cells as a factory to produce adeno-associated virus type 2 vectors. *Hum. Gene Ther.* **2002**, *13*, 1935–1943. [CrossRef] [PubMed]

48. Virag, T.; Cecchini, S.; Kotin, R.M. Producing recombinant adeno-associated virus in foster cells: Overcoming production limitations using a baculovirus-insect cell expression strategy. *Hum. Gene Ther.* **2009**, *20*, 807–817. [CrossRef]

49. Meghrous, J.; Aucoin, M.G.; Jacob, D.; Chahal, P.S.; Arcand, N.; Kamen, A.A. Production of recombinant adeno-associated viral vectors using a baculovirus/insect cell suspension culture system: From shake flasks to a 20-L bioreactor. *Biotechnol. Prog.* **2005**, *21*, 154–160. [CrossRef]

50. Cecchini, S.; Virag, T.; Kotin, R.M. Reproducible high yields of recombinant adeno-associated virus produced using invertebrate cells in 0.02- to 200-liter cultures. *Hum. Gene Ther.* **2011**, *22*, 1021–1030. [CrossRef]

51. Negrete, A.; Yang, L.C.; Mendez, A.F.; Levy, J.R.; Kotin, R.M. Economized large-scale production of high yield of rAAV for gene therapy applications exploiting baculovirus expression system. *J. Gene Med.* **2007**, *9*, 938–948. [CrossRef]

52. Negrete, A.; Kotin, R.M. Production of recombinant adeno-associated vectors using two bioreactor configurations at different scales. *J. Virol. Methods* **2007**, *145*, 155–161. [CrossRef]

53. Kotin, R.M. Large-scale recombinant adeno-associated virus production. *Hum. Mol. Genet.* **2011**, *20*, R2–R6. [CrossRef] [PubMed]

54. Kotin, R.M.; Snyder, R.O. Manufacturing clinical grade recombinant adeno-associated virus using invertebrate cell lines. *Hum. Gene Ther.* **2017**, *28*, 350–360. [CrossRef]

55. Grosse, S.; Penaud-Budloo, M.; Herrmann, A.K.; Borner, K.; Fakhiri, J.; Laketa, V.; Kramer, C.; Wiedtke, E.; Gunkel, M.; Menard, L.; et al. Relevance of assembly-activating protein for adeno-associated virus vector production and capsid protein stability in mammalian and insect cells. *J. Virol.* **2017**, *91*, e01198-17. [CrossRef]

56. Smith, R.H.; Levy, J.R.; Kotin, R.M. A simplified baculovirus-AAV expression vector system coupled with one-step affinity purification yields high-titer rAAV stocks from insect cells. *Mol. Ther.* **2009**, *17*, 1888–1896. [CrossRef] [PubMed]

57. Mou, H.; Vinarsky, V.; Tata, P.R.; Brazauskas, K.; Choi, S.H.; Crooke, A.K.; Zhang, B.; Solomon, G.M.; Turner, B.; Bihler, H.; et al. Dual SMAD signaling inhibition enables long-term expansion of diverse epithelial basal cells. *Cell Stem Cell* **2016**, *19*, 217–231. [CrossRef] [PubMed]

58. Cecchini, S.; Negrete, A.; Virag, T.; Graham, B.S.; Cohen, J.I.; Kotin, R.M. Evidence of prior exposure to human bocavirus as determined by a retrospective serological study of 404 serum samples from adults in the United States. *Clin. Vaccine Immunol.* **2009**, *16*, 597–604. [CrossRef]

59. Deng, X.; Yan, Z.; Cheng, F.; Engelhardt, J.F.; Qiu, J. Replication of an autonomous human parvovirus in non-dividing human airway epithelium is facilitated through the DNA damage and repair pathways. *PLoS Pathog.* **2016**, *12*, e1005399. [CrossRef]

60. Guan, W.; Wong, S.; Zhi, N.; Qiu, J. The genome of human parvovirus B19 virus can replicate in non-permissive cells with the help of adenovirus genes and produces infectious virus. *J. Virol.* **2009**, *83*, 9541–9553. [CrossRef]

61. Ponnazhagan, S.; Weigel, K.A.; Raikwar, S.P.; Mukherjee, P.; Yoder, M.C.; Srivastava, A. Recombinant human parvovirus B19 vectors: Erythroid cell-specific delivery and expression of transduced genes. *J. Virol.* **1998**, *72*, 5224–5230. [CrossRef]

62. Yan, Z.; McCray, P.B., Jr.; Engelhardt, J.F. Advances in gene therapy for cystic fibrosis lung disease. *Hum. Mol. Genet.* **2019**, *28*, R88–R94. [CrossRef]

63. Urabe, M.; Nakakura, T.; Xin, K.Q.; Obara, Y.; Mizukami, H.; Kume, A.; Kotin, R.M.; Ozawa, K. Scalable generation of high-titer recombinant adeno-associated virus type 5 in insect cells. *J. Virol.* **2006**, *80*, 1874–1885. [CrossRef] [PubMed]

64. Aloor, A.; Zhang, J.; Gashash, E.A.; Parameswaran, A.; Chrzanowski, M.; Ma, C.; Diao, Y.; Wang, P.G.; Xiao, W. Site-specific N-glycosylation on the AAV8 capsid protein. *Viruses* **2018**, *10*, 644. [CrossRef] [PubMed]

65. King, J.A.; Dubielzig, R.; Grimm, D.; Kleinschmidt, J.A. DNA helicase-mediated packaging of adeno-associated virus type 2 genomes into preformed capsids. *EMBO J.* **2001**, *20*, 3282–3291. [CrossRef]

66. Aslanidi, G.; Lamb, K.; Zolotukhin, S. An inducible system for highly efficient production of recombinant adeno-associated virus (rAAV) vectors in insect Sf9 cells. *Proc. Natl. Acad. Sci. USA* **2009**, *106*, 5059–5064. [CrossRef] [PubMed]

67. Mietzsch, M.; Grasse, S.; Zurawski, C.; Weger, S.; Bennett, A.; Agbandje-McKenna, M.; Muzyczka, N.; Zolotukhin, S.; Heilbronn, R. OneBac: Platform for scalable and high-titer production of AAV serotype 1-12 vectors for gene therapy. *Hum. Gene Ther.* **2014**, *25*, 212–222. [CrossRef] [PubMed]

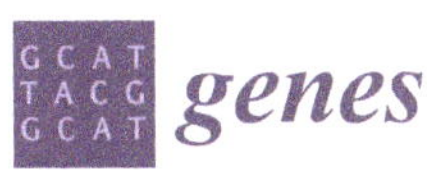 *genes*

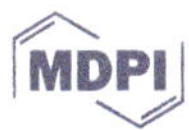

Article

Extracellular Vesicle-Mediated siRNA Delivery, Protein Delivery, and CFTR Complementation in Well-Differentiated Human Airway Epithelial Cells

Brajesh K. Singh *, Ashley L. Cooney, Sateesh Krishnamurthy and Patrick L. Sinn

Stead Family Department of Pediatrics, Carver College of Medicine, The University of Iowa,
Iowa City, IA 52242, USA; Ashley-peterson@uiowa.edu (A.L.C.); sateesh-krishnamurthy@uiowa.edu (S.K.);
patrick-sinn@uiowa.edu (P.L.S.)
* Correspondence: brajesh-singh@uiowa.edu; Tel.: +1-(319)-335-6933

Received: 2 March 2020; Accepted: 24 March 2020; Published: 26 March 2020

Abstract: Extracellular vesicles (EVs) are a class of naturally occurring secreted cellular bodies that are involved in long distance cell-to-cell communication. Proteins, lipids, mRNA, and miRNA can be packaged into these vesicles and released from the cell. This information is then delivered to target cells. Since EVs are naturally adapted molecular messengers, they have emerged as an innovative, inexpensive, and robust method to deliver therapeutic cargo in vitro and in vivo. Well-differentiated primary cultures of human airway epithelial cells (HAE) are refractory to standard transfection techniques. Indeed, common strategies used to overexpress or knockdown gene expression in immortalized cell lines simply have no detectable effect in HAE. Here we use EVs to efficiently deliver siRNA or protein to HAE. Furthermore, EVs can deliver CFTR protein to cystic fibrosis donor cells and functionally correct the Cl^- channel defect in vitro. EV-mediated delivery of siRNA or proteins to HAE provides a powerful genetic tool in a model system that closely recapitulates the in vivo airways.

Keywords: exosomes; microvesicles; cystic fibrosis; lung; primary cells

---

1. Introduction

Primary cultures of well-differentiated human airway epithelial cells (HAE) are a robust model for studying epithelial cell biology. Cells grown at an air–liquid interface form a polarized, pseudostratified columnar epithelium that closely resembles the morphology of the in vivo surface epithelium of the conducting airways [1–3]. This model provides an opportunity to study cell biology, disease progression, pathogenesis, and treatments for lung diseases like cystic fibrosis [4]. However, well-differentiated HAE are refractory to transfection techniques for delivering expression plasmids, small interfering RNA molecules (siRNA) [5–8], and single-stranded oligonucleotides [5,6]. Transfection is possible at the time of seeding when the cells are still poorly differentiated [9]. Transfecting siRNA into poorly differentiated airway cells leads to knockdown of target genes; however, this strategy has its limitations because poorly differentiated HAE are simply less representative of the in vivo airways. As a result, viral-based vectors (such as adenovirus, lentivirus, or adeno-associated virus) are typically employed to deliver genetic material to HAE. Viral vectors can be expensive and time consuming to generate. To date, many effector molecules and approaches have been investigated to increase the transfection efficiency in HAE [7,9]; yet despite much effort, there remains a need to identify an efficient delivery strategy in this in vitro model system. The ability to efficiently transfect well-differentiated HAE would open the doors to wide-ranging experimental questions that are currently not feasible, such as probing novel gene targets for therapeutic rescue of cells lacking cystic fibrosis transmembrane conductance regulator (CFTR) function [9–12].

Extracellular vesicles (EVs) are a family of lipid-bound cellular bodies that are secreted by most cells in the body, including T cells, B cells, dendritic cells, mast cells, and epithelial cells [13–16]. EVs can be purified from several types of extracellular body fluids including blood, urine, amniotic fluid, breast milk, saliva, and cerebrospinal fluid [17]. EVs are also readily collected from the supernatant of various cultured cell types in vitro [18]. The two main types of EVs are microvesicles (MVs) and exosomes, which are classified based upon their biogenesis, release pathways, size, content, and function [19,20]. These vesicles were once thought to be a mechanism for removing unwanted proteins, but many studies show that EVs are involved in intercellular communications. For example, they package highly variable cargo and facilitate transfer of proteins, lipids, microRNAs, and mRNAs from donor cells to target cells [21–26]. Exosomes bind a wide range of surface receptors (tetraspanins, integrins, CD11b and CD18 receptors) and are internalized by phagocytosis or endocytosis [27]. MVs endocytose or potentially fuse to the cell surface; thereby, integrating lipids and proteins directly into the plasma membrane of target cells [19]. Both MVs and exosomes are involved in many cellular processes and evolved to deliver multiple types of genetic and other cargo to a wide range of cellular targets [27–31].

Here we demonstrate the utility and functional impact of exosome-mediated delivery of siRNA and MV-mediated delivery of CFTR protein in well-differentiated HAE. Our data provide evidence that EVs can provide a rapid, inexpensive, and robust tool to deliver small RNAs and proteins into an important model system.

2. Materials and Methods

2.1. Cell Culture

Primary cultures of human airway epithelia were cultured from trachea and bronchi as described previously [2]. Briefly, epithelial cells suspensions were enzymatically dissociated and seeded at a density of 5×10^5 cells/cm^2 onto collagen-coated, Transwell inserts (Corning Costar polycarbonate filters) with 0.6 cm^2 semipermeable support membranes. The cells were then incubated for 24 h at 37 °C and 5% CO_2. The apical medium was removed and the cells were maintained in Ultroser G (Biosepra SA, Cedex, France) medium for more than 4 weeks at an air-liquid interface. All studies described in this article received Institutional Review Board approval (IRB ID 9507432).

2.2. Isolation of Extracellular Vesicles (EVs)

To avoid contamination with fetal bovine serum (FBS) derived EVs, FBS was centrifuged at 110,000× *g* for 2 h and the pellet was discarded. The cell culture media of HEK-293T or A549 cells was replaced with DMEM supplemented with EV cleared FBS one day before supernatant collection. The cell culture supernatants were collected and the EVs were isolated by differential centrifugation as previously described [18,32]. EVs are typically isolated from 60–80 mL of culture supernatant. We collect this supernatant from ~1.5×10^8 cells growing at confluency from 4×150 mm culture dishes. Briefly, the cell supernatants were cleared of intact cells and cell debris by centrifugation at 300× *g* for 10 min and 10,000× *g* for 10 min at 4 °C, before the first ultracentrifugation at 30,000× *g* for 70 min at 4 °C to pellet MVs (Figure 1A). The supernatant was then filtered through a 0.22 μm Amicon filter before the second round of ultracentrifugation at 110,000× *g* for 70 min at 4 °C to pellet exosomes. The MV and exosome pellets were washed in phosphate buffered saline (PBS) once and re-suspended in 200 μl of PBS or culture media with gentle mixing and stored at −80 °C. The recovery of EVs was estimated by measuring the protein concentration using a Bradford assay. The protein concentrations varied from 0.25 to 0.5 μg/μL.

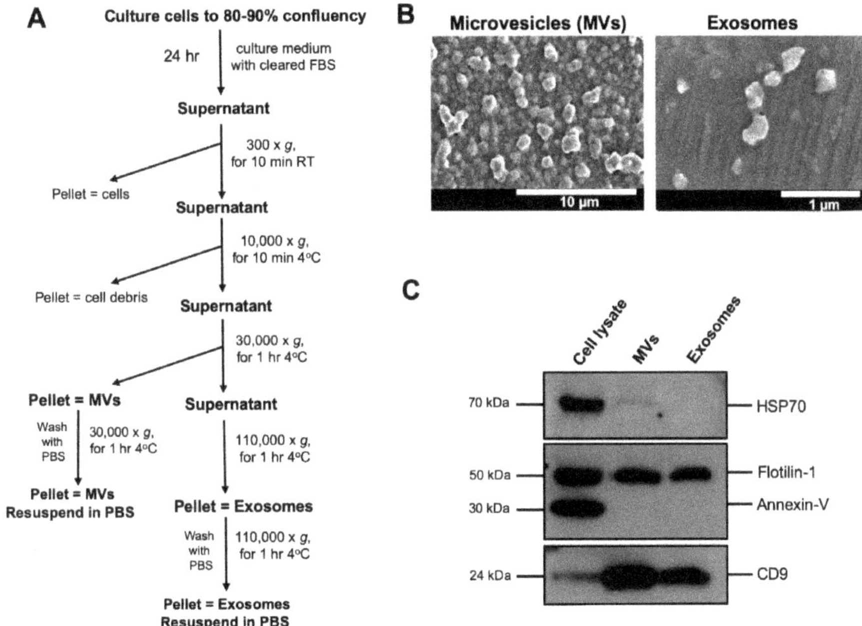

Figure 1. Isolation and characterization of extracellular vesicles (EVs) from A549 cells. (**A**) The workflow of differential ultracentrifugation for extracellular vesicles isolation is shown. (**B**) Scanning electron microscopy of microvesicles (MVs) (left panel) (scale bar = 10 μm) and exosomes (right panel). Scale bar = 1 μm. EVs were isolated from A549 cells cell culture medium by differential ultracentrifugation at 30,000× *g* and 110,000× *g*, respectively, and negatively stained for observation under the EM. (**C**) Proteins from whole cell lysates, MVs, and exosomes from cultured cells were separated on SDS-PAGE, followed by Western blotting using antibodies against CD9, HSP70, Flotilin-1, and Annexin V.

2.3. Electron Microscopy

Isolated EVs were fixed with 2.5% glutaraldehyde in 0.1 M sodium cacodylate buffer for 2 h at room temperature. Fixed exosomes suspensions were deposited on formvar/carbon-coated grids (Ted Pella Inc, Redding, CA, USA) for 20 min. Grids were then washed with two rinses of buffer and post-fixed with 1% osmium tetroxide for 1 h. The grids were dehydrated through ascending grades of ethanol (25%, 50%, 75%, 95% and 100% ethanol). Grids were rinsed two times with hexamethyldisilazane (HMDS) for 15 min each and then air dried overnight. The grids were placed on aluminum stubs, sputter coated and visualized under a Hitachi S-4800 scanning electron microscope (Hitachi High Technologies America Inc., Pleasanton, CA, USA).

2.4. SDS-PAGE and Immunoblot Analysis

Total protein lysates were prepared from HAE and EVs in freshly prepared lysis buffer (1% Triton, 25 mmol/L Tris pH 7.4, 150 mmol/L NaCl) containing protease inhibitors (complete; mini, EDTA-free; Roche Biochemicals, Mannheim, Germany) for 30 min at 4 °C. Five μg of prepared lysates were solubilized in Laemmli reducing sample buffer (Bio-Rad, Hercules, USA) and separated on a 10% precast Mini-PROTEAN TGX gel (Bio-Rad, Hercules, CA, USA). Proteins were electro transferred onto PVDF membrane (Millipore, Burlington, MA, USA), and the membranes were blocked in 5% (*w/v*) skim milk powder in Tris-buffered saline with 0.05% (*v/v*) Tween-20 (TBST) for 1 h at RT. Membranes were probed with anti-flotilin-1, anti-CD9, anti-HSP70, and anti-annexin V from the Exosomal Marker

Antibody Sampler Kit (Cell Signaling Technology, Danvers, MA, USA) diluted in TBST for 1 h. Blots were rinsed and incubated in horseradish peroxidase-conjugated goat anti-sheep IgG (Bio-Rad, Hercules, MA, USA; 1:10,000) or goat anti-mouse IgG (Bio-Rad, Hercules, MA, USA; 1:10,000) for 1 h at RT with shaking. Antibody staining was visualized by chemiluminescence (ECL Plus Western blotting detection reagents, GE Healthcare, Pittsburgh, PA, USA).

2.5. Dicer-Substrate Short Interfering RNA (DsiRNA) Oligonucleotides

The 27-mer DsiRNAs and digoxigenin (DIG)-labeled DsiRNA were designed and synthesized by Integrated DNA Technologies (IDT, Coralville, IA, USA) as described earlier [33–35]. The DIG label was internally coupled to an amino-dT base in a 2-O′ methyl modified DsiRNA against hypoxanthine-guanine phosphoribosyltransferase (HPRT). The sequences of DsiRNAs used in the study are provided in Table 1.

Table 1. Sequences of DsiRNA used in the study. DNA bases are in bold and 2 O′ methyl bases are underlined. Amino dT bases coupled to DIG are in italics.

DsiRNA	Target mRNA	DsiRNA Target Sequence
hHPRT	human HPRT	5′ pGCCAGACUUUGUUGGAUUUGAA**TT**
		3′ UCGGUCUGAAACAACCUAAACUUUAA
DIG-HPRT	human HPRT	5′ pCCAGUAAAGUUA*T*CACAUGUUCUAG
		3′ GUGGUCAUUUCAAUAGUGUACAAGAUC
Scrambled	Not applicable	5′ pCGUUAAUCGCGUAUAAUACGCGU**AT**
		3′ CAGCAAUUAGCGCAUAUUAUGCCGCAUA

2.6. Loading of DsiRNA into Exosomes

Exosomes were loaded with DsiRNA or DIG-labelled DsiRNA by electroporation as previously described [36]. Briefly, exosomes and DsiRNA were mixed in a 1:1 ratio (wt/wt) in electroporation buffer to a final concentration of 250 ng/µL. The exosome-DsiRNA mixtures were electroporated in a 400 µL volume using 0.4-mm cuvettes at 400 mV and 125 µF capacitance with pulse time of 10–15 ms. To remove non-electroporated DsiRNA, electroporated exosomes first treated with RNase and then washed in 1.5 mL of PBS, ultracentrifuged at 110,000× *g* for 70 min and re-suspended in 50 µL of culture media.

2.7. Exosome Labeling

Exosomes were stained with 1X CellMask Deep Red Plasma Membrane stain (Thermo Fisher Scientific, Waltham, MA, USA) for 10 min at 37 °C. Unbound CellMask stain were then washed by ultracentrifugation at 110,000× *g* for 70 min in TLA 100.3 rotor (Beckman Coulter, Indianapolis, IN, USA). Finally, exosomes were re-suspended in 100 µL of culture media and stored at −80 °C for further analysis.

2.8. Confocal Microscopy and Immunostaining

For confocal microscopy, HAE were fixed in 2% paraformaldehyde, permeabilized with 0.2% Triton-X-100 in Superblock (Thermo Fisher Scientific, Waltham, MA, USA), and then blocked in 1× Superblock for 1 h at RT. F-actin was stained with either rhodamine-phalloidin (1:100, cat. no. R415, Thermo Fisher Scientific, Waltham, MA, USA) or Alexa Fluor 488-phalloidin (1:100, cat. no. A12379, Thermo Fisher Scientific, Waltham, MA, USA) for 30 min at RT. For immunostaining, HAE were incubated with primary antibody against mouse anti-CFTR monoclonal antibody (769, CFFT) or anti-Digoxygenin (cat. no. 11333089001, Roche Biochemicals, Mannheim, Germany) overnight at 4 °C. HAE were then incubated for secondary antibodies was Alexa 488-labeled goat anti-mouse or Alexa 488-labeled goat anti-sheep for 1 h at RT. HAE were mounted on a slide with Vectashield with DAPI (Vector Laboratories Inc., Burlingame, CA, USA). Representative images from three donors are shown. Z-stacks were acquired on a Leica TCS SP3 confocal microscope (Leica Microsystems Inc., Buffalo Grove IL, USA) using a 40× or 63× oil-immersion objective.

2.9. Real-Time Quantitative PCR (RT-qPCR)

Total cellular RNA was isolated using Direct-zol™ RNA MiniPrep kit (Zymo Research, Irvine, CA, USA), according to the manufacturer's protocol. The RNA concentration of samples was quantified using ND-1000 spectrophotometer (Thermo Fisher Scientific, Waltham, USA). 0.5 µg of total RNA was reverse transcribed by a high-capacity reverse transcription kit (Thermo Fisher Scientific, Waltham, MA, USA) according to the manufacturer's instructions. qRT-PCR for HPRT and SFRS9 mRNA were performed in an ABI Prism 7900 HT real-time PCR system (Thermo Fisher Scientific, Waltham, MA, USA). The PCR conditions were as follows: 95 °C for 10 min, 95 °C for 15 s, and 60 °C for 1 min for 40 cycles. The following primers were used in RT-qPCR analysis: For hHPRT AGGATTTGGAAAGGGTGTTTATTC (forward) and CCCATCTCCTTCATCACATCTC (reverse) and for hSFRS9: TGCGTAAACTGGATGACACC (forward) and CCTGCTTTGGTATGGAGAGTC (reverse). The mRNA level of HPRT was calculated with normalization to SFRS9 using the $2^{-\Delta\Delta CT}$ method. Fold change in expression are means of three technical triplicates from three human donors.

2.10. Isolation of CFTR- or mCherry-Loaded EVs and Delivery to HAE

To isolate EVs loaded with either mCherry or CFTR, A549 cells were transfected with an expression plasmid or transduced with an adenovirus expressing mCherry (Ad5-mCherry) or CFTR (Ad5-CFTR) under the direction of a short 183-bp synthetic enhancer/promoter F5tg83 as previously described [37,38]. Briefly, cells were grown to 70–80% confluency and transduced at MOI = 50 for 4 h. After transduction, cells were washed three times with PBS to wash away unbound viral particles. Fresh culture medium (DMEM supplemented with EV-cleared FBS) was added to the cells. After 48 h EVs were isolated as described above.

To treat the airway epithelia with EVs apically, HAE were first treated apically with 0.1% lysophosphatidylcholine (LPC) in PBS for 2 h. HAE were rinsed three times with PBS before EVs were applied in a volume of 100 µL culture media for 4 h at 37 °C. EVs were removed and HAE were incubated at 37 °C under 5% CO_2 for the indicated times. In the case of basolateral application, the cultures were inverted, and the EVs were applied to the basolateral surface for 4 h in 80 µl of culture media at 37 °C, 5% CO_2. Following the treatment, the EVs were removed, and the cultures were turned upright and incubated at 37 °C under 5% CO_2 for the indicated times.

2.11. Ussing Chamber Studies of Well-Differentiated HAE

To measure change in anion channel activity, HAE were mounted into Ussing chambers as described earlier [39]. The apical and basolateral chambers were filled with symmetrical Ringer's solution (135 mM NaCl, 5 mM HEPES, 0.6 mM KH_2PO_4, 2.4 mM K_2HPO_4, 1.2 mM $MgCl_2$, 1.2 mM $CaCl_2$, 5 mM dextrose). Dextrose was added to this solution immediately before the experiments. The protocol was performed as follows: treatment with amiloride (100 µM), followed by DIDS (100 µM), apical solution was replaced with a low Cl^- solution, and CFTR Cl^- current was measured as previously described [40].

3. Results

3.1. Isolation and Characterization of Extracellular Vesicles

EVs were isolated from culture media of HEK-293T or A549 cells. EVs were fractionated into two populations by differential ultracentrifugation. The first fraction, containing microvesicles (MVs), was recovered from the pellet after centrifugation at 30,000× *g*, and the second fraction, containing exosomes, was recovered from the pellet after centrifugation at 110,000× *g* (Figure 1A). We next characterized the two fractions for their morphology/size and protein surface markers (Figure 1B,C). As expected, the MV fraction consisted of large vesicles ranging from 300–1000 nm in diameter (Figure 1B, left panel), whereas the second exosome fraction contained smaller size vesicles ranging from 80–150 nm (Figure 1B, right panel). To further confirm the purity of our fractions, proteins from cell lysates, MVs, and exosomes were characterized by immunoblot analysis for EVs specific protein markers [41] (Figure 1C). Tetraspanin-like CD9 and flotillin-1 were highly enriched in the EVs, whereas HSP70 and annexin V were not enriched in either the MV or exosome fractions. HSP70 was not detectable in the exosome fraction, but faintly present in the MV fraction, suggesting that large vesicles contain cellular proteins. This suggests the probable differences in biogenesis, where exosomes are secreted through the endosome pathway and would present endosome markers, whereas larger vesicles such as MVs are produced by direct budding from the cell membrane and would contain cellular proteins or proteins associated with the plasma membrane. The absence of annexin V from the EV fractions confirms the absence of apoptotic bodies in our EV preparations. Our results are consistent with previous reports that describe the protein composition in exosomes and MVs [19,28].

3.2. Exosomes are Internalized at the Basolateral Surface of HAE

For our initial studies, we asked whether EVs would be taken up by well-differentiated HAE and whether there is a preference for the apical or basolateral surface. Our standard protocol requires the HAE cultures to be grown on polycarbonate Transwell inserts with a pore size of 400 nm. Because this pore size physically limits the access of MVs to the basolateral surface, we focused our efforts on exosomes which are smaller than the pore size of the Transwell insert. To evaluate the efficiency of exosome uptake by HAE, exosomes derived from HEK-293T cells were labeled with CellMask Deep Red Plasma Membrane stain and applied to the apical (Figure 2A) or basolateral (Figure 2B) surface of HAE for 4 h. At the indicated time points post-delivery, confocal microscopy was used to evaluate intracellular uptake of CellMask stain. Following apical exosome delivery, few (estimated <1%) CellMask positive cells were observed (Figure 2A). In contrast, following basolateral exosome delivery, we readily observed abundant CellMask positive HAE (Figure 2B). Exosome internalization was observed as early as 3 h after basolateral application. Regardless of apical or basolateral exosome delivery, the CellMask stain was stable for at least 5 days after delivery and remained localized in perinuclear regions below the apical surface. However, the presence of CellMask is not an indication of the stability of internalized exosomes, only the internalized labeled lipid bilayers. These data suggest that exosomes are an efficient delivery vehicle to HAE and that delivery is more efficient from the basolateral surface than the apical surface.

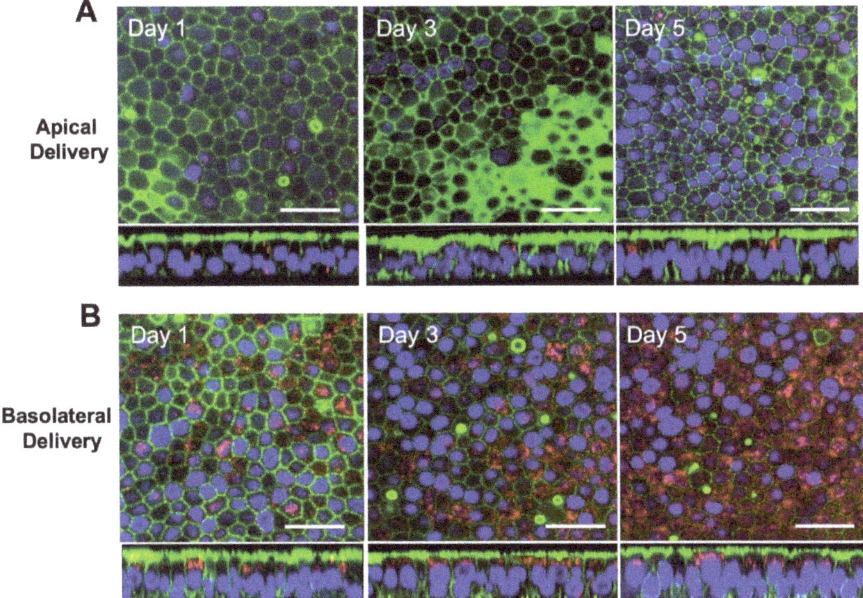

Figure 2. Exosomes can be delivered to well-differentiated HAE. Exosomes (5 µg) were labelled with CellMask Deep Red Plasma Membrane stain and applied apically (**A**) or basolaterally (**B**) to HAE for 4 h. HAE were fixed, permeabilized, and then stained for F-actin (green) and nuclei (blue). HAE were examined by confocal microscopy for internalization of exosomes at the indicated time points. Scale bar = 50 µm.

3.3. Delivery of siRNA into HAE Using Exosomes

To test if EVs could be used to functionally modify gene expression in HAE, we used exosomes to deliver siRNA and quantified the level of knockdown. Because of the clear basolateral preference of exosomes, we focused on basolaterally applied exosomes. Using the previously described protocol (Figure 1A), exosomes were purified from the supernatant of A549 cells. The exosomes were then electroporated in the presence of digoxigenin (DIG)-labeled siRNA. Exosomes containing DIG-siRNA were applied to the basolateral surface of the HAE cultures for 4 hr. Intracellular DIG was imaged 24 h later by confocal microscopy (Figure 3A). DIG-labeled siRNA (green) was readily detected (estimated >80%) of the HAE. No green signal was detected in the HAE cells treated with non-electroporated exosomes (Figure 3B). These results indicate that exosomes are capable of delivering siRNA into HAE.

To verify that exosome delivered siRNA can bring about functional knockdown of its target RNA, we chose the ubiquitously expressed transcript hypoxanthine-guanine phosphoribosyl-transferase (HPRT) [42]. We electroporated exosomes derived from A549 cells with either scrambled or HPRT specific siRNA. The level of knockdown was compared to unelectroporated (control) exosomes. As before, exosomes were applied to the basolateral side of HAE for 4 h. HPRT mRNA levels were quantified 24 h later by qRT-PCR. Compared to controls, HPRT mRNA levels were significantly decreased by ~40% in cells that received HPRT-specific siRNA (Figure 3C). These findings indicate that exosomes can successfully deliver siRNA into HAE.

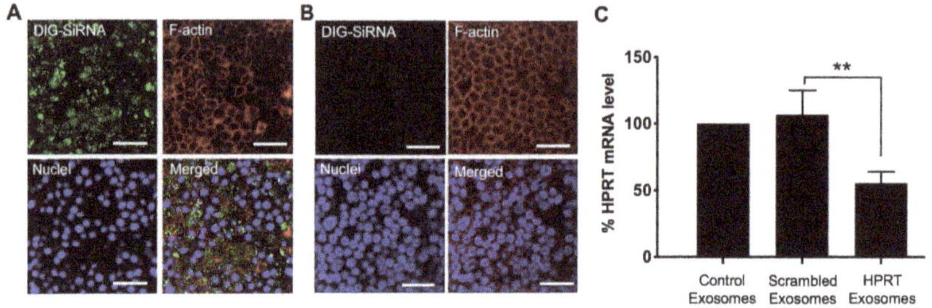

Figure 3. Exosome-mediated delivery of DsiRNA effectively silences target gene in HAE. DsiRNA can be delivered into HAEs using exosomes. HAEs were treated for 4 h with A549 derived exosomes (**A**) electroporated with digoxigenin (DIG) labeled siRNA (green) or (**B**) non-electroporated exosomes. After 24 h, HAE were fixed, permeabilized, and immunostained for DIG-labelled DsiRNA with anti-digoxygenin (green) and for F-actin (red) and nuclei (blue). HAE were examined using confocal microscopy. Scale bar = 50 μm. (**C**) qRT-PCR of HPRT mRNA in exosome treated cells. HAE were treated for 4 h with 10 μg of A549 derived exosomes electroporated with scrambled or siRNA specific to HPRT gene. After 24 h HPRT mRNA levels were measured using qRT-PCR. HPRT mRNA was normalized against reference gene SFRS9 in HAE. All experiments were performed in triplicate from three donors. Each repeat was carried out with a unique exosome preparation. Data are represented as means and s.d. of fold change from 3 donors, ** $p < 0.01$.

3.4. Protein Delivery to HAE Using Exosomes

To evaluate the ability of exosomes to deliver proteins into HAE, we loaded the exosomes with the fluorescent reporter protein mCherry. To do this, HEK-293T cells were transfected with a plasmid expressing mCherry. Three days later, exosomes were collected from the supernatant. HAE were treated basolaterally with purified exosomes for 4 h and the presence of mCherry in HAE was examined 24 h later using confocal microscopy. We readily observed intracellular mCherry signal in treated cells indicating uptake of exosomes by HAE (Figure 4). The mCherry signal remained prominently cytoplasic. Together these data strongly suggest that exosomes are a useful delivery tool in HAE.

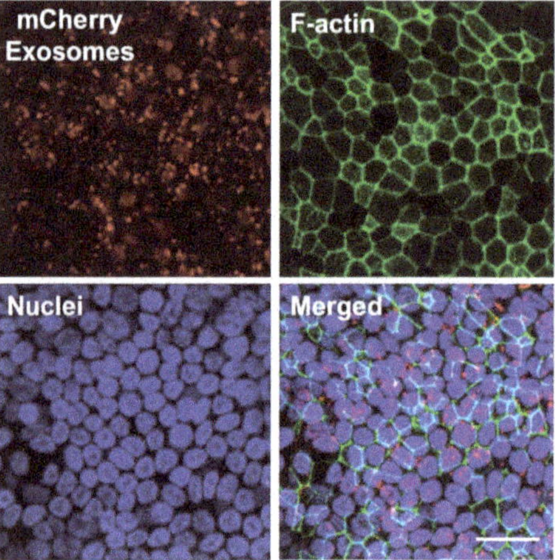

Figure 4. Exosome-mediated protein delivery to well-differentiated HAE. HAE were treated basolaterally for 4 h with exosomes derived from HEK-293T cells that were transfected with a plasmid expressing mCherry protein (red). After 24 h, HAE were fixed, permeabilized, and then stained for F-actin (red) and nuclei (blue). Scale bar = 50 μm.

3.5. MV-Mediated Delivery of CFTR Protein Corrects Anion Defect in HAE from CF Donors

CFTR complementation restores the anion channel defect in well-differentiated human airway epithelial cells derived from CF donors (HAE^{CF}) [43,44]. Typically, viral vectors are required to deliver the *CFTR* cDNA. Here we test whether CFTR protein can be delivered to HAE^{CF} using either exosomes or MVs and functionally correct the Cl$^-$ channel defect. For these experiments, A549 cells were first transduced with Ad-vector (MOI = 50) expressing either mCherry or CFTR. MVs or exosomes were then purified from the A549 supernatant one day later as described (Figure 1A).

Thus, far we focused our efforts on using exosomes to deliver siRNA or protein to HAE. Exosomes are typically 80–150 nm in diameter and will readily pass through the 400 nm pores of the Transwell inserts on which HAE are grown. MVs range in size from 200 to 1000 nm. However, exosomes typically package proteins <150 kDa; whereas, MVs can package proteins as large as ~300 kDa. The fully glycosylated, mature form of CFTR is ~250 kDa. Thus, for CFTR delivery, we sought to contrast exosomes and MVs while allowing equivalent access to the basolateral surface. To achieve basolateral access with an apical application, we pretreated HAE with 0.1% lysophosphatidylcholine (LPC). LPC is a natural airway surfactant that transiently opens tight junctions and allows access to the basolateral surface. LPC treatment is a common strategy to improve transduction efficiencies of viral vectors, such as VSV-G pseudotyped lentivirus [45] or adenovirus [44], with preferences for the basolateral surface of polarized epithelia.

EVs (exosomes or MVs) loaded with mCherry were applied to the apical surface of LPC treated HAE. Intracellular localization of mCherry was examined 24 h later by confocal microscopy (Figure 5A,B). We observed equivalent levels of mCherry expression in HAE treated with MVs or exosomes. We next loaded EVs with CFTR and applied them to the apical surface of LPC treated HAE^{CF}. Cells were fixed and immunohistochemisty was used to detect CFTR protein 24 h after EV application. In this case, CFTR protein was only detected following application of MVs but not exosomes (Figure 5C,D). In addition, the bioelectric properties of epithelia were analyzed in Ussing chambers. HAE^{CF} treated with CFTR MVs showed a significant increase in transepithelial Cl$^-$ current in response to forskolin and 3-isobutyl-1-methylxanthine (F&I) and current was inhibited by the CFTR channel blocker, GlyH-101 (Figure 5E) when compared to cells treated with either mCherry MVs, mCherry exosomes, or CFTR exosomes. These data demonstrated that MV-mediated apical delivery of CFTR protein to primary airway epithelia can correct the anion channel defect in vitro as early as 24 h post treatment.

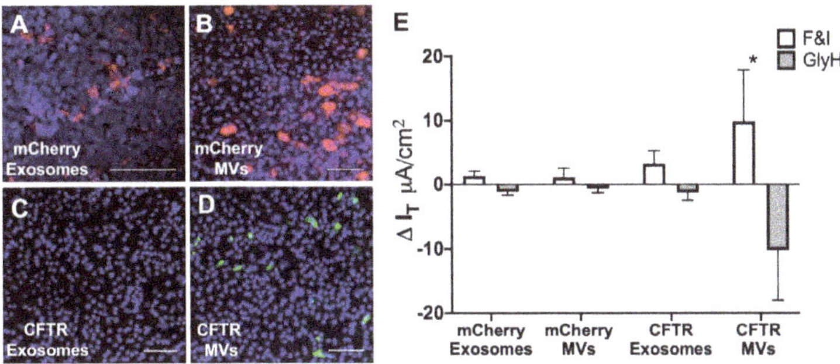

Figure 5. MV-mediated correction of chloride (Cl$^-$) transport in cystic fibrosis (CF) human primary epithelia. HAE^{CF} were treated apically with A549-derived EVs: (**A**) mCherry exosomes, (**B**) mCherry MVs, (**C**) CFTR exosomes, or (**D**) CFTR MVs for 4 h. HAE^{CF} were pretreated with 0.1% LPC for 2 h before EVs treatment. After 24 h, HAE^{CF} were fixed, permeabilized, and examined using confocal microscopy for mCherry (red) or immunostained for CFTR protein (green). Nuclei were stained with DAPI (blue). Scale bar = 100 μm. (**E**) Transepithelial Cl$^-$ current was measured in HAE^{CF} treated with either mCherry-EVs or CFTR-EVs in Ussing chambers. Change in current was measured in response to forskolin and IBMX (F&I) and GlyH-101. Data are represented as means and s.d. of two HAE cultures from three donors, * $p < 0.05$.

4. Discussion

HAE prepared from donor trachea and bronchi are grown at an air–liquid interface and form a pseudostratified columnar epithelium with tight junctions. The cultures include multiple cell types such as ciliated cells, non-ciliated cells, goblet cells, and basal cells that recapitulate the surface cells of the conducting airways [2,46]. These cells provide an excellent model for studying airway cell biology. Indeed, HAE recapitulate many in vivo barriers to gene delivery. In the present study, we investigated the utility of extracellular vesicles (EVs) to deliver different cargos to this model system.

Manipulating genes (either by overexpression or knockdown) is a fundamental strategy for examining gene function. However, the transfection efficiency in well-differentiated HAE is reproducibly below the limit of detection regardless of the transfection or electroporation reagent [7,9,47]. The differentiation process correlates with a highly resistant transfection barrier within 5–6 days after seeding; this prevents the entry of oligonucleotides no matter the formulation of the transfection reagent [7,9,47]. Transfection is only possible when conducted at the time of seeding when the cells are still poorly differentiated [9]. Transfecting siRNA into poorly differentiated airway cells leads to knockdown of target genes; however, this strategy has its limitations because poorly differentiated HAE are simply less representative of the in vivo airways. In the time it takes the epithelia to differentiate (3–4 weeks), the effect of the siRNA gene knockdown will diminish. The established technique for achieving efficient gene transfer in well-differentiated HAE is to use viral vectors such as adenovirus, lentivirus, or AAV. Viral vector can be time consuming and expensive when considering the effort to clone packaging plasmids as well as producing, purifying, and titering the vector.

Due to their small size (~30–100 nm), exosomes are considered nanoparticles. As a class, nanoparticles are used extensively to deliver small molecules, peptides, proteins, DNAs or siRNAs [48]; however, many manufactured lipid-based nanoparticles have associated withxicity and trigger adaptive and innate immune responses [49–52]. Exosomes are naturally adapted to transmit molecular messages between cells without invoking immune responses and are considered a safe means to deliver small therapeutic agents such as siRNA and drugs to specific target tissues in a non-cytotoxic manner [53]. Several studies demonstrate that an exosome-based delivery system can deliver its cargo to multiple cell types in vitro and in vivo. Exosomes offer significant advantages over synthetic drug delivery systems including enhanced serum stability, low immunogenicity, and minimal clearance by lung, liver, and spleen [29,53–55] and have reproducibly been used in vivo to deliver siRNAs or miRNAs [21,56–58]. In addition, exosomes will deliver other therapeutic agents, such as doxorubicin [59], STAT-3 inhibitor JSI-124 (cucurbitacinI) [60], cytosine deaminase (CD) fused with uracil phosphorybosyltransferase (UPRT) [61], curcumin [62], and catalase (exoCAT) [63]. Thus, exosomes are an effective delivery tool for multiple materials into multiple cell types.

Our results suggest that exosomes are readily taken up by the cells in well-differentiated HAE and they can efficiently deliver siRNA. We foresee many applications of this delivery system. For example, siRNAs or proteins that affect the levels of CFTR could be used to screen gene modulators, such as *SIN3A, DERL1, ARF4, CDH1*, et al. In future studies we aim to push the levels of knockdown further by expressing lung epithelial specific peptides (GFE-1 and GFE-2) [64] on the surface of exosomes and/or use a pH-sensitive fusogenic peptide [65] for efficient delivery of the cargo into HAE.

MVs are the class of EVs that are largest in size, and which therefore carry large protein cargo like CFTR and laminin proteins [66]. In this study, we showed MV-mediated delivery of CFTR protein to correct the transepithelial Cl$^-$ current in well-differentiated HAE from CF donors. We used both MVs and exosomes to deliver the CFTR protein, but only MVs were capable of delivering functional CFTR protein to HAE^{CF}. Based on the known size constraints of exosomes, we speculate that the large CFTR protein was more efficiently packaged in MVs. However, the mechanisms of how EVs are differentially produced, released, fused in target cells all may be important for function of a membrane bound channel protein. MVs may be more suitable for delivery of any cell surface channel protein regardless of the size. The mechanism of CFTR incorporation is the subject of future studies and will include western blot and super resolution microscopy analysis. In addition, for our studies we primarily used MVs and exosomes derived from A549 cells. Different EV donor cell lines may lead to different results.

A limitation of EVs purified from cultured cells is the presence of unintentional cellular protein contamination. In general, MVs are more promiscuous for inclusion of cellular proteins than exosomes. In this study, we did not test for the presence of unintentional proteins or nucleotides from the donor cells. However, EV mediated transfer of DNA fragments are shown to be unstable in target cells [29].

We and others have observed that some enveloped viruses, such as measles virus, have a strong preference for basolateral entry into HAE [67]. However, other viruses, such as Rous Sarcoma Virus, preferentially enter the apical surface. Currently it is unclear why EVs have a strong preference for entry at the basolateral surface. We speculate that proteins necessary for EV entry may be basolaterally localized. EVs are likely to play an important role in cell-to-cell communications in lung biology and disease. The lung is a unique organ with a multitude of regionally segregated epithelial cell types; as well as, endothelial and resident immune cells. Exosomes derived from airway cells play a role in innate defense and remodeling [68,69]; however, other cells (such as resident macrophages and neutrophils) are also a significant source of exosomes in the lung. Exchange of EV cargos between these cells can alter gene expression and may reorganize the airway epithelium. It is currently unclear why we observed a clear entry preference for EVs at the basolateral surface of HAE; however, this may represent a bona fide region of interface.

In summary, our study showed the potential use of EVs in manipulating the gene expression in an important in vitro airway model system. Exosomes effectively deliver siRNAs to modulate endogenous gene expression, whereas MVs can be used to deliver large protein cargos. There are many potential applications of this technology in HAE, including: screening of siRNAs and miRNAs to modulate gene expression, delivering sgRNA libraries for screening genetic phenotypes, generating models for rare CFTR mutations, and delivering 100–150 bp single-stranded DNA oligonucleotides.

Author Contributions: Conceptualization, B.K.S. and P.L.S.; methodology, B.K.S., A.L.C. and S.K.; formal analysis: B.K.S., A.L.C. and S.K.; data curation, B.K.S., A.L.C. and S.K.; writing—original draft preparation, B.K.S.; writing—review and editing, B.K.S., A.L.C. and P.L.S.; supervision, B.K.S. and P.L.S.; project administration, B.K.S. and P.L.S.; funding acquisition, B.K.S. and P.L.S. All authors have read and agreed to the published version of the manuscript.

Funding: This work was supported by the Cystic Fibrosis Foundation (SINN15XX1, SINN15XX0, and SINN19XX0) and National Institutes of Health (NIH R01 HL-133089 and NIH R01 AI-132402).

Acknowledgments: We thank Jennifer Bartlett and Miguel Ortiz for critical review of the manuscript. We acknowledge the support of Central Microscopy Research Facility (CMRF), the In Vitro Models and Cell Culture Core, and the Viral Vector Core of The University of Iowa.

Conflicts of Interest: The authors have no financial conflicts of interest. The funders of this study had no role in the design of the study; in the collection, analyses, or interpretation of data; in the writing of the manuscript, or in the decision to publish the results.

References

1. Fulcher, M.L.; Gabriel, S.; Burns, K.A.; Yankaskas, J.R.; Randell, S.H. Well-differentiated human airway epithelial cell cultures. *Methods Mol. Med.* **2005**, *107*, 183–206. [PubMed]
2. Karp, P.H.; Moninger, T.O.; Weber, S.P.; Nesselhauf, T.S.; Launspach, J.L.; Zabner, J.; Welsh, M.J. An in vitro model of differentiated human airway epithelia. Methods for establishing primary cultures. *Methods Mol. Biol.* **2002**, *188*, 115–137. [PubMed]
3. Woodworth, B.A.; Antunes, M.B.; Bhargave, G.; Palmer, J.N.; Cohen, N.A. Murine tracheal and nasal septal epithelium for air-liquid interface cultures: A comparative study. *Am. J. Rhinol.* **2007**, *21*, 533–537. [CrossRef] [PubMed]
4. Zabner, J.; Zeiher, B.G.; Friedman, E.; Welsh, M.J. Adenovirus-mediated gene transfer to ciliated airway epithelia requires prolonged incubation time. *J. Virol.* **1996**, *70*, 6994–7003. [CrossRef] [PubMed]

5. Caci, E.; Melani, R.; Pedemonte, N.; Yueksekdag, G.; Ravazzolo, R.; Rosenecker, J.; Galietta, L.J.; Zegarra-Moran, O. Epithelial sodium channel inhibition in primary human bronchial epithelia by transfected sirna. *Am. J. Respir. Cell Mol. Biol.* **2009**, *40*, 211–216. [CrossRef]

6. Griesenbach, U.; Kitson, C.; Escudero Garcia, S.; Farley, R.; Singh, C.; Somerton, L.; Painter, H.; Smith, R.L.; Gill, D.R.; Hyde, S.C.; et al. Inefficient cationic lipid-mediated sirna and antisense oligonucleotide transfer to airway epithelial cells in vivo. *Respir. Res.* **2006**, *7*, 26. [CrossRef]

7. Krishnamurthy, S.; Behlke, M.A.; Ramachandran, S.; Salem, A.K.; McCray, P.B., Jr.; Davidson, B.L. Manipulation of cell physiology enables gene silencing in well-differentiated airway epithelia. *Mol. Ther. Nucleic Acids* **2012**, *1*, e41. [CrossRef]

8. Platz, J.; Pinkenburg, O.; Beisswenger, C.; Puchner, A.; Damm, T.; Bals, R. Application of small interfering RNA (sirna) for modulation of airway epithelial gene expression. *Oligonucleotides* **2005**, *15*, 132–138. [CrossRef]

9. Ramachandran, S.; Krishnamurthy, S.; Jacobi, A.M.; Wohlford-Lenane, C.; Behlke, M.A.; Davidson, B.L.; McCray, P.B., Jr. Efficient delivery of RNA interference oligonucleotides to polarized airway epithelia in vitro. *Am. J. Physiol. Lung Cell. Mol. Physiol.* **2013**, *305*, L23–L32. [CrossRef]

10. Hutt, D.M.; Herman, D.; Rodrigues, A.P.; Noel, S.; Pilewski, J.M.; Matteson, J.; Hoch, B.; Kellner, W.; Kelly, J.W.; Schmidt, A.; et al. Reduced histone deacetylase 7 activity restores function to misfolded cftr in cystic fibrosis. *Nat. Chem. Biol.* **2010**, *6*, 25–33. [CrossRef] [PubMed]

11. Meacham, G.C.; Patterson, C.; Zhang, W.; Younger, J.M.; Cyr, D.M. The hsc70 co-chaperone chip targets immature cftr for proteasomal degradation. *Nat. Cell Biol.* **2001**, *3*, 100–105. [CrossRef] [PubMed]

12. Okiyoneda, T.; Barriere, H.; Bagdany, M.; Rabeh, W.M.; Du, K.; Hohfeld, J.; Young, J.C.; Lukacs, G.L. Peripheral protein quality control removes unfolded cftr from the plasma membrane. *Science* **2010**, *329*, 805–810. [CrossRef] [PubMed]

13. Blanchard, N.; Lankar, D.; Faure, F.; Regnault, A.; Dumont, C.; Raposo, G.; Hivroz, C. Tcr activation of human t cells induces the production of exosomes bearing the tcr/cd3/zeta complex. *J. Immunol.* **2002**, *168*, 3235–3241. [CrossRef] [PubMed]

14. Raposo, G.; Nijman, H.W.; Stoorvogel, W.; Liejendekker, R.; Harding, C.V.; Melief, C.J.; Geuze, H.J. B lymphocytes secrete antigen-presenting vesicles. *J. Exp. Med.* **1996**, *183*, 1161–1172. [CrossRef]

15. Thery, C.; Regnault, A.; Garin, J.; Wolfers, J.; Zitvogel, L.; Ricciardi-Castagnoli, P.; Raposo, G.; Amigorena, S. Molecular characterization of dendritic cell-derived exosomes. Selective accumulation of the heat shock protein hsc73. *J. Cell Biol.* **1999**, *147*, 599–610. [CrossRef]

16. Van Niel, G.; Raposo, G.; Candalh, C.; Boussac, M.; Hershberg, R.; Cerf-Bensussan, N.; Heyman, M. Intestinal epithelial cells secrete exosome-like vesicles. *Gastroenterology* **2001**, *121*, 337–349. [CrossRef]

17. Lasser, C.; Alikhani, V.S.; Ekstrom, K.; Eldh, M.; Paredes, P.T.; Bossios, A.; Sjostrand, M.; Gabrielsson, S.; Lotvall, J.; Valadi, H. Human saliva, plasma and breast milk exosomes contain RNA: Uptake by macrophages. *J. Transl. Med.* **2011**, *9*, 9. [CrossRef]

18. Thery, C.; Amigorena, S.; Raposo, G.; Clayton, A. Isolation and characterization of exosomes from cell culture supernatants and biological fluids. *Curr. Protoc. Cell Biol.* **2006**, *30*, 3–22. [CrossRef]

19. Raposo, G.; Stoorvogel, W. Extracellular vesicles: Exosomes, microvesicles, and friends. *J. Cell Biol.* **2013**, *200*, 373–383. [CrossRef]

20. Zaborowski, M.P.; Balaj, L.; Breakefield, X.O.; Lai, C.P. Extracellular vesicles: Composition, biological relevance, and methods of study. *Bioscience* **2015**, *65*, 783–797. [CrossRef]

21. Alvarez-Erviti, L.; Seow, Y.; Yin, H.; Betts, C.; Lakhal, S.; Wood, M.J. Delivery of sirna to the mouse brain by systemic injection of targeted exosomes. *Nat. Biotechnol.* **2011**, *29*, 341–345. [CrossRef] [PubMed]

22. El Andaloussi, S.; Lakhal, S.; Mager, I.; Wood, M.J. Exosomes for targeted sirna delivery across biological barriers. *Adv. Drug Deliv. Rev.* **2013**, *65*, 391–397. [CrossRef] [PubMed]

23. Johnstone, R.M. The jeanne manery-fisher memorial lecture 1991. Maturation of reticulocytes: Formation of exosomes as a mechanism for shedding membrane proteins. *Biochem. Cell Biol. Biochim. Et Biol. Cell.* **1992**, *70*, 179–190. [CrossRef] [PubMed]

24. Valadi, H.; Ekstrom, K.; Bossios, A.; Sjostrand, M.; Lee, J.J.; Lotvall, J.O. Exosome-mediated transfer of mrnas and micrornas is a novel mechanism of genetic exchange between cells. *Nat. Cell Biol.* **2007**, *9*, 654–659. [CrossRef] [PubMed]

25. Vlassov, A.V.; Magdaleno, S.; Setterquist, R.; Conrad, R. Exosomes: Current knowledge of their composition, biological functions, and diagnostic and therapeutic potentials. *Biochim. Et Biophys. Acta* **2012**, *1820*, 940–948. [CrossRef]

26. Zomer, A.; Vendrig, T.; Hopmans, E.S.; van Eijndhoven, M.; Middeldorp, J.M.; Pegtel, D.M. Exosomes: Fit to deliver small RNA. *Commun. Integr. Biol.* **2010**, *3*, 447–450. [CrossRef]

27. Thery, C.; Ostrowski, M.; Segura, E. Membrane vesicles as conveyors of immune responses. *Nat. Rev. Immunol.* **2009**, *9*, 581–593. [CrossRef]

28. Doyle, L.M.; Wang, M.Z. Overview of extracellular vesicles, their origin, composition, purpose, and methods for exosome isolation and analysis. *Cells* **2019**, *8*, 727. [CrossRef]

29. Kanada, M.; Bachmann, M.H.; Hardy, J.W.; Frimannson, D.O.; Bronsart, L.; Wang, A.; Sylvester, M.D.; Schmidt, T.L.; Kaspar, R.L.; Butte, M.J.; et al. Differential fates of biomolecules delivered to target cells via extracellular vesicles. *Proc. Natl. Acad. Sci. USA* **2015**, *112*, E1433–E1442. [CrossRef]

30. Sun, D.; Zhuang, X.; Zhang, S.; Deng, Z.B.; Grizzle, W.; Miller, D.; Zhang, H.G. Exosomes are endogenous nanoparticles that can deliver biological information between cells. *Adv. Drug Deliv. Rev.* **2013**, *65*, 342–347. [CrossRef] [PubMed]

31. Kalluri, R.; LeBleu, V.S. The biology, function, and biomedical applications of exosomes. *Science* **2020**, *367*. [CrossRef] [PubMed]

32. Konoshenko, M.Y.; Lekchnov, E.A.; Vlassov, A.V.; Laktionov, P.P. Isolation of extracellular vesicles: General methodologies and latest trends. *Biomed. Res. Int.* **2018**, *2018*, 8545347. [CrossRef] [PubMed]

33. Reynolds, A.; Leake, D.; Boese, Q.; Scaringe, S.; Marshall, W.S.; Khvorova, A. Rational sirna design for RNA interference. *Nat. Biotechnol.* **2004**, *22*, 326–330. [CrossRef]

34. Amarzguioui, M.; Lundberg, P.; Cantin, E.; Hagstrom, J.; Behlke, M.A.; Rossi, J.J. Rational design and in vitro and in vivo delivery of dicer substrate sirna. *Nat. Protoc.* **2006**, *1*, 508–517. [CrossRef] [PubMed]

35. Collingwood, M.A.; Rose, S.D.; Huang, L.; Hillier, C.; Amarzguioui, M.; Wiiger, M.T.; Soifer, H.S.; Rossi, J.J.; Behlke, M.A. Chemical modification patterns compatible with high potency dicer-substrate small interfering rnas. *Oligonucleotides* **2008**, *18*, 187–200. [CrossRef]

36. El-Andaloussi, S.; Lee, Y.; Lakhal-Littleton, S.; Li, J.; Seow, Y.; Gardiner, C.; Alvarez-Erviti, L.; Sargent, I.L.; Wood, M.J. Exosome-mediated delivery of sirna in vitro and in vivo. *Nat. Protoc.* **2012**, *7*, 2112–2126. [CrossRef]

37. Cooney, A.L.; Singh, B.K.; Sinn, P.L. Hybrid nonviral/viral vector systems for improved piggybac DNA transposon in vivo delivery. *Mol. Ther. J. Am. Soc. Gene Ther.* **2015**, *23*, 667–674. [CrossRef]

38. Li, N.; Cooney, A.L.; Zhang, W.; Ehrhardt, A.; Sinn, P.L. Enhanced tropism of species b1 adenoviral-based vectors for primary human airway epithelial cells. *Mol. Methods Clin. Dev.* **2019**, *14*, 228–236. [CrossRef]

39. Li, H.; Sheppard, D.N.; Hug, M.J. Transepithelial electrical measurements with the ussing chamber. *J. Cyst. Fibros* **2004**, *3*, 123–126. [CrossRef]

40. Cooney, A.L.; Abou Alaiwa, M.H.; Shah, V.S.; Bouzek, D.C.; Stroik, M.R.; Powers, L.S.; Gansemer, N.D.; Meyerholz, D.K.; Welsh, M.J.; Stoltz, D.A.; et al. Lentiviral-mediated phenotypic correction of cystic fibrosis pigs. *JCI Insight* **2016**, *1*. [CrossRef]

41. Kowal, J.; Arras, G.; Colombo, M.; Jouve, M.; Morath, J.P.; Primdal-Bengtson, B.; Dingli, F.; Loew, D.; Tkach, M.; Thery, C. Proteomic comparison defines novel markers to characterize heterogeneous populations of extracellular vesicle subtypes. *Proc. Natl. Acad. Sci. USA* **2016**, *113*, E968–E977. [CrossRef]

42. Stout, J.T.; Caskey, C.T. Hprt: Gene structure, expression, and mutation. *Annu. Rev. Genet.* **1985**, *19*, 127–148. [CrossRef]

43. Olsen, J.C.; Johnson, L.G.; Stutts, M.J.; Sarkadi, B.; Yankaskas, J.R.; Swanstrom, R.; Boucher, R.C. Correction of the apical membrane chloride permeability defect in polarized cystic fibrosis airway epithelia following retroviral-mediated gene transfer. *Hum. Gene* **1992**, *3*, 253–266. [CrossRef]

44. Cooney, A.L.; Singh, B.K.; Loza, L.M.; Thornell, I.M.; Hippee, C.E.; Powers, L.S.; Ostedgaard, L.S.; Meyerholz, D.K.; Wohlford-Lenane, C.; Stoltz, D.A.; et al. Widespread airway distribution and short-term phenotypic correction of cystic fibrosis pigs following aerosol delivery of piggybac/adenovirus. *Nucleic Acids Res.* **2018**, *46*, 9591–9600. [CrossRef]

45. Sinn, P.L.; Cooney, A.L.; Oakland, M.; Dylla, D.E.; Wallen, T.J.; Pezzulo, A.A.; Chang, E.H.; McCray, P.B., Jr. Lentiviral vector gene transfer to porcine airways. *Mol. Ther. Nucleic Acids* **2012**, *1*, e56. [CrossRef]

46. Pezzulo, A.A.; Starner, T.D.; Scheetz, T.E.; Traver, G.L.; Tilley, A.E.; Harvey, B.G.; Crystal, R.G.; McCray, P.B., Jr.; Zabner, J. The air-liquid interface and use of primary cell cultures are important to recapitulate the transcriptional profile of in vivo airway epithelia. *Am. J. Physiol. Lung Cell. Mol. Physiol.* **2011**, *300*, L25–L31. [CrossRef]

47. Ramachandran, S.; Karp, P.H.; Jiang, P.; Ostedgaard, L.S.; Walz, A.E.; Fisher, J.T.; Keshavjee, S.; Lennox, K.A.; Jacobi, A.M.; Rose, S.D.; et al. A microrna network regulates expression and biosynthesis of wild-type and deltaf508 mutant cystic fibrosis transmembrane conductance regulator. *Proc. Natl. Acad. Sci. USA* **2012**, *109*, 13362–13367. [CrossRef]

48. Toumey, C. In the footsteps of biotech. *Nat. Nanotechnol.* **2010**, *5*, 475. [CrossRef]

49. Bakand, S.; Hayes, A.; Dechsakulthorn, F. Nanoparticles: A review of particle toxicology following inhalation exposure. *Inhal. Toxicol.* **2012**, *24*, 125–135. [CrossRef]

50. Dobrovolskaia, M.A.; Aggarwal, P.; Hall, J.B.; McNeil, S.E. Preclinical studies to understand nanoparticle interaction with the immune system and its potential effects on nanoparticle biodistribution. *Mol. Pharm.* **2008**, *5*, 487–495. [CrossRef]

51. Iavicoli, I.; Leso, V.; Fontana, L.; Bergamaschi, A. Toxicological effects of titanium dioxide nanoparticles: A review of in vitro mammalian studies. *Eur. Rev. Med Pharmacol. Sci.* **2011**, *15*, 481–508. [PubMed]

52. Maynard, A.D. Don't define nanomaterials. *Nature* **2011**, *475*, 31. [CrossRef] [PubMed]

53. Johnsen, K.B.; Gudbergsson, J.M.; Skov, M.N.; Pilgaard, L.; Moos, T.; Duroux, M. A comprehensive overview of exosomes as drug delivery vehicles—Endogenous nanocarriers for targeted cancer therapy. *Biochim. Et Biophys. Acta* **2014**, *1846*, 75–87. [CrossRef] [PubMed]

54. Chaput, N.; Thery, C. Exosomes: Immune properties and potential clinical implementations. *Semin. Immunopathol.* **2011**, *33*, 419–440. [CrossRef]

55. Marcus, M.E.; Leonard, J.N. Fedexosomes: Engineering therapeutic biological nanoparticles that truly deliver. *Pharmaceuticals* **2013**, *6*, 659–680. [CrossRef]

56. Chen, T.S.; Lim, S.K. Measurement of precursor mirna in exosomes from human esc-derived mesenchymal stem cells. *Methods Mol. Biol.* **2013**, *1024*, 69–86.

57. Munoz, J.L.; Bliss, S.A.; Greco, S.J.; Ramkissoon, S.H.; Ligon, K.L.; Rameshwar, P. Delivery of functional anti-mir-9 by mesenchymal stem cell-derived exosomes to glioblastoma multiforme cells conferred chemosensitivity. *Mol. Ther. Nucleic Acids* **2013**, *2*, e126. [CrossRef]

58. Wahlgren, J.; De, L.K.T.; Brisslert, M.; Vaziri Sani, F.; Telemo, E.; Sunnerhagen, P.; Valadi, H. Plasma exosomes can deliver exogenous short interfering RNA to monocytes and lymphocytes. *Nucleic Acids Res.* **2012**, *40*, e130. [CrossRef]

59. Tian, Y.; Li, S.; Song, J.; Ji, T.; Zhu, M.; Anderson, G.J.; Wei, J.; Nie, G. A doxorubicin delivery platform using engineered natural membrane vesicle exosomes for targeted tumor therapy. *Biomaterials* **2014**, *35*, 2383–2390. [CrossRef]

60. Zhuang, X.; Xiang, X.; Grizzle, W.; Sun, D.; Zhang, S.; Axtell, R.C.; Ju, S.; Mu, J.; Zhang, L.; Steinman, L.; et al. Treatment of brain inflammatory diseases by delivering exosome encapsulated anti-inflammatory drugs from the nasal region to the brain. *Mol. Ther. J. Am. Soc. Gene Ther.* **2011**, *19*, 1769–1779. [CrossRef]

61. Mizrak, A.; Bolukbasi, M.F.; Ozdener, G.B.; Brenner, G.J.; Madlener, S.; Erkan, E.P.; Strobel, T.; Breakefield, X.O.; Saydam, O. Genetically engineered microvesicles carrying suicide mrna/protein inhibit schwannoma tumor growth. *Mol. Ther. J. Am. Soc. Gene Ther.* **2013**, *21*, 101–108. [CrossRef] [PubMed]

62. Sun, D.; Zhuang, X.; Xiang, X.; Liu, Y.; Zhang, S.; Liu, C.; Barnes, S.; Grizzle, W.; Miller, D.; Zhang, H.G. A novel nanoparticle drug delivery system: The anti-inflammatory activity of curcumin is enhanced when encapsulated in exosomes. *Mol. Ther. J. Am. Soc. Gene Ther.* **2010**, *18*, 1606–1614. [CrossRef] [PubMed]

63. Haney, M.J.; Klyachko, N.L.; Zhao, Y.; Gupta, R.; Plotnikova, E.G.; He, Z.; Patel, T.; Piroyan, A.; Sokolsky, M.; Kabanov, A.V.; et al. Exosomes as drug delivery vehicles for parkinson's disease therapy. *J. Control. Release* **2015**, *207*, 18–30. [CrossRef] [PubMed]

64. Laakkonen, P.; Vuorinen, K. Homing peptides as targeted delivery vehicles. *Integr. Biol. Quant. Biosci. Nano Macro* **2010**, *2*, 326–337. [CrossRef]

65. Nakase, I.; Futaki, S. Combined treatment with a ph-sensitive fusogenic peptide and cationic lipids achieves enhanced cytosolic delivery of exosomes. *Sci. Rep.* **2015**, *5*, 10112. [CrossRef]

66. Pathan, M.; Fonseka, P.; Chitti, S.V.; Kang, T.; Sanwlani, R.; Van Deun, J.; Hendrix, A.; Mathivanan, S. Vesiclepedia 2019: A compendium of RNA, proteins, lipids and metabolites in extracellular vesicles. *Nucleic Acids Res.* **2019**, *47*, D516–D519. [CrossRef]
67. Sinn, P.; Williams, G.; Vongpunsawad, S.; Cattaneo, R.; McCray, P. Measles virus preferentially transduces the basolateral surface of well-differentiated human airway epithelia. *J. Virol.* **2002**, *76*, 2403–2409. [CrossRef]
68. Gupta, R.; Radicioni, G.; Abdelwahab, S.; Dang, H.; Carpenter, J.; Chua, M.; Mieczkowski, P.A.; Sheridan, J.T.; Randell, S.H.; Kesimer, M. Intercellular communication between airway epithelial cells is mediated by exosome-like vesicles. *Am. J. Respir. Cell Mol. Biol.* **2019**, *60*, 209–220. [CrossRef]
69. Kesimer, M.; Scull, M.; Brighton, B.; DeMaria, G.; Burns, K.; O'Neal, W.; Pickles, R.J.; Sheehan, J.K. Characterization of exosome-like vesicles released from human tracheobronchial ciliated epithelium: A possible role in innate defense. *FASEB J.* **2009**, *23*, 1858–1868. [CrossRef]

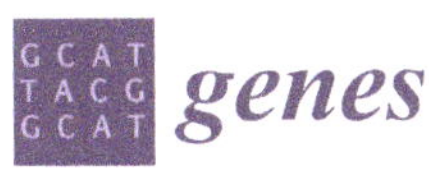 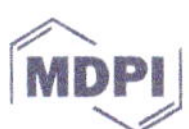

Article

High Prevalence of *Staphylococcus aureus* Enterotoxin Gene Cluster Superantigens in Cystic Fibrosis Clinical Isolates

Anthony J. Fischer [1,*], Samuel H. Kilgore [2], Sachinkumar B. Singh [1], Patrick D. Allen [1], Alexis R. Hansen [1], Dominique H. Limoli [2] and Patrick M. Schlievert [2]

[1] Stead Family Department of Pediatrics, University of Iowa Carver College of Medicine, Iowa City, IA 52242, USA; sachinkumar-singh@uiowa.edu (S.B.S.); Patrick.D.Allen@dmu.edu (P.D.A.); alexis-hansen@uiowa.edu (A.R.H.)
[2] Department of Microbiology and Immunology, University of Iowa Carver College of Medicine, Iowa City, IA 52242, USA; samuel-kilgore@uiowa.edu (S.H.K.); dominique-limoli@uiowa.edu (D.H.L.); patrick-schlievert@uiowa.edu (P.M.S.)
* Correspondence: anthony-fischer@uiowa.edu

Received: 7 November 2019; Accepted: 9 December 2019; Published: 12 December 2019

Abstract: Background: *Staphylococcus aureus* is a highly prevalent respiratory pathogen in cystic fibrosis (CF). It is unclear how this organism establishes chronic infections in CF airways. We hypothesized that *S. aureus* isolates from patients with CF would share common virulence properties that enable chronic infection. Methods: 77 *S. aureus* isolates were obtained from 45 de-identified patients with CF at the University of Iowa. We assessed isolates phenotypically and used genotyping assays to determine the presence or absence of 18 superantigens (SAgs). Results: We observed phenotypic diversity among *S. aureus* isolates from patients with CF. Genotypic analysis for SAgs revealed 79.8% of CF clinical isolates carried all six members of the enterotoxin gene cluster (EGC). MRSA and MSSA isolates had similar prevalence of SAgs. We additionally observed that EGC SAgs were prevalent in *S. aureus* isolated from two geographically distinct CF centers. Conclusions: *S. aureus* SAgs belonging to the EGC are highly prevalent in CF clinical isolates. The greater prevalence in these SAgs in CF airway specimens compared to skin isolates suggests that these toxins confer selective advantage in the CF airway.

Keywords: cystic fibrosis; *Staphylococcus aureus*; superantigen; enterotoxin gene cluster; MRSA

---

1. Introduction

Cystic fibrosis (CF) is a common lethal genetic disease, which results in chronic airway infections, irreversible bronchiectasis, and respiratory failure. *Staphylococcus aureus* is the most prevalent bacterial pathogen in children with CF [1], and is present in ≈70% of all individuals with CF in the United States. Although *Pseudomonas aeruginosa* is the predominant pathogen in older patients, *S. aureus* is the most common bacterial species in patients with CF under age 24 [2]. Unlike *P. aeruginosa*, which has multiple effective treatments to eradicate early infections and control chronic infections [3–5], *S. aureus* infections can be difficult to control with antibiotics [6]. CFTR modulator drugs may help prevent incident infections with *S. aureus*, but they are unlikely to eliminate chronic *S. aureus* infections [7,8]. Understanding how *S. aureus* infects and persists in the CF airway is critically important, as these infections may increase the risk of subsequent disease progression [9,10].

We hypothesized that *S. aureus* isolates in the CF airway would share common virulence properties. Some readily visible phenotypes such as hemolysis, pigmentation, and protease secretion could enable *S. aureus* to elude host defenses. People with CF are commonly treated with antibiotics; resistance to antibiotics may be occur under the selective pressure of antibiotic exposure. Another potential mechanism enabling *S. aureus* to establish chronic infection is the secretion of toxins that misdirect the immune response. *S. aureus* produces a large number of secreted toxins that may be critical for establishing infections [11]. These include 18 unique superantigens (SAgs), secreted toxins that bind both the T cell receptor and major histocompatibility complex molecules on antigen presenting cells [12,13].

Some SAgs are well known for their roles in acute infection. In the extreme example of toxic shock syndrome, the SAg TSST-1 cross-links T cells and antigen presenting cells, stimulating massive cytokine release and blocking the immune system from developing lasting immunity [12,13]. By contrast, the enterotoxin gene cluster (EGC), an element encoding six staphylococcal enterotoxin (SE) and SE-like SAgs G, I, M, N, O, and U, is generally associated with long term mucosal colonization. The EGC is present in between 50% to 70% of isolates from individuals with nasal carriage of *S. aureus* [14,15]. These EGC toxins can stimulate T cell proliferation [16], yet neutralizing antibody response to these toxins is surprisingly poor [17]. While these toxins have been associated with asymptomatic colonization, experimental studies in rabbits show that EGC SAgs may play crucial for infections such as endocarditis [18].

It is not clear what role SAgs play in CF respiratory infections. EGC SAgs are prevalent in clinical isolates of *S. aureus*; a recent European study showed that 57% of CF isolates harbored at least one gene belonging to the EGC [19]. This is similar to the prevalence of EGC in isolates from a cohort of patients with atopic dermatitis in the United States and Europe [20,21]. Our study had two goals: To determine whether these SAgs are as prevalent in CF isolates in the United States, and to determine if the superantigens were associated with methicillin resistance, which is common in the United States and has been linked to worse outcomes [10,22].

2. Materials and Methods

Ethics Statements: All bacterial isolates examined in this study were de-identified when they were supplied to the research team. The University of Iowa Institutional Review Board (IRB) approved specimen collection after obtaining informed consent under approval numbers 200311016 and 200803708.

Sources of Clinical Isolates: *University of Iowa Cystic Fibrosis Biobank*. 77 de-identified *S. aureus* clinical isolates were obtained from the University of Iowa Hospitals and Clinics clinical laboratory following CF clinic visits made between 12 December 2011 and 20 July 2012. Specimens were obtained from both adult and pediatric patients.

CF Biospecimen Registry (CFBR) at Emory and Children's Center for Cystic Fibrosis: 20 *S. aureus* isolates from people with CF were collected between 1 January 2012 and 31 December 2013. These human subject samples were provided by the CF Biospecimen Registry at the Children's Healthcare of Atlanta and Emory University CF Discovery Core courtesy of Arlene Stecenko. The Emory University IRB has approved collecting and banking of these specimens after obtaining informed consent.

The Geisel School of Medicine at Dartmouth University: The Hogan laboratory at the Geisel School of Medicine at Dartmouth University graciously provided 12 deidentified *S. aureus* isolates from the Dartmouth CF Translational Research Core. These isolates were obtained from adult patients with CF between 1 January 2015 and 31 December 2017 with support by the CF Foundation RDP grant STANTO15R0.

Bacterial Phenotypes: Clinical isolates of *S. aureus* were streaked onto tryptic soy agar (TSA) and blood agar to examine colony size, color, and hemolysis pattern. We streaked colonies onto milk agar to score for secreted protease. Beta-toxin was scored by partial lysis on sheep blood agar; alpha-toxin by complete lysis on rabbit blood agar. Oxacillin resistance was determined by growth on Mueller–Hinton agar with 4% NaCl in the presence or absence of 6 µg/mL oxacillin at 33–35 °C. We examined for chloramphenicol, tetracycline, or erythromycin resistance by presence or absence of growth with 10 µg/mL of each antibiotic.

Superantigen Testing: Clinical isolates of *S. aureus* were tested for the presence or absence of SAg genes using PCR of genomic DNA preparations following a published protocol with appropriate positive and negative controls for each of the SAgs [23]. PCR primers are listed in supplemental materials.

Statistical Analysis: We determined the prevalence of SAgs as the number of subjects positive for a given SAg divided by the total number of subjects analyzed. In subgroup analysis, we compared SAg prevalence in subjects with a single culture vs. those with multiple cultures using Fisher's exact test. We compared the proportions of MRSA and MSSA isolates that were positive for each of the SAgs using Fisher's exact test. To measure the strength of the association, we calculated an odds ratio to determine the increase in odds that the individual SAg would be present in MRSA compared to MSSA. Odds ratios were calculated using conditional maximum likelihood estimate with the fisher.test command in R. $P < 0.05$ was considered statistically significant. We did not adjust for multiple comparisons. To determine whether MRSA and MSSA have distinct complements of SAgs, we performed unsupervised hierarchical clustering of the University of Iowa Biobank isolates based on the presence of SAg genes. We used R Studio version 0.98.1085 or SAS version 9.4 for statistical testing.

3. Results

3.1. S. aureus Specimens From Patients With CF Are Heterogeneous in Phenotypic Appearance

We obtained 77 clinical isolates of *S. aureus* from adult and pediatric patients with CF at the University of Iowa. These specimens were obtained from $N = 45$ patients in visits between 12 December 2011 and 20 July 2012. The median age of these patients was 15.75 years as of the date of their last culture (IQR 8.34–26.89, range 5.27–58.66). Between 1 and 7 specimens were obtained per subject (Supplemental Figure S1), with 28 subjects having a single culture. 44 of these specimens were from sputum samples and 33 were from oropharyngeal swabs.

3.1.1. Colony Morphology

In chronic airway infections, CF pathogens like *Pseudomonas aeruginosa* diversify through genetic mutations [24]. However, if phenotypes are required for survival in the CF airway, these features may be found with increased frequency. Therefore, we examined the *S. aureus* isolates from patients with CF for colony phenotypes (Table 1). *S. aureus* normally expresses staphyloxanthin, a golden pigment that protects against host-derived oxidants [25]. We found that many isolates were hypopigmented: 13 were white, 37 were yellow, and 27 were gold.

Table 1. Phenotypes of *S. aureus* isolated from individuals with cystic fibrosis.

Characteristic	Number of Isolates (Total = 77)	%
Clinical Source		
Sputum	44	57.1%
Throat culture	33	42.9%
Antibiotic Resistance		
Oxacillin	28	36.4%
Chloramphenicol	0	0.0%
Tetracycline	12	15.6%
Erythromycin	75	97.4%
Hemolysis		
Complete, rabbit blood agar (α-toxin)	63	81.8%
Partial, sheep blood agar (β-toxin)	41	53.2%
Color		
White	13	16.9%
Yellow	37	48.1%
Gold	27	35.1%
Secreted Protease		
Not detected	41	53.2%
Faint	13	16.9%
Present	23	29.9%

Protease secretion is considered a virulence factor in skin infections [26], and protease production could be damaging to airways. Therefore, we tested for secreted protease by examining milk agar plates for zones of clearance. 23 of the isolates had distinct zones of clearance consistent with protease secretion, 13 had small or faint zones of clearance, and 41 isolates exhibited no clearance of milk agar in this assay. There was a strong correlation between hypopigmentation and protease activity. Protease activity, as determined by clearance of milk agar, was detected in 85% of white colonies but 7.5% of gold colonies ($P < 0.001$).

Another characteristic of *S. aureus* is hemolysis, a phenotype that is linked to alpha and beta hemolysin toxins. Previous studies of bacteria deficient in alpha toxin reveal its importance in cellular and animal models of CF [27,28]. We tested for the activity of these toxins by hemolysis patterns on sheep and rabbit blood agar plates. Alpha toxin (encoded by *hla*) activity was observed in the majority of specimens, whereas beta-toxin (*hlb*) activity was observed in 40% of specimens.

3.1.2. Antibiotic Resistance

CF pathogens are under selective pressure from antibiotic treatment. We determined MRSA status of these isolates by growth on Mueller–Hinton agar in the presence of 6 μg/mL of oxacillin. 28 isolates derived from 19 individuals were phenotypically resistant to oxacillin. 49 isolates from 30 individuals were methicillin-susceptible *S. aureus* (MSSA). Four subjects had isolates of both MRSA and MSSA. Because macrolides and tetracyclines are commonly prescribed to patients with CF [2], we hypothesized that the *S. aureus* isolates would be resistant to these antibiotic classes, but remain susceptible to antibiotics that are not routinely given. Each isolate was grown on TSA containing either erythromycin, tetracycline, or chloramphenicol. Chronic azithromycin is routinely prescribed at the University of Iowa CF center [8]. The vast majority of isolates from the University of Iowa (75/77) exhibited erythromycin resistance, but tetracycline resistance was less common (12/77). Within the University of Iowa collection, the two isolates susceptible to erythromycin were obtained as oropharyngeal cultures.

3.2. High Prevalence of Enterotoxin Gene Cluster Genes in S. aureus Isolated From Patients With Cystic Fibrosis

S. aureus encodes a variety of secreted toxins, including bacterial superantigens (SAgs). We hypothesized that there would be similar heterogeneity in *S. aureus* secreted toxins. Using previously described methods [23], we assessed for the presence of 18 unique SAgs. Among these toxins, the most common were genes belonging to the enterotoxin gene cluster (EGC), including *seg, sel-i, sel-m, sel-n, sel-o,* and *sel-u*. These genes were highly prevalent in isolates of *S. aureus* from patients with CF. All six EGC genes were identified in 37 of the 45 patients examined. 97.8% of patients within this cohort grew *S. aureus* that encoded at least one member of the EGC (Table 2). The genes encoding EGC toxins were significantly more prevalent in CF specimens compared to the classic *S. aureus* SAg toxic shock syndrome toxin-1(TSST-1; gene *tstH*), which was present in 11.7% of isolates.

Because some subjects within the University of Iowa cohort had multiple cultures, there may be greater opportunities to identify specific bacterial genes within these subjects. Therefore, we compared the prevalence of each toxin in subjects with multiple cultures vs. those with one culture. We identified *sea* and more frequently in patients with repeated cultures. Genes encoding EGC toxins were highly prevalent in both groups. We observed no statistically significant differences in age or culture source between groups.

3.2.1. EGC Prevalence in MRSA and MSSA

We hypothesized that the genes encoding secreted toxins may be associated with either methicillin susceptibility or resistance. To determine whether MRSA isolates had specific toxin signature(s), we performed hierarchical clustering based on the presence or absence of toxins (Figure 1). MRSA isolates were distributed widely in this analysis and often shared the same toxin profile as MSSA isolates. We separately tested whether individual toxins were associated with MRSA or MSSA (Table 3). None of the MRSA isolates were positive for *tstH*, consistent with previous observations that TSST-1 is generally associated with MSSA [29]. MSSA was more likely than MRSA to be positive for *sel-p* (P = 0.03). While *sel-p* and *tstH* were more common in MSSA, *sel-x* was more common in MRSA. However, no combination of SAgs was perfectly predictive of methicillin resistance, and genes encoding EGC toxins were prevalent in both MSSA and MRSA isolates.

Table 2. Prevalence of *S. aureus* superantigen genes detected from individuals with cystic fibrosis.

Toxin	Iowa Subjects with CF Total = 45		Single Culture Total = 28		Multiple Cultures Total = 17		P[†]
	N	%	N	%	N	%	
sea	19	42.2%	8	28.6%	11	64.7%	0.03
seb	2	4.4%	1	3.6%	1	5.9%	1.00
sec	4	8.9%	2	7.1%	2	11.8%	0.63
sed	6	13.3%	2	7.1%	4	23.5%	0.18
see	3	6.7%	0	0.0%	3	17.6%	0.05
seg	42	93.3%	25	89.3%	17	100.0%	0.28
sel-h	0	0.0%	0	0.0%	0	0.0%	-
sel-i	42	93.3%	25	89.3%	17	100.0%	0.28
sel-k	4	8.9%	2	7.1%	2	11.8%	0.63
sel-l	3	6.7%	1	3.6%	2	11.8%	0.55
sel-m	39	86.7%	23	82.1%	16	94.1%	0.38
sel-n	41	91.1%	25	89.3%	16	94.1%	1.00
sel-o	43	95.6%	26	92.9%	17	100.0%	0.52
sel-p	30	66.7%	15	53.6%	15	88.2%	0.02
sel-q	15	33.3%	8	28.6%	7	41.2%	0.52
sel-u	41	91.1%	24	85.7%	17	100.0%	0.28
sel-x	39	86.7%	23	82.1%	16	94.1%	0.38
tstH	8	17.8%	3	10.7%	5	29.4%	0.23
≥1 of *egc*	44	97.8%	27	96.4%	17	100.0%	1.00
6 of *egc*	37	82.2%	21	75.0%	16	94.1%	0.13

[†]P values compare subjects with single culture to subjects with multiple cultures using Fisher's exact test. Bold font indicates genes belonging to the enterotoxin gene cluster.

Table 3. Association of *S. aureus* toxin genes with methicillin susceptibility or resistance.

Toxin	S. aureus Total = 77		MSSA Total = 49		MRSA Total = 28		OR *	P[†]
	N	%	N	%	N	%		
sea	25	32.5%	17	34.7%	8	28.6%	0.76	0.62
seb	3	3.9%	3	6.1%	0	0.0%	-	0.30
sec	5	6.5%	5	10.2%	0	0.0%	-	0.15
sed	8	10.4%	3	6.1%	5	17.9%	3.28	0.13
see	5	6.5%	4	8.2%	1	3.6%	0.42	0.65
seg	69	89.6%	45	91.8%	24	85.7%	0.54	0.45
sel-h	0	0.0%	0	0.0%	0	0.0%	-	-
sel-i	69	89.6%	44	89.8%	25	89.3%	0.95	1.00
sel-k	5	6.5%	3	6.1%	2	7.1%	1.18	1.00
sel-l	3	3.9%	3	6.1%	0	0.0%	-	0.30
sel-m	67	87.0%	42	85.7%	25	89.3%	1.38	0.74
sel-n	68	88.3%	43	87.8%	25	89.3%	1.16	1.00
sel-o	71	92.2%	46	93.9%	25	89.3%	0.55	0.66
sel-p	46	59.7%	34	69.4%	12	42.9%	0.34	0.03
sel-q	17	22.1%	11	22.4%	6	21.4%	0.94	1.00
sel-u	69	89.6%	45	91.8%	24	85.7%	0.54	0.45
sel-x	61	79.2%	33	67.3%	28	100.0%	-	0.0003
tstH	9	11.7%	9	18.4%	0	0.0%	-	0.02
hla	63	81.8%	37	75.5%	26	92.9%	4.15	0.07
hlb	41	53.2%	19	38.8%	22	78.6%	5.65	0.001

* OR = Odds ratio, values > 1 indicate increased odds of the toxin being encoded in MRSA versus methicillin-susceptible *S. aureus* (MSSA). [†]P values calculated by Fisher's exact test. Bold font indicates genes belonging to the enterotoxin gene cluster.

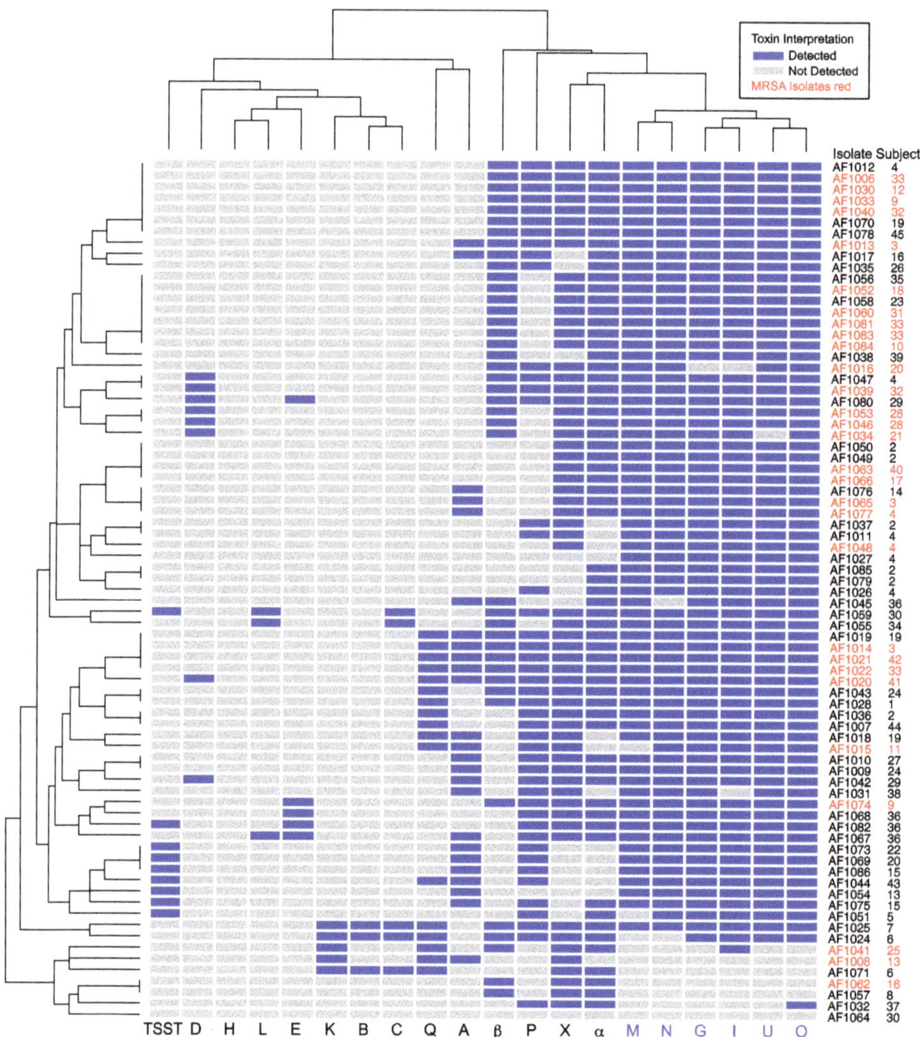

Figure 1. Unsupervised hierarchical clustering of cystic fibrosis (CF) clinical isolates based on presence of *S. aureus* toxin genes. Isolate numbers and subjects are indicated at right. Toxin genes are on the bottom margin, with members of the enterotoxin gene cluster (EGC) in blue. Letters A, B, C, D, E, and G are staphylococcal enterotoxin (SE) superantigens characterized as causing emesis after oral administration. Letters H, I, K, L, M–Q, and X are SE-like superantigens. TSST is toxic shock syndrome toxin-1 superantigen. α and β are cytotoxins. Blue shading represents toxin presence. MRSA isolates are indicated with red font. Dendrograms at left and top show relatedness of the isolates and toxins, respectively. The EGC was prevalent in both MRSA and MSSA isolates.

3.2.2. EGC Prevalence in *S. aureus* From Other U.S. CF Centers

We considered the possibility that the high prevalence of *S. aureus* encoding EGC was due to geographic sampling. To address this possibility, we obtained 12 *S. aureus* isolates from adults with CF at Dartmouth University and 20 *S. aureus* isolates from Emory University. We genotyped these isolates for the same set of toxins (Table 4). Notably, there were no significant differences between isolates obtained in Iowa compared to Dartmouth or Emory, suggesting that the high prevalence of the EGC is not related to geographic sampling of one region of the United States.

Table 4. *S. aureus* toxin genes identified in CF clinical isolates from geographically separate regions. Bold font indicates genes belonging to the enterotoxin gene cluster.

Toxin	Iowa Total = 77		Emory Total = 20		Dartmouth Total = 12	
	N	**%**	**N**	**%**	**N**	**%**
sea	25	32.5%	0	0.0%	2	16.7%
seb	3	3.9%	0	0.0%	0	0.0%
sec	5	6.5%	1	5.0%	0	0.0%
sed	8	10.4%	3	15.0%	0	0.0%
see	5	6.5%	4	20.0%	0	0.0%
seg	**69**	**89.6%**	**16**	**80.0%**	**10**	**83.3%**
sel-h	0	0.0%	0	0.0%	0	0.0%
sel-i	**69**	**89.6%**	**16**	**80.0%**	**10**	**83.3%**
sel-k	5	6.5%	1	5.0%	2	16.7%
sel-l	3	3.9%	1	5.0%	0	0.0%
sel-m	**67**	**87.0%**	**15**	**75.0%**	**9**	**75.0%**
sel-n	**68**	**88.3%**	**16**	**80.0%**	**10**	**83.3%**
sel-o	**71**	**92.2%**	**15**	**75.0%**	**9**	**75.0%**
sel-p	46	59.7%	5	25.0%	0	0.0%
sel-q	17	22.1%	2	10.0%	2	16.7%
sel-u	**69**	**89.6%**	**16**	**80.0%**	**10**	**83.3%**
sel-x	61	79.2%	19	95.0%	11	91.7%
tstH	9	11.7%	1	5.0%	2	16.7%

4. Discussion

S. aureus isolates from patients with CF displayed heterogeneity of color and protease secretion. However, the majority of these diverse *S. aureus* isolates encoded the EGC. The heterogeneity of *S. aureus* colony phenotypes suggests that putative virulence factors such as staphyloxanthin and protease may not be under strong selective pressure to remain in the CF airway. By contrast, alpha-toxin mediated hemolysis was routinely observed. Chronic antibiotic exposure represents a strong selective pressure; most of the isolates from the University of Iowa were resistant to erythromycin. The high prevalence of EGC toxins suggests that *S. aureus* is under pressure to maintain these genes during infection of the CF airway.

We considered the possibility that high prevalence of EGC was related to geographic exposure. Using three geographically distinct collections of *S. aureus* isolated from U.S. patients with cystic fibrosis, we found that EGC toxins had similarly high prevalence. This is similar to a recent study of *S. aureus* isolates from Europe patients with CF, in which EGC toxins were present in ≈57% of isolates [19]. The EGC prevalence within this U.S. collection is even higher, suggesting the continued emergence of strains encoding this locus, possibly through the spread of one or more clones. *S. aureus* clonality is common in CF. In the European study, 5 *spa* types accounted for 25.6% of all *S. aureus* isolates. However, EGC-positive *S. aureus* isolates were not limited to a single clonal group [19].

Most of the CF isolates in the current study were obtained in 2011 and 2012, a time period similar to when specimens were collected for a study of atopic dermatitis that used the same genotyping methodology [21]. We compared the prevalence of each of the SAgs in CF versus atopic dermatitis. All of the SAgs belonging to the EGC (*seg*, *sel-i*, *sel-m*, *sel-n*, *sel-o*, and *sel-u*) were significantly more prevalent in CF as compared to atopic dermatitis collection. Among subjects with atopic dermatitis, three distinct genotypes of *S. aureus* were apparent. The first of these *S. aureus* genotypes, which nearly always encoded all EGC toxins, appears highly similar to the prevailing *S. aureus* within the CF population. Longitudinal studies are needed to determine whether or not the EGC associates with persistence of *S. aureus* in diseases like CF and atopic dermatitis.

In comparing the prevalence of the EGC in these CF isolates to *S. aureus* isolates derived from other anatomic sites, we find that CF has a uniquely high prevalence for this group of SAg toxins. The EGC is more prevalent in CF than in atopic dermatitis, diabetic foot ulcer, and significantly more prevalent than in vaginal mucosa [30] and in patients with menstrual toxic shock syndrome (TSS) [12]. The enrichment of EGC-positive isolates in these CF airway isolates suggests that the EGC may confer selective advantage for *S. aureus* strains in adapting to its role as a chronic pathogen in the airway. Typically, members of the EGC are considered colonization SAgs, due to low-level production [31].

In striking contrast to the CF, *S. aureus* isolated from acute inflammatory infections such as TSS and post-influenza necrotizing pneumonia have very high prevalence of *tstH* and produce SAgs in higher concentration [12,18]. We observed that a minority of CF clinical isolates encode *tstH*; it is unknown what effect this SAg may have on progression of CF lung disease.

It is unclear whether patients with CF develop intact immune responses to *S. aureus* [32,33]. Compared to *P. aeruginosa*, patients with CF may have attenuated antibody production [33]. We hypothesize that this could be a consequence of immune misdirection by *S. aureus* SAgs. Moreover, these SAgs could facilitate increased inflammation, an important factor in CF disease progression. Future studies should examine the immune response to these prevalent *S. aureus* SAgs.

S. aureus SAgs represent a possible target for vaccination. Given the high prevalence of EGC SAgs in CF, future attempts at immunizing patients with CF against *S. aureus* may use these antigens as vaccine targets. Notably, a recent study has shown that immunization of rabbits against the SAgs TSST-1 and SEC, and the cytotoxin α-toxin protected 87/88 animals after intra-pulmonary challenge [34]. This vaccination strategy depended on formation of cross-protective neutralizing antibodies. For example, antibodies raised against SEC protect against both SEB and the EGC SAg SEl-U. That study also suggested that vaccination against toxoids may be a more effective strategy than vaccination against cell surface *S. aureus* virulence factors. In keeping with this notion, a group has recently performed a first-in-humans vaccine trial against the TSST-1 toxoid [35].

4.1. Advantages

This study establishes that enterotoxin gene cluster members are highly prevalent in *S. aureus* isolates in American patients with CF, independent of methicillin resistance. Because we used consistent methodology for genotyping, we can compare respiratory isolates of *S. aureus* from patients with CF to cutaneous isolates from patients with atopic dermatitis that were obtained at a similar time. This comparison reveals that genes encoding EGC toxins are enriched in respiratory isolates. We have also confirmed the high prevalence of EGC toxins using *S. aureus* isolates from geographically distinct CF centers.

4.2. Limitations

Because these data are cross-sectional, it is unknown how long these strains have been present in the CF airway. Many of these patients were sputum-producing. Thus, these infections may represent chronic infection rather than initial infection. We are unable to correlate the presence or absence of secreted toxins with pulmonary outcomes such as FEV_1, since the specimens are de-identified. Although many strains encode secreted toxins, we cannot determine whether these genes are actively expressed in the CF airway. Because of de-identification, we are also unable to determine whether there is adaptive host response to presence or absence of these toxins. We intend to address these limitations in future studies with a larger number of fully identified specimens.

5. Conclusions

S. aureus remains a prevalent pathogen in CF. Improvements in the prevention and treatment of *S. aureus* infection remain a major goal in this disease. This study reveals the SAg ECG gene cluster is highly prevalent in *S. aureus* CF isolates, revealing a potential vaccination target for this organism in CF.

Supplementary Materials: The following are available online at http://www.mdpi.com/2073-4425/10/12/1036/s1, Supplemental Methods: Genotyping assay. Figure S1: Frequency of repeated cultures within University of Iowa Biobank.

Author Contributions: Conceptualization, A.J.F. and P.M.S.; methodology, A.J.F., S.H.K., S.B.S., D.H.L., P.D.A., A.R.H.; formal analysis, A.J.F., S.H.K., D.H.L., P.M.S.; resources, S.B.S. and D.H.L.; data curation, A.J.F., S.H.K., S.B.S., P.M.S.; writing—original draft preparation, A.J.F.; writing—review and editing, A.J.F., D.H.L., S.B.S., P.M.S.; visualization, A.J.F.; supervision, A.J.F., P.M.S.; project administration, A.J.F. and P.M.S.; funding acquisition, A.J.F. and P.M.S.

Funding: A.J.F. was supported in part by the University of Iowa Department of Pediatrics, the Cystic Fibrosis Foundation CFF FISCHE16I0, and NHLBI K08 HL136927. S.H.K. and P.M.S. were supported by University of Iowa start-up funds. D.H.L. is supported by CFF Post-doc to Faculty Transition Award LIMOLI18F5 and University of Iowa start-up funds.

Acknowledgments: We acknowledge Timothy Starner for assistance with University of Iowa CF Biobank isolates, Arlene Stecenko for assistance with Emory University isolates, and Deborah Hogan and Alex Crocker for assistance with Dartmouth isolates.

Conflicts of Interest: P.M.S. has received patent protection regarding *S. aureus* secreted toxins, including methods to induce immune response to *S. aureus* with novel toxoids. The remaining authors have no financial conflicts of interest. The funders of this study had no role in the design of the study; in the collection, analyses, or interpretation of data; in the writing of the manuscript, or in the decision to publish the results.

References

1. Salsgiver, E.L.; Fink, A.K.; Knapp, E.A.; LiPuma, J.J.; Olivier, K.N.; Marshall, B.C.; Saiman, L. Changing epidemiology of the respiratory bacteriology of patients with cystic fibrosis. *Chest* **2016**, *149*, 390–400. [CrossRef] [PubMed]

2. Cystic Fibrosis Foundation 2016 Patient Registry Annual Data Report. 2017. Available online: https://www.cff.org/research/researcher-resources/patient-registry/2016-patient-registry-annual-data-report.pdf (accessed on 4 November 2019).

3. Ramsey, B.W.; Pepe, M.S.; Quan, J.M.; Otto, K.L.; Montgomery, A.B.; Williams-Warren, J.; Vasiljev, K.M.; Borowitz, D.; Bowman, C.M.; Marshall, B.C.; et al. Intermittent administration of inhaled tobramycin in patients with cystic fibrosis. Cystic fibrosis inhaled tobramycin study group. *N. Engl. J. Med.* **1999**, *340*, 23–30. [CrossRef] [PubMed]

4. Gibson, R.L.; Emerson, J.; McNamara, S.; Burns, J.L.; Rosenfeld, M.; Yunker, A.; Hamblett, N.; Accurso, F.; Dovey, M.; Hiatt, P.; et al. Significant microbiological effect of inhaled tobramycin in young children with cystic fibrosis. *Am. J. Respir. Crit. Care Med.* **2003**, *167*, 841–849. [CrossRef] [PubMed]

5. Tiddens, H.A.; De Boeck, K.; Clancy, J.P.; Fayon, M.; Arets, H.G.M.; Bresnik, M.; Derchak, A.; Lewis, S.A.; Oermann, C.M. Open label study of inhaled aztreonam for *Pseudomonas* eradication in children with cystic fibrosis: The alpine study. *J. Cyst. Fibros.* **2015**, *14*, 111–119. [CrossRef]

6. Dezube, R.; Jennings, M.T.; Rykiel, M.; Diener-West, M.; Boyle, M.P.; Chmiel, J.F.; Dasenbrook, E.C. Eradication of persistent methicillin-resistant *Staphylococcus aureus* infection in cystic fibrosis. *J. Cyst. Fibros.* **2018**. [CrossRef]

7. Heltshe, S.L.; Mayer-Hamblett, N.; Burns, J.L.; Khan, U.; Baines, A.; Ramsey, B.W.; Rowe, S.M. *Pseudomonas aeruginosa* in cystic fibrosis patients with G551D-CFTR treated with ivacaftor. *Clin. Infect. Dis.* **2015**, *60*, 703–712. [CrossRef]

8. Singh, S.B.; McLearn-Montz, A.J.; Milavetz, F.; Gates, L.K.; Fox, C.; Murry, L.T.; Sabus, A.; Porterfield, H.S.; Fischer, A.J. Pathogen acquisition in patients with cystic fibrosis receiving ivacaftor or lumacaftor/ivacaftor. *Pediatr. Pulmonol.* **2019**. [CrossRef]

9. Caudri, D.; Turkovic, L.; Ng, J.; de Klerk, N.H.; Rosenow, T.; Hall, G.L.; Ranganathan, S.C.; Sly, P.D.; Stick, S.M. The association between *Staphylococcus aureus* and subsequent bronchiectasis in children with cystic fibrosis. *J. Cyst. Fibros.* **2018**, *17*, 462–469. [CrossRef]

10. Dasenbrook, E.C.; Merlo, C.A.; Diener-West, M.; Lechtzin, N.; Boyle, M.P. Persistent methicillin-resistant *Staphylococcus aureus* and rate of FEV$_1$ decline in cystic fibrosis. *Am. J. Respir. Crit. Care Med.* **2008**, *178*, 814–821. [CrossRef]

11. Dinges, M.M.; Orwin, P.M.; Schlievert, P.M. Exotoxins of *Staphylococcus aureus*. *Clin. Microbiol. Rev.* **2000**, *13*, 16–34. [CrossRef]

12. Spaulding, A.R.; Salgado-Pabon, W.; Kohler, P.L.; Horswill, A.R.; Leung, D.Y.; Schlievert, P.M. Staphylococcal and streptococcal superantigen exotoxins. *Clin. Microbiol. Rev.* **2013**, *26*, 422–447. [CrossRef] [PubMed]

13. McCormick, J.K.; Yarwood, J.M.; Schlievert, P.M. Toxic shock syndrome and bacterial superantigens: An update. *Annu. Rev. Microbiol.* **2001**, *55*, 77–104. [CrossRef] [PubMed]

14. Jarraud, S.; Peyrat, M.A.; Lim, A.; Tristan, A.; Bes, M.; Mougel, C.; Etienne, J.; Vandenesch, F.; Bonneville, M.; Lina, G. *egc*, a highly prevalent operon of enterotoxin gene, forms a putative nursery of superantigens in *Staphylococcus aureus*. *J. Immunol.* **2001**, *166*, 669–677. [CrossRef] [PubMed]

15. Becker, K.; Friedrich, A.W.; Peters, G.; von Eiff, C. Systematic survey on the prevalence of genes coding for staphylococcal enterotoxins SELM, SELO, and SELN. *Mol. Nutr. Food Res.* **2004**, *48*, 488–495. [CrossRef] [PubMed]

16. Grumann, D.; Scharf, S.S.; Holtfreter, S.; Kohler, C.; Steil, L.; Engelmann, S.; Hecker, M.; Volker, U.; Broker, B.M. Immune cell activation by enterotoxin gene cluster (*egc*)-encoded and non-*egc* superantigens from *Staphylococcus aureus*. *J. Immunol.* **2008**, *181*, 5054–5061. [CrossRef]

17. Holtfreter, S.; Bauer, K.; Thomas, D.; Feig, C.; Lorenz, V.; Roschack, K.; Friebe, E.; Selleng, K.; Lovenich, S.; Greve, T.; et al. *egc*-Encoded superantigens from *Staphylococcus aureus* are neutralized by human sera much less efficiently than are classical staphylococcal enterotoxins or toxic shock syndrome toxin. *Infect. Immun.* **2004**, *72*, 4061–4071. [CrossRef]

18. Stach, C.S.; Vu, B.G.; Merriman, J.A.; Herrera, A.; Cahill, M.P.; Schlievert, P.M.; Salgado-Pabon, W. Novel tissue level effects of the *Staphylococcus aureus* enterotoxin gene cluster are essential for infective endocarditis. *PLoS ONE* **2016**, *11*, e0154762. [CrossRef]

19. Garbacz, K.; Piechowicz, L.; Podkowik, M.; Mroczkowska, A.; Empel, J.; Bania, J. Emergence and spread of worldwide *Staphylococcus aureus* clones among cystic fibrosis patients. *Infect. Drug Res.* **2018**, *11*, 247–255. [CrossRef]

20. Mempel, M.; Lina, G.; Hojka, M.; Schnopp, C.; Seidl, H.P.; Schafer, T.; Ring, J.; Vandenesch, F.; Abeck, D. High prevalence of superantigens associated with the *egc* locus in *Staphylococcus aureus* isolates from patients with atopic eczema. *Eur. J. Clin. Microbiol. Infect. Dis.* **2003**, *22*, 306–309. [CrossRef]

21. Merriman, J.A.; Mueller, E.A.; Cahill, M.P.; Beck, L.A.; Paller, A.S.; Hanifin, J.M.; Ong, P.Y.; Schneider, L.; Babineau, D.C.; David, G.; et al. Temporal and racial differences associated with atopic dermatitis *Staphylococcus aureus* and encoded virulence factors. *mSphere* **2016**, *1*. [CrossRef]

22. Dasenbrook, E.C.; Checkley, W.; Merlo, C.A.; Konstan, M.W.; Lechtzin, N.; Boyle, M.P. Association between respiratory tract methicillin-resistant *Staphylococcus aureus* and survival in cystic fibrosis. *JAMA J. Am. Med. Assoc.* **2010**, *303*, 2386–2392. [CrossRef] [PubMed]

23. Salgado-Pabon, W.; Case-Cook, L.C.; Schlievert, P.M. Molecular analysis of staphylococcal superantigens. *Methods Mol. Biol.* **2014**, *1085*, 169–185. [CrossRef] [PubMed]

24. Smith, E.E.; Buckley, D.G.; Wu, Z.; Saenphimmachak, C.; Hoffman, L.R.; D'Argenio, D.A.; Miller, S.I.; Ramsey, B.W.; Speert, D.P.; Moskowitz, S.M.; et al. Genetic adaptation by *Pseudomonas aeruginosa* to the airways of cystic fibrosis patients. *Proc. Natl. Acad. Sci. USA* **2006**, *103*, 8487–8492. [CrossRef] [PubMed]

25. Clauditz, A.; Resch, A.; Wieland, K.P.; Peschel, A.; Gotz, F. Staphyloxanthin plays a role in the fitness of *Staphylococcus aureus* and its ability to cope with oxidative stress. *Infect. Immun.* **2006**, *74*, 4950–4953. [CrossRef]

26. Kolar, S.L.; Ibarra, J.A.; Rivera, F.E.; Mootz, J.M.; Davenport, J.E.; Stevens, S.M.; Horswill, A.R.; Shaw, L.N. Extracellular proteases are key mediators of *Staphylococcus aureus* virulence via the global modulation of virulence-determinant stability. *MicrobiologyOpen* **2013**, *2*, 18–34. [CrossRef]

27. Jarry, T.M.; Memmi, G.; Cheung, A.L. The expression of alpha-haemolysin is required for *Staphylococcus aureus* phagosomal escape after internalization in CFT-1 cells. *Cell. Microbiol.* **2008**, *10*, 1801–1814. [CrossRef]

28. Keitsch, S.; Riethmuller, J.; Soddemann, M.; Sehl, C.; Wilker, B.; Edwards, M.J.; Caldwell, C.C.; Fraunholz, M.; Gulbins, E.; Becker, K.A. Pulmonary infection of cystic fibrosis mice with *Staphylococcus aureus* requires expression of alpha-toxin. *Biol. Chem.* **2018**, *399*, 1203–1213. [CrossRef]

29. Schlievert, P.M.; Strandberg, K.L.; Lin, Y.C.; Peterson, M.L.; Leung, D.Y. Secreted virulence factor comparison between methicillin-resistant and methicillin-sensitive *Staphylococcus aureus*, and its relevance to atopic dermatitis. *J. Allergy Clin. Immunol.* **2010**, *125*, 39–49. [CrossRef]

30. Vu, B.G.; Stach, C.S.; Salgado-Pabon, W.; Diekema, D.J.; Gardner, S.E.; Schlievert, P.M. Superantigens of *Staphylococcus aureus* from patients with diabetic foot ulcers. *J. Infect. Dis.* **2014**, *210*, 1920–1927. [CrossRef]

31. Roetzer, A.; Gruener, C.S.; Haller, G.; Beyerly, J.; Model, N.; Eibl, M.M. Enterotoxin gene cluster-encoded *sei* and *seln* from *Staphylococcus aureus* isolates are crucial for the induction of human blood cell proliferation and pathogenicity in rabbits. *Toxins* **2016**, *8*, 314. [CrossRef]

32. Hollsing, A.E.; Granstrom, M.; Strandvik, B. Prospective study of serum staphylococcal antibodies in cystic fibrosis. *Arch. Dis. Child.* **1987**, *62*, 905–911. [CrossRef] [PubMed]

33. Moss, R.B.; Hsu, Y.P.; Lewiston, N.J. ^{125}I-Clq-binding and specific antibodies as indicators of pulmonary disease activity in cystic fibrosis. *J. Pediatr.* **1981**, *99*, 215–222. [CrossRef]

34. Spaulding, A.R.; Salgado-Pabon, W.; Merriman, J.A.; Stach, C.S.; Ji, Y.; Gillman, A.N.; Peterson, M.L.; Schlievert, P.M. Vaccination against *Staphylococcus aureus* pneumonia. *J. Infect. Dis.* **2014**, *209*, 1955–1962. [CrossRef] [PubMed]

35. Roetzer, A.; Jilma, B.; Eibl, M.M. Vaccine against toxic shock syndrome in a first-in-man clinical trial. *Expert Rev. Vaccines* **2017**, *16*, 81–83. [CrossRef]

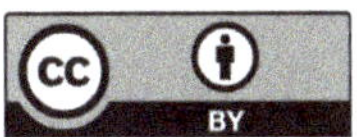

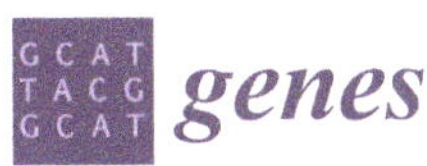 *genes*

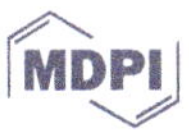

Review

Molecular Diagnosis and Genetic Counseling of Cystic Fibrosis and Related Disorders: New Challenges

Thierry Bienvenu, Maureen Lopez and Emmanuelle Girodon *

Molecular Genetics Laboratory, Cochin Hospital, APHP.Centre–Université de Paris, 75014 Paris, France; thierry.bienvenu@inserm.fr (T.B.); maureen.lopez@aphp.fr (M.L.)
* Correspondence: emmanuelle.girodon@aphp.fr; Tel.: +33-015-841-1924

Received: 9 May 2020; Accepted: 2 June 2020; Published: 4 June 2020

Abstract: Identification of the cystic fibrosis transmembrane conductance regulator *(CFTR)* gene and its numerous variants opened the way to fantastic breakthroughs in diagnosis, research and treatment of cystic fibrosis (CF). The current and future challenges of molecular diagnosis of CF and CFTR-related disorders and of genetic counseling are here reviewed. Technological advances have enabled to make a diagnosis of CF with a sensitivity of 99% by using next generation sequencing in a single step. The detection of heretofore unidentified variants and ethnic-specific variants remains challenging, especially for newborn screening (NBS), CF carrier testing and genotype-guided therapy. Among the criteria for assessing the impact of variants, population genetics data are insufficiently taken into account and the penetrance of CF associated with *CFTR* variants remains poorly known. The huge diversity of diagnostic and genetic counseling indications for *CFTR* studies makes assessment of variant disease-liability critical. This is especially discussed in the perspective of wide genome analyses for NBS and CF carrier screening in the general population, as future challenges.

Keywords: cystic fibrosis; CFTR; CFTR-related disorders; molecular diagnosis; CFTR variants; Next Generation Sequencing (NGS); disease liability; interpretation; penetrance; genotype-guided therapy

1. Introduction

Cystic fibrosis (CF) is one of the most frequent life-limiting autosomal recessive diseases, characterized in its classical form by chronic pulmonary obstruction and infections, pancreatic insufficiency, male infertility, sweat chloride concentrations ≥60 mmol/L and two loss-of-function variants in the cystic fibrosis transmembrane conductance regulator *(CFTR)* gene (NM_000492.4; LRG_663t1) [1]. With the implementation of newborn screening (NBS) for CF, an increasing number of diagnoses are now made in asymptomatic patients. *CFTR* variants have diverse effects on expression and function of the CFTR protein, which principally acts as an ATP-gated chloride channel. Its absence or dysfunction leads to ion flux perturbations in the epithelial cells of various organs involved in CF [2].

Since the discovery of the *CFTR* gene more than thirty years ago, considerable scientific advances have made CF a model in terms of comprehensive knowledge of a genetic disease, molecular diagnosis, genetic counseling and personalized medicine. Technical milestones have led to identify a huge number of *CFTR* gene variants and a variety of molecular mechanisms responsible for CF [3], which contribute to the wide phenotype variability, and to achieve one of the highest sensitivities in the diagnosis of a hereditary disease, more than 99% of CF-causing variants being identified in newborns with CF [4]. The advent of next generation sequencing (NGS)-based technologies has deeply modified laboratory's practice, improved genotyping coverage and questioned screening policy. Specific molecular tools have also been developed for preimplantation genetic diagnosis [5] and non-invasive prenatal diagnosis of CF [6]. Other clinical entities related to *CFTR* variants have been described since the early 90s, with a continuum of CFTR dysfunction, from CFTR-related disorders (CFTR-RD), which are defined by evidence of CFTR dysfunction but do not meet the criteria for a CF diagnosis [7], to a number of conditions associated with a higher proportion of CF carriers compared to the general population, such as asthma or bronchopulmonary allergic aspergillosis [8]. Very recently, Miller et al. reported an increased risk for 57 CF-related symptoms in CF carriers in a study that questions the relevance of detecting CF carriers for preventive care [9]. CFTR-RDs principally include isolated male infertility by congenital bilateral absence of the vas deferens, idiopathic pancreatitis, disseminated bronchiectasis and chronic rhinosinusitis. The contribution of *CFTR* variants however varies from one condition to another, and may act in a multifactorial context, with other genes being potentially involved, such as *ADGRG2* in male infertility by the absence of vas deferens [10] or *PRSS1*, *SPINK1* and *CTRC* in pancreatitis [11]. There is thus a huge diversity of diagnostic and genetic counseling indications for searching *CFTR* variants, and appropriate tools should be used to answer clinical questions [1,12,13]. A great challenge in 2020 remains to accurately assess the disease liability of *CFTR* variants in the appropriate clinical context and to determine whether a variant should be reported as disease-causing, whether a genotype is compatible with the phenotype or which phenotype is compatible with the genotype identified in the context of NBS for CF, and whether a variant should be considered for genetic counseling purposes. The availability of genotype-guided therapy has also brought a renewed interest in deciphering the impact of *CFTR* variants.

In the present article, we review the current and future challenges of molecular diagnosis and genetic counseling. Despite a very high sensitivity of molecular tools, characterization of heretofore unidentified disease-causing variants in patients remains a technical challenge. We will also focus on ethnic-specific variants, the detection of which being challenging for NBS, CF carrier testing and genotype-guided therapy. We will then emphasize on the importance to consider population genetics and penetrance data in the process to evaluate the impact of variants. These data will eventually be discussed in the perspective of implementation of wide genome analyses for NBS and preconception CF carrier screening in the general population in an increasing number of countries.

2. Molecular Diagnosis

The following section reviews the process to achieve a molecular diagnosis of CF or CFTR-RD, by using a panel of tools in successive stages and also covers the indications of prenatal diagnosis and carrier testing.

2.1. Molecular Diagnosis of CF and CFTR-RD

A CF diagnosis is suggested by characteristic symptoms, a family history of CF (most often in a sibling) or a positive CF NBS result and is confirmed by evidence of CFTR dysfunction, most often by abnormal sweat chloride test results or by identification of two CF-causing alleles, one on each parental gene [1]. Diagnostic algorithms also include other CFTR functional investigations such as trans-epithelial nasal potential difference measurement or intestinal current measurement on rectal biopsies [1]. The diagnosis of CFTR-RD is established in the event of symptoms suggestive for CFTR dysfunction but when the biological criteria for CF are not met. These clinical entities essentially include monosymptomatic disorders in adults but the distinction between a mild CF and a CFTR-RD with multiorgan involvement may be artificial. Despite limitations, as for all tests, and the number of inconclusive situations, *CFTR* genetic analysis is a cornerstone for the diagnosis of CF and CFTR-RD. In adult patients having a monosymptomatic disease suggestive of a CFTR-RD, the proportion of homozygotes or compound heterozygotes is lower than in CF patients. It was shown to be as high as 82% in male infertility by absence of vas deferens [14] but low in other entities [7], e.g., 6.3% in aquagenic palmoplantar keratoderma [15]. Diagnostic sensitivies also vary between studies, depending on inclusion criteria and investigations for other causes, such as for disseminated bronchiectasis or pancreatitis. Provision of clinical and biological information prior to *CFTR* testing is thus essential to ensure that appropriate studies are carried out and that accurate interpretation is given.

More than 2000 *CFTR* variants have been reported to the Cystic Fibrosis Mutation Database [16], identified in patients with CF, a CFTR-RD or various other clinical presentations and in healthy individuals. Beside frequent variants that account for 50%–90% CF alleles worldwide, the majority of *CFTR* variants are as rare as to be called "private", as they are only present in individual families, or could be specific of an ethnic population. *CFTR* variants have been classified into five categories according to their clinical consequence: CF-causing variants, which are responsible for CF when combined in *trans* with a known CF-causing variant; CFTR-RD-causing variants, which are observed in patients with a CFTR-RD when combined in *trans* with a CF-causing variant; variants of varying clinical consequences (VVCC), which are reported as well in CF patients as in patients with a CFTR-RD when in *trans* with a CF-causing variant; variants of unproven or uncertain clinical significance (VUS) and variants with no clinical consequences [12]. Molecular diagnosis of CF and CFTR-RD is thus challenging especially due to the high heterogeneity of variants and genotypes and the difficulty to accurately evaluate their impact.

2.2. Tools and Strategies Used for the Molecular Diagnosis of CF and CFTR-RD

Robust strategies and cutting-edge methods have been steadily developed to identify *CFTR* variants, to study their impact and to predict their pathogenicity. A diagnosis may be achieved in three successive molecular steps, the implementation of which depending on the results of each previous step (Figure 1). The first step still often starts with the detection of the most frequent disease-causing variants using different commercially available kits, very often CE-marked for in vitro diagnosis. The sensitivity of variant panels greatly varies according to geographic/ethnic origins. For example, the sensitivity (or variant detection rate) of the Elucigene® CF-EU2v1 kit (Elucigene®, Delta Diagnostics, Manchester, UK) targeting 51 *CFTR* variants, varies from 93% in Ireland [17] to 49% in Turkey [18]. Whenever necessary, according to various strategies depending on the clinical situations and to national algorithms for CF NBS, which mostly include a prior step of sweat testing, rare variants are then searched by Sanger sequencing or NGS analysis of the 27 coding regions of the *CFTR* gene, targeted intronic regions containing known deep-intronic disease-causing variants, and part of the promoter. The NGS-based approach enables the simultaneous detection of single nucleotide variants and large deletions or duplications encompassing one or several exons [19]. For practical, organizational and economic reasons, some laboratories have now applied NGS as the single technique in their routine practice, possibly in two steps, as implemented in a few CF NBS programs, notably considering multi-ethnic populations [20]. Variant detection rate of this comprehensive step proved to be as high as 99% in CF newborns [4].

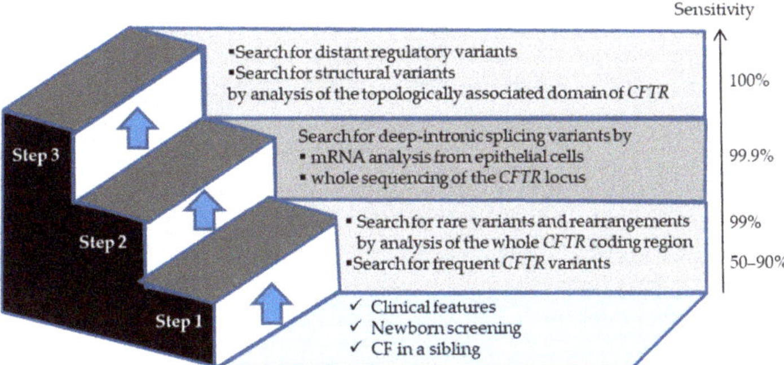

Figure 1. Molecular investigation for the diagnosis of cystic fibrosis (CF) and cystic fibrosis transmembrane conductance regulator related disorders (CFTR-RD) in three steps. Sensitivity refers to variant detection rate in patients with CF.

The second step concerns about 2% of patients with a high clinical suspicion of CF who carry only one CF-causing variant, and theoretically 0.01% of CF patients who carry no CF-causing variant. It is focused on the identification of rare or unknown deep-intronic variants, which may affect the structure, the size and/or the sequence of the *CFTR* messenger RNA (mRNA). This can be done either by studying *CFTR* mRNA of patients' epithelial cells, which are easily obtained by nasal brushing [21,22], or by analyzing the whole *CFTR* locus by NGS [23,24]. The disadvantages of mRNA studies are the requirement of another sample from a specific tissue and the instability of abnormal transcripts containing stop codons, which may thus be hardly or not detected. The limitations of sequencing the whole gene are the cost to analyze the large-sized introns and the complexity to evaluate the impact of numerous identified variants [23].

After the second step, very few patients with CF still have an incomplete genotype. The third step, which is not performed in a clinical setting yet, aims to search for variants in the distant regulatory elements that may quantitatively alter CFTR expression [25], as well as large structural variants (such as duplications, deletions, inversions and translocations of blocks of DNA sequence). This can be achieved by resequencing a large genomic region including the entire topologically associated domain of *CFTR* on NGS specific platforms.

2.3. Prenatal and Preimplantation Diagnoses of CF

When applied to couples at-risk of ¼ or ½ of having a child with CF, the molecular strategy applied for prenatal diagnosis is simpler and consists of the detection of the known CF-causing variants that were previously identified in the index case or the parents. Considerable progress has been made in the field of preimplantation genetic diagnosis [5] and non-invasive prenatal diagnosis. Early detection of paternal CF variants in maternal blood has been routinely available for a few years [6,26] and, in the very near future, non-invasive procedures should be available to all at-risk couples through NGS haplotype-based approaches [27].

Prenatal diagnosis of CF may also be performed in the absence of family history of CF if ultrasound digestive abnormalities such as fetal echogenic bowel, fetal intestinal loop dilatation and non-visualization of the fetal gallbladder are observed during pregnancy [28]. Depending on national regulations, the term of pregnancy and ultrasound signs, the strategy followed and extent of the study may be the same as for diagnosis. Ensuring coverage of population-specific variants in this context is critical.

2.4. Recommendations for Population-Based CF Carrier Screening

Identification of CF-causing variants among all *CFTR* variants is of utmost importance, as only they are considered for CF carrier testing and prenatal diagnosis with subsequent termination of pregnancy. In 2002, the American College of Medical Genetics defined guidelines for clinical genetics laboratories [29]. Although over 900 variants were already described, a minimum variant panel for population-based carrier screening purposes was defined, consisting of 25 variants, restricted to 23 two years later, based on a frequency above 0.1% in CF chromosomes in a pan-ethnic population [30] (Table S1). These recommendations were needed to focus on true CF-causing variants and establish a rapid CF carrier diagnosis but presented limitations for specific ethnics groups, so that variant panels had to be tailored accordingly and many of them were considerably expanded. In order to document the highly variable variant distribution and frequency among populations, a systematic search in PubMed was made using keywords "CFTR", "cystic fibrosis", "variant" or "CFTR", "cystic fibrosis" and "mutation". Recent data in specific ethnic populations for which little was known were chosen to illustrate the variable representativeness of the 23 variant panel, with cumulated frequencies varying from 3% to 91% depending on the ethnic groups (Table S1). Moreover, in some of them, the majority of CF patients carried at least one population-specific variant, such as c.3276C>G (Y1092X) in Cameroon, c.3310G>T (E1104X) in Tunisia [31] or c.3700A>G (I1234V) in Qatar and in certain Arab tribes [32]. Although ethnicity-based genetic testing may appear obsolete with the wide implementation of NGS, the challenge remains to ensure the coverage of population-specific CF-causing variants wherever appropriate, especially as the NGS-based approach is not affordable in all countries.

2.5. Impact of Variant Heterogeneity on Personalized Medicine

Development of drugs to correct, enhance and stabilize the CFTR protein has made *CFTR* genotyping crucial to optimize therapy. It has renewed interest for the original variant classification that was based on functional data, six classes being recognized according to the CFTR protein defect in: I. synthesis, II. processing and maturation, III. gating, IV. conductance, V. abundance due to reduced amount of normal mRNA and VI. stability at the membrane [33–35]. However, clinical trials have showed that numerous variants caused pleiotropic defects, such as the most frequent CF-causing variant worldwide, c.1521_1523del (F508del) [36], thus justifying the use of drug combinations. Ivacaftor was the first drug to be US Food and Drug Administration approved for the treatment of CF, efficiently targeting the gating defect of class III variants, and it was further extended to class IV variants (Table S2). The list may however differ with that approved by the European Medicines Agency. These variants represent only 2%–10% of CF-causing variants in several populations and are totally absent in other ethnic groups (Table S2). Moreover, the clinical significance of several of them is questionable. Since then, combinations of ivacaftor with other molecules that aim to increase CFTR protein trafficking to the plasma membrane have been approved for specific variants: lumacaftor/ivacaftor in F508del homozygous patients; tezacaftor/ivacaftor in patients carrying F508del and a variant associated with residual CFTR function and elexacaftor/tezacaftor/ivacaftor in patients carrying at least one copy of F508del. The monumental interest of the triple-combination is that a large proportion of patients with CF are eligible for treatment in numerous populations. However, in specific ethnic groups, F508del is absent (such as Iraq, Sudan, Qatar, Japan and China) or extremely rare (Jordan 6%–7%, Bahrain 8%) [37] (Table S1). The challenge is thus to make personalized therapy accessible to all patients. Other strategies are still under development, such as amplifiers that increase the amount of CFTR available for modulators, readthrough agents targeting in frame premature termination codons and gene therapy [38].

3. How to Assess the Impact of *CFTR* Variants—The Challenge of Penetrance

Assessing the impact of *CFTR* variants is a comprehensive process, which allows one to answer clinical questions that cover diagnostic, genetic counseling and therapeutic issues. It is a daily challenge in specialized CF molecular laboratories, especially when dealing with rare or unknown variants. It relies on a good dialogue between clinicians, electrophysiologists and molecular geneticists, with appropriate clinical information provided by the clinicians, and occasionally requires the expertise of researchers (Figure 2). In 2015, international recommendations for interpretation and classification of sequence variations were published [39], based on diverse criteria including population, computational, segregation and functional data. They are reviewed in the present section. The recommended phenotypic classification into five categories, that is, "pathogenic", "likely pathogenic", "uncertain significance", "likely benign" and "benign" is however not completely equivalent as that used for *CFTR* variants and does not take into account phenotypic diversity, as "pathogenic" may be used for CF-causing and CFTR-RD-causing variants. As an example, variant c.1210-34TG[12]T[5] (TG12T5) may be considered pathogenic in the context of male infertility by absence of vas deferens but not in the context of CF.

3.1. Population Data (Clinical)

Assessing the impact and potential clinical consequence of a *CFTR* variant starts with search for clinical observations related to this variant in laboratory's own database, publicly available databases and the literature. Considering the class of variants in *trans* is essential in the context of a recessive disorder as CF. Beside the original CF Mutation Database, which most often describes the original observation and provides links to literature in PubMed, two other locus specific databases provide substantial and complementary information on variants and also provide links to epidemiological, computational, functional and literature data (Table 1). CFTR2 collects data from North American and European national CF patient registries [40], i.e., only from patients diagnosed with CF. *CFTR*-France is dedicated to the interpretation of rare variants and is built on data from genetics laboratories and the French CF patient registry [41]. It collects genetic and clinical data from patients with CF and CFTR-RD and from asymptomatic individuals who are compound heterozygous for two *CFTR* variants. Due to different designs, these two databases may provide discordant information and variant classification one should be aware of. In particular, the class of CFTR-RD-causing variants is not referenced in CFTR2 and variants classified as CFTR-RD in *CFTR*-France may be found either as VVCC or not CF-causing in CFTR2. Other general databases such as ClinVar [42], and Human Gene Mutation Database® [43], also provide clinical information and variant classification, mostly based on literature data, but numerous variants have been overclassified as "pathogenic" [44].

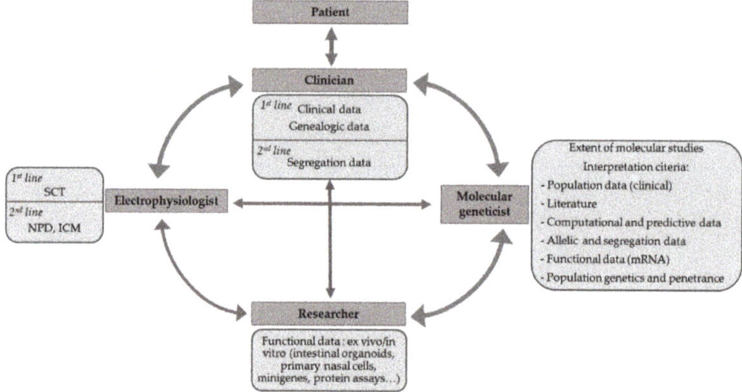

Figure 2. Links between health care professionals for carrying out appropriate *CFTR* studies and accurate interpretation of *CFTR* genetic test results. NPD: nasal potential difference; ICM: intestinal chloride measurement; SCT: sweat chloride testing.

Table 1. Data available in *CFTR*-France and CFTR2 according to categories of evidence of variant pathogenicity.

Categories of Evidence		*CFTR*-France		CFTR2
Population data: general population	+	Link to dbSNP and gnomAD	+	Reference to general population and CF carriers analysis for incomplete penetrance of *CFTR* variants
Population data: clinical observations	+	- 853 variants in about 5000 CF and CFTR-RD patients, and asymptomatic compound heterozygous individuals (data collected in molecular genetics laboratories, cross-reference with the French CF Registry) - Per patient: Age at diagnosis, symptoms, pancreatic status, meconium ileus, sweat chloride values, NBS - Link to CF Mutation Database and CFTR2	+	- 432 variants in about 89,000 CF patients (data collected from national registries) - Aggregated data for a given variant or genotype: age, lung and pancreatic function, *Pseudomonas aeruginosa* infection, sweat chloride values - Reference to ClinVar and LOVD
Literature	+	Link to PubMed for functional data	+	Link to PubMed for clinical and functional data
Computational predictions	+	AGVGD, MAPP, SIFT, PolyPhen-2, CYSMA	-	
Allelic and segregation data	+	- Data on variants identified in *trans* - Data on complex alleles	+	- Data provided on specific genotypes - No data on complex alleles
Functional data	+	Link to PubMed (transcript and protein studies)	+	- Data on CFTR protein maturation, folding, quantity and function in different cell lines - Link to PubMed

+: data available in the locus specific databases; -: data unavailable in the locus specific databases; LOVD: Leiden Open Variant Database [45]; NBS: newborn screening.

3.2. Literature Data

The literature review may provide valuable information for clinical, population genetics and functional data.

3.3. Computational and Predictive Data

In silico bioinformatics tools help predict the impact of variants at the mRNA level or the protein level, based on conservation of amino acids within different proteins of the same family, evolutionary conservation within species and biochemical distance between amino acids. Importantly, any intronic or exonic variant, even synonymous, may alter splicing. There are some limitations with using in silico tools, notably because of challenges in prioritizing one tool over the other and the lack of reliable standard interpretation guidelines [19]. Cystic fibrosis missense analysis (CYSMA) is a recently developed website dedicated to *CFTR* missense variants based on integrated in-house bioinformatics tools, which proved efficient to predict the impact of *CFTR* variants [46].

With the advent of wide genome analysis, aggregators that combine multiple evaluation tools have been implemented, such as Varsome [47] or Intervar [48]. They may be of help but exhibit significant limitations for *CFTR* variants, displaying a high degree of uncertainty for numerous variants [44].

3.4. Allelic and Segregation Data

Genetic studies in the parents of a patient are necessary to confirm the status of homozygous for a variant or compound heterozygous for two variants. Inheritance of two variants from the same parent (in *cis*) indicates the presence of a complex allele and numerous frequent or rare complex alleles have been described in the *CFTR* gene [41,49,50]. Complex alleles increase the complexity of *CFTR* variant classification, as illustrated for the c.445G>A (G149R) CF-causing variant and the c.1327G>T (D443Y) CFTR-RD-causing variant, each of them being described in *cis* with an already frequent complex allele c.[1727G>C;2002C>T] (G576A;R668C) [51]. *Cis*-variants may also affect the response to CFTR modulators, which impacts on reporting genetic test results [52]. De novo occurrence of variants is extremely rare in CF but has been described [53], also justifying parents' study. Abnormal segregation during parents' study may also unmask the presence of a deletion that would have escaped detection, depending on the techniques used [54].

3.5. Functional Data

Evidence of CFTR dysfunction may be brought by different categories of investigation, including in vivo, ex vivo and in vitro tests. While sweat testing is most often performed before comprehensive genetic testing in children, it may be performed after identification of *CFTR* variants in newborns, depending on NBS programs, or in adults with a possible CFTR-RD or CF. Nasal potential difference or intestinal current measurements are often used in the second line in case of inconclusive sweat test results or to help variant interpretation for patients carrying VUS. Likewise, other tests may be of help, such as sweat secretion after β-adrenergic stimulation, also called evaporimetry [55]. Ex vivo assessment of CFTR function on miniaturized versions of organs called organoids, from minimally invasive rectal biopsies [56] or on bronchial or nasal cells [57,58], is based on sophisticated and comprehensive techniques implemented in a few expert laboratories, which help diagnose, understand mechanistic defects and better predict organ-specific drug responses [59].

In vitro assays implemented to evaluate the impact of variants on *CFTR* mRNA or protein are also usually performed in a research setting. Minigene systems most often reproduce one or several exons in cloned plasmids, which are then transfected in human cells. They interrogate the impact of intronic or exonic variants on splicing [60,61] and are useful alternative tools when patients' epithelial cells are not available for mRNA study. Importantly, they have allowed demonstration of a splicing impact of variants heretofore considered as missense, such c.2908G>C (G970R), which escapes CFTR modulator therapy [62] or c.3700A>G (I1234V) [63], or as nonsense, like c.2491G>T (E831X) [64]. Functional in vitro studies that focus on CFTR protein synthesis, maturation and function, are invaluable investigation tools. However, as noted above, many *CFTR* variants impair more than one single cellular process, as F508del [36]. Virtually no assay reflects the full biological function of the CFTR protein, so that the absence of defect observed does not rule out an impact on CFTR protein function. Eventually, numerous studies performed on presumed missense variants have also neglected a potential impact on splicing and should thus be considered cautiously.

3.6. Population Genetics and Penetrance Associated to CFTR *Variants*

Looking at variant frequencies in the general population has long been used to assess potential variant pathogenicity. A greater frequency of a variant in the ethnic-matched general population than in the population of CF patients, or greater than expected considering the frequency of CF, is a strong support for a benign interpretation. Data from the general population, globally and in specific population groups, are available on large reference datasets such as gnomAD [65]. Indeed, some variants are rarely found in our routine practice but are frequent in specific general populations, such as c.1666A>G (I556V), which allelic frequency in the Asian population reaches 4.7%, and c.2620-26A>G, which allelic frequency in the Ashkenazi Jewish population is 2.7%. These variants, which may have been overclassified in locus specific databases, should definitely be considered non-disease-causing. The occurrence of a rare or previously undescribed variant in *trans* of a known CF-causing variant in a healthy individual is also in favor of benignity.

Population genetics data proved useful to get an insight into the penetrance associated with *CFTR* variants. The penetrance of a phenotype is defined as the proportion of patients carrying a given genotype who develop this phenotype. For a recessive disease as CF, homozygous or compound heterozygous genotypes are most often detected in symptomatic patients and are described in clinical databases, which means that potential cases in healthy individuals are rarely taken into account, unless through family testing. CFTR2 thus represents the tip of the iceberg of all possible phenotypes associated with a variant. Few studies have shown an unexpectedly low penetrance associated with some *CFTR* variants, such as the c.1210-34TG[11]T[5] (TG11T5) variant [66], c.350G>A (R117H) [67] and other variants [40,68]. As an illustration, taking into account clinical observations and epidemiological data, a French collaborative study showed that the penetrance of CF in individuals compound heterozygous for R117H;T7 and F508del was as low as 0.03% and that of CFTR-RD was 3% [67] (Figure 3). Such comprehensive data are however not available for the huge amount of *CFTR* variants but incomplete penetrance may be supported by other lines of evidence. First, clinical observations and comparison of disease phenotypes in CFTR2 and *CFTR*-France databases suggest an incomplete penetrance of CF for variants that have been classified as CF-causing in CFTR2 but milder in *CFTR*-France, such as c.328G>C (D110H), c.349C>T (R117C) or c.617T>G (L206W). Second, the higher frequency of variants in the general population than in the population of CF patients is strongly against a severe deleterious effect, as for variants c.1210-12T[5] (T5), c.2991G>C (L997F) or R117H. Eventually, based on variant frequencies in the general population and results of the French NBS program over the 2002–2017 period, a recent study strongly suggested incomplete penetrance for 10 *CFTR* variants found in inconclusive cases after CF NBS [68]. The low penetrance associated with some variants such as the T5 variants might help clinicians to adapt medical care and follow-up of newborns carrying these variants, as well as genetic counseling given to families.

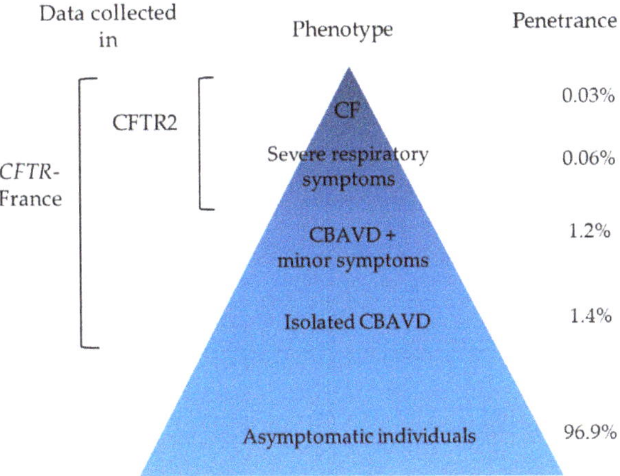

Figure 3. Penetrance of phenotypes in individuals who are compound heterozygous for c.[350G>A;1210-12T[7]];[1521_1523del] (R117H;T7/F508del) from Thauvin et al. [67].

4. The Challenges of Genetic Counseling—When Genetic Counseling Meets Diagnosis

Genetic counseling for CF is a very important part of medical consultation and laboratory activities, which has become complex over the years (Figure 4). It has long been focused on the identification of CF carriers in the family of patients having CF and on provision of counseling services to couples in order to ensure informed reproductive decision-making [69]. Once a CF carrier is identified, testing for the most frequent CF-causing variants according to his/her geographic origins is recommended in the partner in a prenatal or preconception setting [13]. Extended *CFTR* sequencing analysis in the partners is however more and more performed, at least in partners of CF patients, because of the prior risk for the couple of having a child with CF (1/70, provided a CF carrier frequency of 1/35) [69]. Genetic counseling should also be considered for all symptomatic patients who carry *CFTR* variants, due to the potential risk of CF in the patients' offspring and relatives. The identification of a CF variant leads to recommend CF carrier testing in the relatives and the partner in case of a parental project. While cascade testing for known CFTR-RD variants is not recommended, the identification of VVCC or VUS makes genetic counseling delicate and may be discussed on a case-by-case basis. Occasionally, *CFTR* testing in healthy adult siblings of a patient leads to identify the same genotype as in the patient. These individuals might develop symptoms related to a CFTR-RD or a mild form of CF, and thus need clinical investigation. On the other hand, such findings contribute to documenting the variable penetrance associated with some *CFTR* variants.

Identification of CF carriers may also occur in the absence of any family history of CF, during the process of NBS, or during preconception carrier screening or during wide genome analysis as an unsolicited or secondary finding (Figure 4). Expanded preconception carrier screening for CF and other recessive disorders is also under consideration in countries according to an overall positive attitude of the general population [70,71]. Preconception CF carrier screening has already been implemented in the US, Israël and Northeast Italy [72]. In most countries however, for practical reasons variant panels used for diagnostic purposes are also used for carrier testing. Again, it is important to discriminate true CF-causing variants from those that are CFTR-RD-causing, VVCC or non disease-causing. The wide implementation of NGS-based *CFTR* analysis in various clinical settings has increased this concern, with the identification of rare VUS or variants for which discrepant interpretation is found in databases or the literature. For genetic counseling purposes, the question of penetrance associated with variants is even more critical. Contrary to the diagnostic setting where the main question to answer is "does the genotype account for the phenotype?", which may already be difficult with inconclusive genotypes, a challenging question in genetic counseling is to predict the phenotype resulting from the combination of a VUS or a VVCC with a known CF-causing variant.

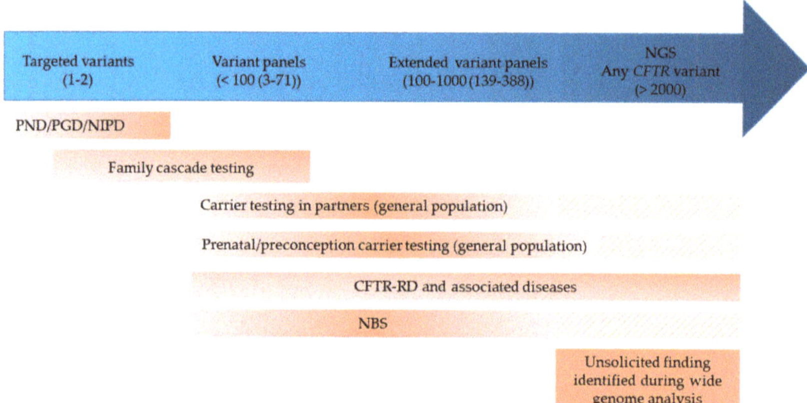

Figure 4. Genetic counseling situations (in orange), with potential identification of CF carriers, according to variable practices of molecular analysis (in blue). The number of variants tested is indicated in brackets. CFTR-RD: CFTR-related disorder; NBS: newborn screening; NIPD: non-invasive prenatal diagnosis; PND: prenatal diagnosis; PGD: preimplantation genetic diagnosis. Hatched lines: expected practice in the near future.

Identification of carriers of CF-causing variants is also of particular concern in the context of CF NBS. On one hand, testing the parents may lead to identify another *CFTR* variant, possibly outside the NBS panel depending on laboratory's practice. This result then raises the question of looking for this second variant in the infant who has a negative sweat test result. On the other hand, extended *CFTR* gene sequencing is being considered as part of the core strategy in an increasing number of programs [73,74]. Moreover, the relevance of implementing extended NBS for numerous genetic diseases is currently debated [74–77], also taking into account economical aspects. The introduction of NGS, with or without prior immunoreactive trypsinogen measurement and without filtering CF variants would lead to detect not only a higher number of carriers of known CF-causing variants but a much higher number of carriers of VVCC and VUS. The risk would be to consider neonates as carriers of a CF-causing variant and to offer inappropriate genetic counseling and testing in the family, and eventually inappropriate prenatal diagnosis.

The face of genetic counseling for CF will inevitably deeply change in the coming years. Health public policies of CF carrier screening in the general population aim to detect most CF carrier couples and prenatal requests may increase, especially with the availability of non-invasive procedures. This would ineluctably impact on the prevalence of CF births, which then would raise the question of the relevance of NBS if the incidence of CF is getting very low. In other respects, due to formidable progress in genotype-guided therapy, parents at risk of having a child with CF could prefer the option of continuation of pregnancy over that of termination. Prediction of changing attitudes and practices is a delicate business.

Very recently, a study conducted on 19,802 CF carriers who were matched each with five controls, reported a higher prevalence of 57 out of 59 CF-related symptoms or conditions in CF carriers than in the general population. These conditions included already known CFTR-RDs, conditions where a higher prevalence of *CFTR* variants has already been reported, such as allergic bronchopulmonary aspergillosis, asthma, primary sclerosing cholangitis [8] or pancreatic cancer [78] and others that were not previously described associated with CFTR dysfunction, such as cirrhosis or intestina atresia [9]. Despite a number of limitations of this study, notably the absence of any data about *CFTR* testing (the number and kind of variants is not known, a number of CF carriers might have a CFTR-RD or bear a second *CFTR* variant), and the low absolute risk for a carrier to develop each condition, the results of the study, if confirmed, would challenge the status of "healthy carrier" and open a new era in personalized preventive medicine. This would also lead to dramatically modify the message given to the parents of a so-called "healthy" carrier detected through NBS, both for the child and the carrier parent, as well as to all carriers identified through family cascade testing or preconception carrier screening. Genetic counseling should be very cautious with such data, which should also be discussed keeping in mind the presumed heterozygote selective advantage, at least for carriers of F508del [79]. Especially in the perspective of expanded carrier screening in the general population, the risk is again to overestimate *CFTR* variants as CF-causing, hence overpredict healthy individuals at risk for developing a number of diseases. As long as the penetrance associated with *CFTR* variants is not known, implementation of genomic analysis for CF NBS and genetic counseling purposes appear detrimental. An optimal compromise would be to perform NGS with bioinformatics targeting a wide panel of fully penetrant CF-causing variants, as recently implemented for CF NBS [73,74]. It seems we are moving from a technological challenge towards a societal, political and ethical challenge.

Supplementary Materials: The following are available online at http://www.mdpi.com/2073-4425/11/6/619/s1, Table S1. Sensitivity of the ACMG recommended CF-causing variant panel for CF carrier screening in different countries and ethnic populations. ACMG: American College of Medical Genetics. Allelic frequencies among CF alleles are indicated in percentage. 0 (cells in grey) indicates that the variant was absent in the population tested. Table S2: Frequency in different countries of non-F508del variants approved for CFTR modulator therapy. * Variants approved by Food and Drug Administration (FDA) for ivacaftor in a first list and ** in the second list. Variants approved by European Medicines Agency (EMA) are in grey; £ Variants approved by FDA for tezacaftor/ivacaftor when in combination with F508del; § Variants approved by EMA for tezacaftor/ivacaftor; 0 indicates that the variant was absent in the population tested; nd*: frequency < 0.01%. The total does not reflect the approval in each country.

Author Contributions: Conception and design of the study, T.B. and E.G.; Review of literature data, writing of the manuscript, T.B., M.L. and E.G. All authors have read and agreed to the published version of the manuscript.

Funding: This research received no external funding.

Acknowledgments: Vaincre La Mucoviscidose is acknowledged for supporting our activities.

Conflicts of Interest: The authors declare no conflict of interest.

References

1. Farrell, P.M.; White, T.B.; Ren, C.L.; Hempstead, S.E.; Accurso, F.; Derichs, N.; Howenstine, M.; McColley, S.A.; Rock, M.; Rosenfeld, M.; et al. Diagnosis of cystic fibrosis: Consensus guidelines from the cystic fibrosis foundation. *J. Pediatr.* **2017**, *181*, S4–S15. [CrossRef] [PubMed]

2. Schwiebert, E.M.; Egan, M.E.; Hwang, T.H.; Fulmer, S.B.; Allen, S.S.; Cutting, G.R.; Guggino, W.B. CFTR regulates outwardly rectifying chloride channels through an autocrine mechanism involving ATP. *Cell* **1995**, *81*, 1063–1073. [CrossRef]

3. Bareil, C.; Bergougnoux, A. *CFTR* gene variants, epidemiology and molecular pathology. *Arch. Pédiatrie* **2020**, *27*, eS8–eS12. [CrossRef]

4. Audrézet, M.P.; Munck, A.; Scotet, V.; Claustres, M.; Roussey, M.; Delmas, D.; Férec, C.; Desgeorges, M. Comprehensive *CFTR* gene analysis of the French cystic fibrosis screened newborn cohort: Implications for diagnosis, genetic counseling, and mutation-specific therapy. *Genet. Med.* **2015**, *17*, 108–116. [CrossRef] [PubMed]

5. Girardet, A.; Viart, V.; Plaza, S.; Daina, G.; De Rycke, M.; Des Georges, M.; Fiorentino, F.; Harton, G.; Ishmukhametova, A.; Navarro, J.; et al. The improvement of the best practice guidelines for preimplantation genetic diagnosis of cystic fibrosis: Toward an international consensus. *Eur. J. Hum. Genet.* **2016**, *24*, 469–478. [CrossRef]

6. Gruber, A.; Pacault, M.; El Khattabi, L.A.; Vaucouleur, N.; Orhant, L.; Bienvenu, T.; Girodon, E.; Vidaud, D.; Leturcq, F.; Costa, C.; et al. Non-invasive prenatal diagnosis of paternally inherited disorders from maternal plasma: Detection of *NF1* and *CFTR* mutations using droplet digital PCR. *Clin. Chem. Lab. Med.* **2018**, *56*, 728–738. [CrossRef]

7. Bombieri, C.; Claustres, M.; De Boeck, K.; Derichs, N.; Dodge, J.; Girodon, E.; Sermet, I.; Schwarz, M.; Tzetis, M.; Wilschanski, M.; et al. Recommendations for the classification of diseases as CFTR-related disorders. *J. Cyst. Fibros.* **2011**, *10*, S86–S102. [CrossRef]

8. Pagin, A.; Sermet-Gaudelus, I.; Burgel, P.-R. Genetic diagnosis in practice: From cystic fibrosis to CFTR-related disorders. *Arch. Pédiatrie* **2020**, *27*, eS25–eS29. [CrossRef]

9. Miller, A.C.; Comellas, A.P.; Hornick, D.B.; Stoltz, D.A.; Cavanaugh, J.E.; Gerke, A.K.; Welsh, M.J.; Zabner, J.; Polgreen, P.M. Cystic fibrosis carriers are at increased risk for a wide range of cystic fibrosis-related conditions. *Proc. Natl. Acad. Sci. USA* **2020**, *117*, 1621–1627. [CrossRef]

10. Pagin, A.; Bergougnoux, A.; Girodon, E.; Reboul, M.; Willoquaux, C.; Kesteloot, M.; Raynal, C.; Bienvenu, T.; Humbert, M.; Lalau, G.; et al. Novel *ADGRG2* truncating variants in patients with X-linked congenital absence of vas deferens. *Andrology* **2020**, *8*, 618–624. [CrossRef]

11. Masson, E.; Chen, J.-M.; Audrézet, M.-P.; Cooper, D.N.; Férec, C. A conservative assessment of the major genetic causes of idiopathic chronic pancreatitis: Data from a comprehensive analysis of *PRSS1*, *SPINK1*, *CTRC* and *CFTR* genes in 253 young French patients. *PLoS ONE* **2013**, *8*, e73522. [CrossRef] [PubMed]

12. Castellani, C.; Cuppens, H.; Macek, M.; Cassiman, J.J.; Kerem, E.; Durie, P.; Tullis, E.; Assael, B.M.; Bombieri, C.; Brown, A.; et al. Consensus on the use and interpretation of cystic fibrosis mutation analysis in clinical practice. *J. Cyst. Fibros.* **2008**, *7*, 179–196. [CrossRef] [PubMed]

13. Dequeker, E.; Stuhrmann, M.; Morris, M.A.; Casals, T.; Castellani, C.; Claustres, M.; Cuppens, H.; des Georges, M.; Ferec, C.; Macek, M.; et al. Best practice guidelines for molecular genetic diagnosis of cystic fibrosis and CFTR-related disorders—Updated European recommendations. *Eur. J. Hum. Genet.* **2009**, *17*, 51–65. [CrossRef] [PubMed]

14. Ratbi, I.; Legendre, M.; Niel, F.; Martin, J.; Soufir, J.-C.; Izard, V.; Costes, B.; Costa, C.; Goossens, M.; Girodon, E. Detection of cystic fibrosis transmembrane conductance regulator (*CFTR*) gene rearrangements enriches the mutation spectrum in congenital bilateral absence of the vas deferens and impacts on genetic counselling. *Hum. Reprod.* **2007**, *22*, 1285–1291. [CrossRef] [PubMed]

15. Raynal, C.; Girodon, E.; Audrezet, M.P.; Cabet, F.; Pagin, A.; Reboul, M.P.; Dufernez, F.; Fergelot, P.; Bergougnoux, A.; Fanen, P.; et al. *CFTR* gene variants: A predisposition factor to aquagenic palmoplantar keratoderma. *Br. J. Dermatol.* **2019**, *181*, 1097–1099. [CrossRef] [PubMed]

16. Cystic Fibrosis Mutation Data Base (CFMDB). Available online: http://www.genet.sickkids.on.ca/ (accessed on 7 May 2020).

17. The Molecular Genetic Epidemiology of Cystic Fibrosis: Report of a Joint Meeting of WHO/ECFTN/ICF(M)A/ECFS, Genoa, Italy, 19 June 2002. Available online: https://apps.who.int/iris/handle/10665/68702 (accessed on 7 May 2020).

18. Kılınç, M.O.; Ninis, V.N.; Dağlı, E.; Demirkol, M.; Özkınay, F.; Arıkan, Z.; Çoğulu, Ö.; Hüner, G.; Karakoç, F.; Tolun, A. Highest heterogeneity for cystic fibrosis: 36 mutations account for 75% of all CF chromosomes in Turkish patients. *Am. J. Med. Genet.* **2002**, *113*, 250–257. [CrossRef]

19. Bergougnoux, A.; Taulan-Cadars, M.; Claustres, M.; Raynal, C. Current and future molecular approaches in the diagnosis of cystic fibrosis. *Expert Rev. Respir. Med.* **2018**, *12*, 415–426. [CrossRef]

20. Kharrazi, M.; Yang, J.; Bishop, T.; Lessing, S.; Young, S.; Graham, S.; Pearl, M.; Chow, H.; Ho, T.; Currier, R.; et al. Newborn screening for cystic fibrosis in California. *Pediatrics* **2015**, *136*, 1062–1072. [CrossRef]

21. Faà, V.; Incani, F.; Meloni, A.; Corda, D.; Masala, M.; Baffico, A.M.; Seia, M.; Cao, A.; Rosatelli, M.C. Characterization of a disease-associated mutation affecting a putative splicing regulatory element in intron 6b of the Cystic Fibrosis Transmembrane Conductance Regulator (*CFTR*) Gene. *J. Biol. Chem.* **2009**, *284*, 30024–30031. [CrossRef]

22. Costa, C.; Pruliere-Escabasse, V.; de Becdelievre, A.; Gameiro, C.; Golmard, L.; Guittard, C.; Bassinet, L.; Bienvenu, T.; Georges, M.D.; Epaud, R.; et al. A recurrent deep-intronic splicing CF mutation emphasizes the importance of mRNA studies in clinical practice. *J. Cyst. Fibros.* **2011**, *10*, 479–482. [CrossRef]

23. Bonini, J.; Varilh, J.; Raynal, C.; Thèze, C.; Beyne, E.; Audrezet, M.-P.; Ferec, C.; Bienvenu, T.; Girodon, E.; Tuffery-Giraud, S.; et al. Small-scale high-throughput sequencing–based identification of new therapeutic tools in cystic fibrosis. *Genet. Med.* **2015**, *17*, 796–806. [CrossRef] [PubMed]

24. Bergougnoux, A.; Délétang, K.; Pommier, A.; Varilh, J.; Houriez, F.; Altieri, J.P.; Koenig, M.; Férec, C.; Claustres, M.; Lalau, G.; et al. Functional characterization and phenotypic spectrum of three recurrent disease-causing deep intronic variants of the *CFTR* gene. *J. Cyst. Fibros.* **2019**, *18*, 468–475. [CrossRef]

25. Moisan, S.; Berlivet, S.; Ka, C.; Gac, G.L.; Dostie, J.; Férec, C. Analysis of long-range interactions in primary human cells identifies cooperative *CFTR* regulatory elements. *Nucleic Acids Res.* **2016**, *44*, 2564–2576. [CrossRef]

26. Guissart, C.; Dubucs, C.; Raynal, C.; Girardet, A.; Tran Mau Them, F.; Debant, V.; Rouzier, C.; Boureau-Wirth, A.; Haquet, E.; Puechberty, J.; et al. Non-invasive prenatal diagnosis (NIPD) of cystic fibrosis: An optimized protocol using MEMO fluorescent PCR to detect the p.Phe508del mutation. *J. Cyst. Fibros.* **2017**, *16*, 198–206. [CrossRef]

27. Guissart, C.; Them, F.T.M.; Debant, V.; Viart, V.; Dubucs, C.; Pritchard, V.; Rouzier, C.; Boureau-Wirth, A.; Haquet, E.; Puechberty, J.; et al. A broad test based on fluorescent-multiplex PCR for noninvasive prenatal diagnosis of Cystic Fibrosis. *Fetal Diagn. Ther.* **2019**, *45*, 403–412. [CrossRef] [PubMed]

28. Bergougnoux, A.; Jouannic, J.-M.; Verneau, F.; Bienvenu, T.; Gaitch, N.; Raynal, C.; Girodon, E. Isolated nonvisualization of the fetal gallbladder should be considered for the prenatal diagnosis of Cystic Fibrosis. *Fetal Diagn. Ther.* **2019**, *45*, 312–316. [CrossRef]

29. Richards, C.S.; Bradley, L.A.; Amos, J.; Allitto, B.; Grody, W.W.; Maddalena, A.; McGinnis, M.J.; Prior, T.W.; Popovich, B.W.; Watson, M.S. Standards and Guidelines for *CFTR* Mutation Testing. *Genet. Med.* **2002**, *4*, 379–391. [CrossRef] [PubMed]

30. Watson, M.S.; Cutting, G.R.; Desnick, R.J.; Driscoll, D.A.; Klinger, K.; Mennuti, M.; Palomaki, G.E.; Popovich, B.W.; Pratt, V.M.; Rohlfs, E.M.; et al. Cystic fibrosis population carrier screening: 2004 revision of American college of medical genetics mutation panel. *Genet. Med.* **2004**, *6*, 387–391. [CrossRef] [PubMed]

31. Stewart, C.; Pepper, M.S. Cystic fibrosis on the African continent. *Genet. Med.* **2016**, *18*, 653–662. [CrossRef] [PubMed]

32. Hammoudeh, S.; Gadelhak, W.; AbdulWahab, A.; Al-Langawi, M.; Janahi, I.A. Approaching two decades of cystic fibrosis research in Qatar: A historical perspective and future directions. *Multidiscip. Respir. Med.* **2019**, *14*, 29. [CrossRef]

33. Welsh, M.J.; Smith, A.E. Molecular mechanisms of CFTR chloride channel dysfunction in cystic fibrosis. *Cell* **1993**, *73*, 1251–1254. [CrossRef]

34. Highsmith, W.E.; Burch, L.H.; Zhou, Z.; Olsen, J.C.; Boat, T.E.; Spock, A.; Gorvoy, J.D.; Quittell, L.; Friedman, K.J.; Silverman, L.M.; et al. A novel mutation in the cystic fibrosis gene in patients with pulmonary disease but normal sweat chloride concentrations. *N. Engl. J. Med.* **1994**, *331*, 974–980. [CrossRef]

35. Haardt, M.; Benharouga, M.; Lechardeur, D.; Kartner, N.; Lukacs, G.L. C-terminal truncations destabilize the Cystic Fibrosis Transmembrane Conductance Regulator without impairing its biogenesis. A novel class of mutation. *J. Biol. Chem.* **1999**, *274*, 21873–21877. [CrossRef] [PubMed]

36. Veit, G.; Avramescu, R.G.; Chiang, A.N.; Houck, S.A.; Cai, Z.; Peters, K.W.; Hong, J.S.; Pollard, H.B.; Guggino, W.B.; Balch, W.E.; et al. From CFTR biology toward combinatorial pharmacotherapy: Expanded classification of cystic fibrosis mutations. *Mol. Biol. Cell* **2016**, *27*, 424–433. [CrossRef] [PubMed]

37. Al-Sadeq, D.; Abunada, T.; Dalloul, R.; Fahad, S.; Taleb, S.; Aljassim, K.; Al Hamed, F.A.; Zayed, H. Spectrum of mutations of cystic fibrosis in the 22 Arab countries: A systematic review. *Respirology* **2019**, *24*, 127–136. [CrossRef] [PubMed]

38. Fajac, I.; Girodon, E. Genomically-guided therapies: A new era for cystic fibrosis. *Arch. Pédiatrie* **2020**, *27*, eS41–eS44. [CrossRef]

39. Richards, S.; Aziz, N.; Bale, S.; Bick, D.; Das, S.; Gastier-Foster, J.; Grody, W.W.; Hegde, M.; Lyon, E.; Spector, E.; et al. Standards and guidelines for the interpretation of sequence variants: A joint consensus recommendation of the American college of medical genetics and genomics and the association for molecular pathology. *Genet. Med.* **2015**, *17*, 405–423. [CrossRef]

40. Sosnay, P.R.; Siklosi, K.R.; Van Goor, F.; Kaniecki, K.; Yu, H.; Sharma, N.; Ramalho, A.S.; Amaral, M.D.; Dorfman, R.; Zielenski, J.; et al. Defining the disease liability of variants in the cystic fibrosis transmembrane conductance regulator gene. *Nat. Genet.* **2013**, *45*, 1160–1167, CFTR2. Available online: https://www.cftr2.org/ (accessed on 7 May 2020). [CrossRef]

41. Claustres, M.; Thèze, C.; des Georges, M.; Baux, D.; Girodon, E.; Bienvenu, T.; Audrezet, M.-P.; Dugueperoux, I.; Férec, C.; Lalau, G.; et al. *CFTR*-France, a national relational patient database for sharing genetic and phenotypic data associated with rare *CFTR* variants. *Hum. Mutat.* **2017**, *38*, 1297–1315. Available online: https://cftr.iurc.montp.inserm.fr/cgi-bin/home.cgi (accessed on 7 May 2020). [CrossRef]

42. Landrum, M.J.; Lee, J.M.; Benson, M.; Brown, G.; Chao, C.; Chitipiralla, S.; Gu, B.; Hart, J.; Hoffman, D.; Hoover, J.; et al. ClinVar: Public archive of interpretations of clinically relevant variants. *Nucleic Acids Res.* **2016**, *44*, D862–D868. Available online: https://www.ncbi.nlm.nih.gov/clinvar/ (accessed on 7 May 2020). [CrossRef]

43. Stenson, P.D.; Mort, M.; Ball, E.V.; Evans, K.; Hayden, M.; Heywood, S.; Hussain, M.; Phillips, A.D.; Cooper, D.N. The Human Gene Mutation Database: Towards a comprehensive repository of inherited mutation data for medical research, genetic diagnosis and next-generation sequencing studies. *Hum. Genet.* **2017**, *136*, 665–677. Available online: http://www.hgmd.cf.ac.uk/ac/index.php (accessed on 7 May 2020). [CrossRef] [PubMed]

44. Boussaroque, A.; Bergougnoux, A.; Raynal, C.; Audrézet, M.-P.; Sasorith, S.; Férec, C.; Bienvenu, T.; Girodon, E. Pitfalls in the interpretation of *CFTR* variants in the context of incidental findings. *Hum. Mutat.* **2019**, *40*, 2239–2246. [CrossRef]

45. Leiden Open Version Database (LOVD). Available online: https://www.lovd.nl/ (accessed on 7 May 2020).

46. Sasorith, S.; Baux, D.; Bergougnoux, A.; Paulet, D.; Lahure, A.; Bareil, C.; Taulan-Cadars, M.; Roux, A.; Koenig, M.; Claustres, M.; et al. The CYSMA web server: An example of integrative tool for in silico analysis of missense variants identified in Mendelian disorders. *Hum. Mutat.* **2020**, *41*, 375–386. [CrossRef] [PubMed]

47. Kopanos, C.; Tsiolkas, V.; Kouris, A.; Chapple, C.E.; Albarca Aguilera, M.; Meyer, R.; Massouras, A. VarSome: The human genomic variant search engine. *Bioinformatics* **2019**, *35*, 1978–1980. Available online: http://varsome.com/ (accessed on 7 May 2020). [CrossRef] [PubMed]

48. Li, Q.; Wang, K. InterVar: Clinical interpretation of genetic variants by the 2015 ACMG-AMP Guidelines. *Am. J. Hum. Genet.* **2017**, *100*, 267–280. Available online: http://wintervar.wglab.org/ (accessed on 7 May 2020). [CrossRef] [PubMed]

49. Vecchio-Pagán, B.; Blackman, S.M.; Lee, M.; Atalar, M.; Pellicore, M.J.; Pace, R.G.; Franca, A.L.; Raraigh, K.S.; Sharma, N.; Knowles, M.R.; et al. Deep resequencing of *CFTR* in 762 F508del homozygotes reveals clusters of non-coding variants associated with cystic fibrosis disease traits. *Hum. Genome Var.* **2016**, *3*, 16038. [CrossRef]

50. Bergougnoux, A.; Boureau-Wirth, A.; Rouzier, C.; Altieri, J.-P.; Verneau, F.; Larrieu, L.; Koenig, M.; Claustres, M.; Raynal, C. A false positive newborn screening result due to a complex allele carrying two frequent CF-causing variants. *J. Cyst. Fibros.* **2016**, *15*, 309–312. [CrossRef]

51. El-Seedy, A.; Girodon, E.; Norez, C.; Pajaud, J.; Pasquet, M.-C.; de Becdelièvre, A.; Bienvenu, T.; des Georges, M.; Cabet, F.; Lalau, G.; et al. *CFTR* mutation combinations producing frequent complex alleles with different clinical and functional outcomes. *Hum. Mutat.* **2012**, *33*, 1557–1565. [CrossRef]

52. Chevalier, B.; Hinzpeter, A. The influence of *CFTR* complex alleles on precision therapy of cystic fibrosis. *J. Cyst. Fibros.* **2020**, *19*, S15–S18. [CrossRef]

53. Křenková, P.; Piskáčková, T.; Holubová, A.; Balaščaková, M.; Krulišová, V.; Čamajová, J.; Turnovec, M.; Libik, M.; Norambuena, P.; Štambergová, A.; et al. Distribution of *CFTR* mutations in the Czech population: Positive impact of integrated clinical and laboratory expertise, detection of novel/de novo alleles and relevance for related/derived populations. *J. Cyst. Fibros.* **2013**, *12*, 532–537. [CrossRef]

54. Niel, F.; Legendre, M.; Bienvenu, T.; Bieth, E.; Lalau, G.; Sermet, I.; Bondeux, D.; Boukari, R.; Derelle, J.; Levy, P.; et al. A new large *CFTR* rearrangement illustrates the importance of searching for complex alleles. *Hum. Mutat.* **2006**, *27*, 716–717. [CrossRef] [PubMed]

55. Quinton, P.; Molyneux, L.; Ip, W.; Dupuis, A.; Avolio, J.; Tullis, E.; Conrad, D.; Shamsuddin, A.K.; Durie, P.; Gonska, T. β-Adrenergic sweat secretion as a diagnostic test for Cystic Fibrosis. *Am. J. Respir. Crit. Care Med.* **2012**, *186*, 732–739. [CrossRef] [PubMed]

56. Dekkers, J.F.; Wiegerinck, C.L.; de Jonge, H.R.; Bronsveld, I.; Janssens, H.M.; de Winter-de Groot, K.M.; Brandsma, A.M.; de Jong, N.W.M.; Bijvelds, M.J.C.; Scholte, B.J.; et al. A functional CFTR assay using primary cystic fibrosis intestinal organoids. *Nat. Med.* **2013**, *19*, 939–945. [CrossRef] [PubMed]

57. Awatade, N.T.; Wong, S.L.; Hewson, C.K.; Fawcett, L.K.; Kicic, A.; Jaffe, A.; Waters, S.A. Human primary epithelial cell models: Promising tools in the era of cystic fibrosis personalized medicine. *Front. Pharmacol.* **2018**, *9*, 1429. [CrossRef]

58. Pranke, I.M.; Hatton, A.; Simonin, J.; Jais, J.P.; Le Pimpec-Barthes, F.; Carsin, A.; Bonnette, P.; Fayon, M.; Stremler-Le Bel, N.; Grenet, D.; et al. Correction of CFTR function in nasal epithelial cells from cystic fibrosis patients predicts improvement of respiratory function by CFTR modulators. *Sci. Rep.* **2017**, *7*, 7375. [CrossRef]

59. Amaral, M.D.; de Boeck, K.; Amaral, M.; Davies, J.C.; de Boeck, K.; Drevinek, P.; Elborn, S.; Kerem, E.; Lee, T. Theranostics by testing CFTR modulators in patient-derived materials: The current status and a proposal for subjects with rare *CFTR* mutations. *J. Cyst. Fibros.* **2019**, *18*, 685–692. [CrossRef]

60. Raynal, C.; Baux, D.; Theze, C.; Bareil, C.; Taulan, M.; Roux, A.-F.; Claustres, M.; Tuffery-Giraud, S.; des Georges, M. A classification model relative to splicing for variants of unknown clinical significance: Application to the *CFTR* gene. *Hum. Mutat.* **2013**, *34*, 774–784. [CrossRef]

61. Sharma, N.; Sosnay, P.R.; Ramalho, A.S.; Douville, C.; Franca, A.; Gottschalk, L.B.; Park, J.; Lee, M.; Vecchio-Pagan, B.; Raraigh, K.S.; et al. Experimental assessment of splicing variants using expression Minigenes and comparison with in Silico predictions. *Hum. Mutat.* **2014**, *35*, 1249–1259. [CrossRef]

62. Amato, F.; Scudieri, P.; Musante, I.; Tomati, V.; Caci, E.; Comegna, M.; Maietta, S.; Manzoni, F.; Di Lullo, A.M.; Wachter, E.; et al. Two *CFTR* mutations within codon 970 differently impact on the chloride channel functionality. *Hum. Mutat.* **2019**, *40*, 742–748. [CrossRef]

63. Ramalho, A.S.; Clarke, L.A.; Sousa, M.; Felicio, V.; Barreto, C.; Lopes, C.; Amaral, M.D. Comparative ex vivo, in vitro and in silico analyses of a *CFTR* splicing mutation: Importance of functional studies to establish disease liability of mutations. *J. Cyst. Fibros.* **2016**, *15*, 21–33. [CrossRef]

64. Hinzpeter, A.; Aissat, A.; Sondo, E.; Costa, C.; Arous, N.; Gameiro, C.; Martin, N.; Tarze, A.; Weiss, L.; de Becdelièvre, A.; et al. Alternative splicing at a NAGNAG acceptor site as a novel phenotype modifier. *PLoS Genet.* **2010**, *6*, e1001153. [CrossRef]

65. Karczewski, K.J.; Francioli, L.C.; Tiao, G.; Cummings, B.B.; Alföldi, J.; Wang, Q.; Collins, R.L.; Laricchia, K.M.; Ganna, A.; Birnbaum, D.P.; et al. The mutational constraint spectrum quantified from variation in 141,456 humans. *Nature* **2020**, *581*, 434–443. [CrossRef]

66. Groman, J.D.; Hefferon, T.W.; Casals, T.; Bassas, L.; Estivill, X.; Des Georges, M.; Guittard, C.; Koudova, M.; Fallin, M.D.; Nemeth, K.; et al. Variation in a repeat sequence determines whether a common variant of the cystic fibrosis transmembrane conductance regulator gene is pathogenic or benign. *Am. J. Hum. Genet.* **2004**, *74*, 176–179. [CrossRef] [PubMed]

67. Thauvin-Robinet, C.; Munck, A.; Huet, F.; Génin, E.; Bellis, G.; Gautier, E.; Audrézet, M.-P.; Férec, C.; Lalau, G.; Des Georges, M.; et al. The very low penetrance of cystic fibrosis for the R117H mutation: A reappraisal for genetic counselling and newborn screening. *J. Med. Genet.* **2009**, *46*, 752–758. [CrossRef] [PubMed]

68. Boussaroque, A.; Audrézet, M.-P.; Raynal, C.; Sermet-Gaudelus, I.; Bienvenu, T.; Férec, C.; Bergougnoux, A.; Lopez, M.; Scotet, V.; Munck, A.; et al. Penetrance is a critical parameter for assessing the disease liability of *CFTR* variants. *J. Cyst. Fibros.* **2020**. [CrossRef] [PubMed]

69. Bieth, E.; Nectoux, J.; Girardet, A.; Gruchy, N.; Mittre, H.; Laurans, M.; Guenet, D.; Brouard, J.; Gerard, M. Genetic counseling for cystic fibrosis: A basic model with new challenges. *Arch. Pédiatrie* **2020**, *27*, eS30–eS34. [CrossRef]

70. Nijmeijer, S.C.M.; Conijn, T.; Lakeman, P.; Henneman, L.; Wijburg, F.A.; Haverman, L. Attitudes of the general population towards preconception expanded carrier screening for autosomal recessive disorders including inborn errors of metabolism. *Mol. Genet. Metab.* **2019**, *126*, 14–22. [CrossRef] [PubMed]

71. Van Steijvoort, E.; Chokoshvili, D.; Cannon, J.W.; Peeters, H.; Peeraer, K.; Matthijs, G.; Borry, P. Interest in expanded carrier screening among individuals and couples in the general population: Systematic review of the literature. *Hum. Reprod. Update* **2020**, *26*, 335–355. [CrossRef]

72. Delatycki, M.B.; Alkuraya, F.; Archibald, A.; Castellani, C.; Cornel, M.; Grody, W.W.; Henneman, L.; Ioannides, A.S.; Kirk, E.; Laing, N.; et al. International perspectives on the implementation of reproductive carrier screening. *Prenat. Diagn.* **2020**, *40*, 301–310. [CrossRef]

73. Bergougnoux, A.; Lopez, M.; Girodon, E. The role of extended *CFTR* gene sequencing in newborn screening for Cystic Fibrosis. *Int. J. Neonatal Screen.* **2020**, *6*, 23. [CrossRef]

74. Farrell, P.M.; Rock, M.J.; Baker, M.W. The impact of the *CFTR* gene discovery on Cystic Fibrosis diagnosis, counseling, and preventive therapy. *Genes* **2020**, *11*, 401. [CrossRef] [PubMed]

75. Ceyhan-Birsoy, O.; Murry, J.B.; Machini, K.; Lebo, M.S.; Yu, T.W.; Fayer, S.; Genetti, C.A.; Schwartz, T.S.; Agrawal, P.B.; Parad, R.B.; et al. Interpretation of genomic sequencing results in healthy and ill newborns: Results from the BabySeq Project. *Am. J. Hum. Genet.* **2019**, *104*, 76–93. [CrossRef]

76. Kingsmore, S.F. Newborn testing and screening by whole-genome sequencing. *Genet. Med.* **2016**, *18*, 214–216. [CrossRef] [PubMed]

77. Wilcken, B.; Wiley, V. Fifty years of newborn screening. *J. Paediatr. Child Health* **2015**, *51*, 103–107. [CrossRef] [PubMed]

78. Cazacu, I.M.; Farkas, N.; Garami, A.; Balaskó, M.; Mosdósi, B.; Alizadeh, H.; Gyöngyi, Z.; Rakonczay, Z.; Vigh, É.; Habon, T.; et al. Pancreatitis-Associated Genes and pancreatic cancer risk: A systematic review and meta-analysis. *Pancreas* **2018**, *47*, 1078–1086. [CrossRef] [PubMed]

79. Farrell, P.; Férec, C.; Macek, M.; Frischer, T.; Renner, S.; Riss, K.; Barton, D.; Repetto, T.; Tzetis, M.; Giteau, K.; et al. Estimating the age of p.(Phe508del) with family studies of geographically distinct European populations and the early spread of cystic fibrosis. *Eur. J. Hum. Genet.* **2018**, *26*, 1832–1839. [CrossRef] [PubMed]

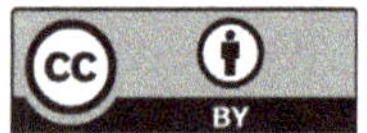

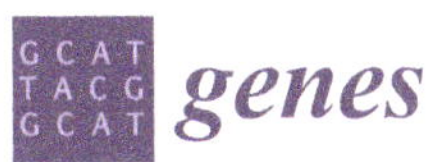 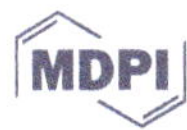

Review

The Changing Epidemiology of Cystic Fibrosis: Incidence, Survival and Impact of the *CFTR* Gene Discovery

Virginie Scotet [1,*], Carine L'Hostis [1] and Claude Férec [1,2]

[1]   Inserm, University of Brest, EFS, UMR 1078, GGB, F-29200 Brest, France; carine_lhostis@hotmail.com (C.L.);
      claude.ferec@univ-brest.fr (C.F.)

[2]   Department of Molecular Genetics, University Hospital of Brest, F-29200 Brest, France

*   Correspondence: virginie.scotet@inserm.fr; Tel.: +33-298017281

Received: 25 April 2020; Accepted: 18 May 2020; Published: 26 May 2020

Abstract: Significant advances in the management of cystic fibrosis (CF) in recent decades have dramatically changed the epidemiology and prognosis of this serious disease, which is no longer an exclusively pediatric disease. This paper aims to review the changes in the incidence and survival of CF and to assess the impact of the discovery of the responsible gene (the *CFTR* gene) on these changes. The incidence of CF appears to be decreasing in most countries and patient survival, which can be monitored by various indicators, has improved substantially, with an estimated median age of survival of approximately50 years today. Cloning of the *CFTR* gene 30 years ago and efforts to identify its many mutations have greatly improved the management of CF. Implementation of genetic screening policies has enabled earlier diagnosis (via newborn screening), in addition to prevention within families or in the general population in some areas (via prenatal diagnosis, family testing or population carrier screening). In the past decade, in-depth knowledge of the molecular bases of CF has also enabled the emergence of CFTR modulator therapies which have led to major clinical advances in the treatment of CF. All of these phenomena have contributed to changing the face of CF. The advent of targeted therapies has paved the way for precision medicine and is expected to further improve survival in the coming years.

Keywords: cystic fibrosis; *CFTR* gene; incidence; survival; genotype-phenotype correlations; health policies; newborn screening; CFTR modulators

---

1. Introduction

Cystic fibrosis (CF) has traditionally been defined as the most common life-threatening inherited disorder of children in Caucasian populations, with an incidence of 1/2500 live births [1]. This definition is no longer appropriate today. Although CF remains a serious disorder, advances in the treatment and management of the disease have remarkably changed the characteristics of the CF population [2–7].

Epidemiological changes have occurred both in the incidence of CF, which seems to be decreasing in most countries, and in the survival of CF patients, which has greatly improved in recent decades [4–8]. When CF was first described by Dorothy H. Anderson in 1938 [9], the patients usually died in their first year of life. Nowadays, the proportion of adult patients exceeds that of children in developed countries and the estimated median age of survival is close to 50 years [10–12], which means that half of the babies born today with CF may expect to survive into their fifth decade. From an exclusively pediatric disease, CF has gradually also become a disease of the adult, with new associated pathologies to be managed. Such epidemiological changes can be tracked by reliable tools such as CF patient registries, which monitor the demographical and clinical characteristics of the CF population.

The discovery of the gene responsible for CF—the *CFTR* gene—30 years ago [13–15] marked an important milestone in the history of CF. It has upset our knowledge of the pathophysiology of the disease, contributed to improving the diagnosis and treatment of CF patients and paved the way for novel therapeutic approaches and the advent of targeted therapies [16]. This discovery has contributed and will continue to contribute to the epidemiological changes observed in CF, through the implementation of genetic-based health policies that allow early diagnosis or prevention within families and/or populations, and the emergence of CFTR modulator therapies [17].

This paper reviews the changes that have occurred in the epidemiology of CF, focusing on incidence and survival, and reports the impact of the discovery of the *CFTR* gene on these changes.

2. The Incidence of Cystic Fibrosis

2.1. Estimates of the Incidence of CF Worldwide

The incidence of CF has traditionally been estimated at 1/2500 live births in a populations of European descent [1]. However, data from newborn screening (NBS) programs for CF reveal that the incidence appears to be lower than in the past. Today, the incidence of CF is estimated, on average, between 1/3000 and 1/6000 in such populations [18,19], which corresponds to carrier rates of 1/28 and 1/40, respectively.

Previously, the incidence of CF was generally estimated from epidemiological studies, which may have been biased by under diagnosis and/or underreporting of cases. Incidence estimates have become more reliable since the implementation of NBS for CF, which has rapidly expanded worldwide in the last decade [19]. The complete registration of cases at birth has led to an accurate measurement of the incidence and better monitoring of its time trends. Nevertheless, even with NBS data, it remains of upmost importance to ensure that studies include the same type of patients when comparing incidence data between countries (such as inclusion or not of false negatives and of patients with meconium ileus).

In a very recent paper describing why NBS for CF is worthwhile, we reviewed the latest data on the incidence of CF worldwide [19]. In Europe, the incidence ranges from 1/1353 in Ireland [20] to 1/25,000 in Finland [21] and is on average 1/4500 in Western Europe [22–24] and 1/6000 in Northern and Central Europe [25–27]. In Australasia, where a NBS program has been implemented for a long time, the incidence is well established and is on average 1/3000 [28]. The incidence is also approximately1/3300 in Canada [29] and 1/4000 in the USA, where large ethnical variations are observed [30,31].

Very high incidences of CF, probably due to genetic drift and founding effects, have been reported in small isolated populations, such as in the Amish population in Ohio (1/569) [32] or in Saguenay-Lac-Saint-Jean in Quebec (1/902) [33].

The disease is much rarer in other parts of the world. In Latin and South America, the incidence of CF remains difficult to estimate in most countries due to the lack of registries and NBS programs as well as the high ethnic admixture of the population. The average incidence seems to be approximately1/8000 to 1/10,000, ranging from 1/6100 in Argentina to 1/15,000 in Costa Rica [19]. In Asian populations, the existence of CF is now better established, but the incidence remains underestimated in most countries. It appears higher in the Middle East (where consanguinity is common) than in East Asia. The incidence ranges from 1/2560 in Jordan [34] to 1/350,000 in Japan [35] and is estimated between 1/10,000 and 1/100,000 in the Indian population [36,37]. Few data are available in African populations [38].

2.2. Time Trends in the Incidence of CF

Time trends in the incidence of CF have been investigated in several studies, most of which reported a decline [23,39–43] but not all [44,45]. This was the case for example in two American states: in Colorado which observed no decline in incidence over a 24 year period (1983–2006) [44] and in Wisconsin, which analyzed time trends over an 18 year period (1994–2011) and even observed a trending (but not significant) increase in incidence in recent years (in different genotype groups and in all ethnic groups) [45]. In Brittany (western France), we analyzed time trends in the incidence of CF over a 35 year period and observed a significant decline (from 1/1983 in the late 1970s to 1/3268 over the 2005–2009 period) but also a clear breakpoint at the end of the 1980s, which seemed consecutive to the availability of prenatal diagnosis [42].

The temporal trends observed in incidence result from the combination of many factors. They stem from demographic changes (such as larger population admixtures, decreasing consanguinity, and decreasing fertility rates), from implementation of genetic-based health policies allowing prevention within families or populations (such as prenatal diagnosis, genetic preimplantation diagnosis, family testing, prenatal screening, and population carrier screening), but also from cultural behaviors toward use of genetic testing, prenatal diagnosis and pregnancy terminations. The causes of the changes observed in incidence therefore vary by region and by population. Our team has shown that CF health policies implemented in Brittany have reduced the incidence of CF by approximately one-third over the study period [42,46].

The greatest declines in the incidence of CF have been observed in areas where prenatal screening or population carrier screening (aiming at identifying all the couples with a one-in-four risk of having a CF child in a population) is underway [23,39,40,43]. For example, in Massachusetts (USA), where NBS for CF was implemented in 1999, Hale et al. reported a significant decrease in the number of screened CF patients since the publication of the US recommendations for population carrier screening in 2003 [39]. The authors also observed a change in the structure of the screened cohort, with a lower proportion of p.Phe508del homozygous patients. An Italian study, which analyzed time trends in the incidence of CF in the Veneto/Trentino Alto Adige area over a 21 year period (1993–2013), also observed a significant decline in incidence that was higher (~35%) in the eastern part of the area where population carrier screening is underway [23,40]. Similarly, Stafler et al. analyzed the impact of population carrier screening on the incidence of CF in Israel [43]. This country, which has not set up a NBS program for CF but which initiated population carrier screening in 1999, observed a marked decline in the incidence of CF (~60%) over a 22 year period.

However, comparison of time trends in incidence between areas remains complex due to variability in study periods but also in public health policies that are implemented in those areas.

3. The Survival of Cystic Fibrosis Patients

3.1. The Changing Face of CF

Prognosis of CF patients has greatly improved in recent decades. One of the most striking evidences of this change is the substantial growth in the proportion of adult patients, which currently exceeds 50% in most countries, and even 60% in Canada (Table 1) [10–12,47–51]. In this country, the proportion of adult patients has more than doubled in 35 years, increasing from 29.5% in 1984 to 61.5% in 2018 [12]. This growth should continue, as illustrated by a study based on the European CF Registry, which predicted that the number of adult patients living with CF in Europe was expected to increase by 75% between 2010 and 2025 [52].

Cystic fibrosis, long qualified as a pediatric disease, has also gradually become a disease of the adult. The transition to adult care center is now a key step for patients and their family, and new elements have to be taken into account in disease management, such as employability, desire for married life, and parenthood [53]. The number of pregnancies and paternities identified in CF patients has therefore progressively increased and one of the challenges is now to assess the safety of CFTR modulator therapies in pregnancy and breastfeeding [54,55]. As a result of the changing epidemiology, a growing number of studies has also been devoted to patients who reach the age of 40 [56,57]. These "long survivors" now represent 11.9% of the CF population in France and 15.9% in Canada (Table 1). This population, which includes patients carrying mild genotypes but also patients diagnosed in adulthood, is particularly interesting for identifying the predictors of better survival [58].

Table 1. Characteristics of the cystic fibrosis (CF) population and survival estimates presented in various CF registry annual data reports.

CF Registry [ref]	Year	Patients	Median Age	Age ≥ 18 y.	Age ≥ 40 y.	Median Age at Death	Median Age of Survival
		n	y.	%	%	y.	y.
Australia [48]	2017	3151	19.6	53.7%	-	35.6	-
Belgium [49]	2016	1275	22.5	61.2%	-	-	-
Canada [10]	2018	4370	23.5	61.5%	15.9%	33.0	52.1
ECFS [50]	2017	48204	18.5	51.3%	-	29.0	-
France [51]	2017	7114	20.3	55.9%	11.9%	33.8	-
Ireland [52]	2018	1239	20.9	58.5%	11.3%	33.0	44.4
UK [11]	2018	10509	20.0	54.7%	-	32.0	47.3
USA [12]	2018	30775	19.8	54.6%	-	30.8	47.4

This table only presents data from the CF registries for which at least two of the indicators of interest were available. ECFS: CF Registry of the European Cystic Fibrosis Society. y.: years.

Many factors are responsible for these major advances such as standardization of care, with management of patients in specialized centers by multidisciplinary teams, better control of pulmonary infection with the development of new inhaled therapies, better control of *Pseudomonas aeruginosa* colonization, aggressive nutritional supplementation with pancreatic enzymes, early diagnosis through newborn screening, and lung transplantation [5].

Providing up-to-date estimates of survival is crucial for advising patients and their families on life expectancy, planning health care needs and guiding the development of new therapies.

3.2. Better Understanding of Survival Indicators

For many years, changes in prognosis of CF were described by monitoring the proportion of adult patients, the death rates or the median age at death. This last metric, which informs on the distribution of the age of patients at time of their death, is not a survival metric as it does not consider the patients who survived.

Nowadays, time trends in survival can be monitored by additional metrics such as survival probabilities by birth cohort, the estimated median age of survival(also called the predicted median survival age) and the estimated median age of survival conditional on living to a given age (see below). It should be noted that life expectancy, which is often misused in CF, is almost never estimated.

There are several ways to estimate survival in CF and the terminology used in that field is complex and often confusing for patients and their families, but also for the medical community. It is, however, crucial for clinicians to understand the difference between the various metrics, so that they can provide appropriate information to patients. A very comprehensive guide has recently been published by Keogh and Stanojevic [59] in order to facilitate the interpretation of the estimated median age of survival in CF and to standardize the presentation of survival data in CF patient registry reports. One other paper by Sykes et al. explains very well the three methods for estimating survival [60]. Briefly, these methods are:

(1) The birth cohort approach, which is a longitudinal method that consists of following one or several birth cohorts and registering all the deaths that occur in those cohorts over time. This method, which requires time, draws for each birth cohort a Kaplan–Meier survival curve, which looks like a staircase curve that goes down at each death. This enables determination of the median survival when 50% of the patients of the cohort have died.

(2) The period approach, which is a cross-sectional method that is commonly used by registries. It analyzes the structure of the CF population present in a registry on a specified period (usually a 5 year window; for example, the period 2014–2018) and estimates a survival curve by applying the age-specific mortality rates observed among those prevalent cases to a fictive cohort. This method estimates the median age of survival from birth, which corresponds to the age

beyond which half of the babies born today with CF are expected to live. This approach assumes that death rates remain unchanged over time (which is not true) and requires large samples.

(3) The conditional survival approach, which was applied recently in CF [61]. As the estimated median age of survival only applies to babies born today and as some patients have already surpassed the estimated age, another metric has been proposed recently: the estimated median age of survival conditional to surviving to a given age (for example, age of 30 or 40). This metric represents the age at which 50% of the patients who have already survived to the given age are expected to live. It is more relevant for CF patients and is higher than the estimate from birth. Keogh et al. showed, using data from the UK CF Registry, that in p.Phe508del homozygous patients, the estimated median age of survival from birth was 46 years in males and 41 years in females, whereas the estimated median age of survival conditional on surviving to 30 was 6 and 8 years higher, respectively [61].

The prerequisite for a quality survival analysis is to have a well-defined study population with complete registration of CF cases and deaths. Comparisons of survival data between countries require standardization in data processing and analysis.

3.3. Current Survival Estimates in CF

National CF registries are valuable tools for performing quality survival analyzes and have been instrumental in demonstrating improved survival. Examination of the annual CF registry reports shows, however, that the presentation of survival data is not homogeneous [10–12,47–51]. To date, all CF registries show the median age at death, which may be supplemented by a graph representing the distribution of ages at death or the time trends in this median age at death. Four registries (the Canadian, Irish, UK and US ones) determine the estimated median age of survival based on the period approach. The French and Canadian registries show survival probabilities by birth cohort, while the US registry also presents two other metrics: a graph representing the estimates of conditional survival at specific ages (up to 40 years) and another one illustrating time trends in annual mortality rates.

Longitudinal monitoring of registry data shows that the median age at death and the estimated median age of survival continue to increase gradually, while mortality rates decrease. When CF was described for the first time in 1938 [9], patients with CF usually died in their first year of life. In the 1960s, they rarely survived beyond the age of five. The most recent CF registry data (2017 or 2018 annual reports) show that the median age at death ranges from 29.0 years (ECFS registry) to 35.6 years (Australian registry) (Table 1). The estimated median age of survival, which is determined by four registries, is currently 44.4 years in Ireland, 47.3 years in the UK, 47.4 years in the USA and 52.1 years in Canada (Table 1). This metrics has increased by more than 15 years in 30 years in the USA [12]. Regarding conditional survival analysis, the US registry report shows that the estimated median age of survival is close to 55 years for patients who reach the age of 30, and exceeds 60 years for patients who reach the age of 40 [12].

3.4. Prognostic Factors

Although survival estimate has greatly improved globally, it continues to be impacted by various individual factors. Beyond the main predictor of worse survival that is lung function ($FEV_1 < 30\%$ predicted) [62], other factors have been associated with reduced survival such as female sex, higher age at diagnosis, severe *CFTR* genotype, ethnic background, lower socio-economic status, worse nutritional status, pancreatic insufficiency, early colonization with *Pseudomonas aeruginosa*, and presence of diabetes [5]. Prognostic scores based on various variables have thus been developed to predict the risk of death or the risk of lung transplantation [63–66].

Two other factors should have a major impact on the survival of CF, which will have to be measured precisely in the coming years: the expanding implementation of NBS for CF and the emergence of targeted therapies.

3.5. New Statistical Developments and Future Trends in Survival

A survey that was recently carried out to decipher how CF patients access and use information on life expectancy shows that most respondents wanted more personalized survival data [67]. Mathematical developments are therefore underway in order to further improve the modeling of survival by providing personalized estimates. One of the challenges is to develop models based on longitudinal data that are able to consider the current health status of the patients (and not only their baseline characteristics). A dynamic predictive model providing personalized estimates of survival was recently developed using data from the UK CF Registry [68]. This model, which integrates 16 predictors, is able to predict survival up to 10 years for patients up to 50 years of age.

The estimated median age of survival of CF patients, which is close to 50 years today, is expected to continue to improve in the future, with the rapid expanding of NBS for CF worldwide over the past decade and with the recent advent of CFTR modulator therapies. Further work is needed to assess the effect of these factors on the survival of CF. Some studies have suggested that NBS for CF results in a prolonged survival, but few are yet able to assess its long-term effects. The studies performed in that field are presented in the next section.

The increase in survival estimates undeniably changes the population's perception of the disease and leads to ethical reflection on the decisions to be made by couples when CF is diagnosed before birth.

4. The Impact of the Discovery of the *CFTR* Gene on the Epidemiology of the Disease

The discovery of the *CFTR* gene in 1989 marked an important milestone in the history of CF and raised tremendous hope in the medical and scientific community. An exemplary collaboration involving more than 100 laboratories worldwide and carried out through an international consortium for the study of the gene mutations (Cystic Fibrosis Genetic Analysis Consortium) has led to the identification of more than 2000 different *CFTR* mutations to date [69]. The molecular exploration of this gene has enabled a better understanding of the genotype/phenotype correlations, improved the diagnosis and the management of CF patients and their families, and opened up the way to the emergence of mutation-specific therapies, which contribute to modify the epidemiology of CF [16,17]. In a very comprehensive article published in this special issue of *Genes*, Farrell et al. reviews the "impact of the *CFTR* gene discovery on CF diagnosis, genetic counseling and preventive therapy" [16].

4.1. Study of Genotype/Phenotype Correlations

The growing number of mutations identified in the *CFTR* gene and the variability observed in the phenotypic expression of CF have led the researchers to try to establish genotype/phenotype correlations [70,71].

Quickly after the gene discovery, the *CFTR* mutations could be classified into six classes according to their impact on the level of protein function [72]. Schematically, mutations in classes I, II, and III are usually associated with a classical form of CF (severe mutations), while those in classes IV, V, and VI are related to a milder phenotype (mild mutations) characterized by pancreatic sufficiency and later bacterial colonization. The estimated median age of survival of patients carrying at least one mild mutation is generally ten years higher than that of patients with severe mutations.

Various tools are available to help identify the clinical impact of a *CFTR* variant: (1) international mutations databases such as the Cystic Fibrosis Mutation Database (http://www.genet.sickkids.on.ca/), CFTR2 database (https://cftr2.org/) or UMD-CFTR database (http://www.umd.be/CFTR/); (2) CF registries, which may assist genetic counseling by providing aggregated clinical data associated with a given genotype; (3) bioinformatics prediction tools such as Polyphen or SIFT applications.

Despite these tools, it often remains difficult to predict with certainty the phenotype of a given genotype, and it quickly became obvious that the *CFTR* genotype could not explain all the phenotypic variability observed in CF, in particular in lung damage. Further research has been undertaken to identify other factors that influence the severity of the disease, including gene modifiers (such as genes involved in the immune response or in inflammation) [73,74], epigenetic factors and environmental factors (such as tobacco, pollution, socio-economic status, and adherence to therapies) [75].

The study of genotype/phenotype correlations also highlighted the existence of conditions associated with CFTR dysfunction that do not fulfill diagnostic criteria for CF. Those disorders, called *CFTR*-related disorders (*CFTR*-RDs) [76], include congenital bilateral absence of vas deferens, acute recurrent or chronic pancreatitis and disseminated bronchiectasis. Inclusion of patients with such conditions in epidemiological studies dealing with incidence or survival of CF can bias the estimates and the time trends.

4.2. Implementation of Genetic-Based Health Policies

In-depth knowledge of the molecular abnormalities of the *CFTR* gene [77] has enabled genetic screening policies to be implemented, allowing prevention within families (such as prenatal diagnosis for one-in-four at-risk couples or carrier testing in families) or in the general population in some areas (such as population carrier screening). As mentioned above, these health policies have contributed to reducing—in most countries and with varying degrees of importance—the incidence of CF through the identification of cases before birth [23,39–43,46].

The discovery of the *CFTR* gene has also increased the performance of NBS for CF by introducing DNA analysis into the screening protocol, and thus improved the diagnosis and management of CF [16,78,79]. The coupling of the immunereactive trypsinogen assay to the search for *CFTR* mutations has eliminated the need for a second blood sample. This has reduced the anxiety generated in families, leading to an earlier diagnosis and early access to specialized care centers, which prevents malnutrition and lung damage [80]. The positive effects of NBS for CF on short-term and long-term clinical outcomes are widely recognized [80–83] and include better nutritional status, lower pancreatic insufficiency, better lung function, lower infection rates, fewer and shorter hospitalizations. Some studies have shown that NBS for CF results in prolonged survival [84–86], but it is still too early for most countries to assess its long-term impact on survival. This could recently be measured in an Italian area in which NBS for CF has been running for over 40 years [87]. Tridello et al. reported a significantly higher survival probability at 20 years in the screened than in the non-screened group, both in patients with severe (84.9% vs. 63.6%; difference: 21.3%; $p = 0.007$) and moderate disease (94.5% vs. 85.9%; difference: 8.6%; $p = 0.016$). A 9% difference was also observed in the survival probability at 30 years (80.1% vs. 71.0%) but was not significant [87]. Through early diagnosis, NBS for CF maximizes survival in severe CF. The expanding of NBS worldwide in the past decade will inevitably continue to impact survival in the future.

4.3. Advent of CFTR Modulator Therapies

Deciphering of the molecular bases of CF has also led to the development of novel therapeutic approaches and the search for pharmaceutical treatments aiming at correcting the defective CFTR protein. These drugs, called CFTR modulators, search to improve the production, processing or expression of the protein and include correctors, potentiators, stabilizers, amplifiers and read through agents [88,89]. This approach is said to be "targeted" or "mutation specific" because the type of molecules to be administered to patients depends on the type of *CFTR* mutations they carry. Many studies have been carried out in that field over the past decade and have led to major clinical advances in treatment, with significant improvements in biological and clinical endpoints of CF (as sweat chloride concentration orFEV_1) [90].

It was almost 25 years after the discovery of the *CFTR* gene that the first CFTR modulator (ivacaftor—Kalydeco®) could be marketed. This potentialtor was approved in 2012 for the treatment of CF patients aged ≥6 years carrying at least one G551D mutation [91]. This treatment was associated with significant improvements at day 28 in sweat chloride level, nasal potential difference and lung function (median increase of 8.7 points in the percentage of predicted FEV_1). In 2015, the combination of ivacaftor with a corrector (lumacaftor/ivacaftor—Orkambi®) was then approved for patients aged ≥12 years who were p.Phe508del homozygous [92]. This combination significantly increased the percentage of predicted FEV_1 (from 2.6 to 4.0 points) and was associated with a lower rate of pulmonary exacerbations, hospitalizations and use of intravenous antibiotics. In 2018, a second dual combination (tezacaftor/ivacaftor—Symdeko®) appeared [93] and, very recently, a triple combination therapy (elexacaftor/tezacaftor/ivacaftor–Trikafta™) was approved for the treatment of patients aged ≥12 years carrying at least one p.Phe508del mutation [94]. This very promising therapy resulted in an increase up to 14 points in the percentage of predicted FEV_1 but also in significant improvements in sweat chloride concentration, pulmonary exacerbations and quality of life.

While there is variability in response, the targeted therapies are transforming the life of CF patients and their advent is expected to further improve patient survival in the coming years. As these molecules have only been marketed since 2012, it is too early to assess their impact on patient survival. This is why an American team has recently sought to model, through simulations based on data from the US CF Registry, the long-term health outcomes of CF patients treated with the lumacaftor/ivacaftor combination [95]. This treatment is predicted to increase the estimated median age of survival of p.Phe508del homozygous patients by 6.1 years. The increment in survival is further improved by the initiation of treatment at an early age and the persistence of treatment (an increment of 17.7 years if the treatment is started at age 6 and of 3.8 years if it is started at age 25).

Over the past decade, the treatment of CF has therefore shifted from a therapy treating the symptoms to a therapy that also restores the function of the CFTR protein. These targeted therapies have expanded the field of personalized or precision medicine [89].

5. Conclusions

The epidemiological profile of CF has changed considerably in recent decades. This disease is no longer the most common serious illness in children but is now also a serious genetic disease among adults. Today, more than half of the patients are adults and patient survival has substantially increased with an estimated median age of survival close to 50 years today. The incidence of CF appears to be declining in most regions. The discovery of the *CFTR* gene in 1989 upset our knowledge of the pathophysiology of the disease. It has made it possible to better understand phenotypic variability through studies of genotype/phenotype correlations and has led to significant progress in the diagnosis and management of CF patients and their families. It also paved the way for pharmacology work and CFTR modulator therapies have been marketed for 10 years. Such treatments are revolutionizing the treatment of CF and transforming the life of CF patients. All these phenomena have contributed to changing the epidemiology of CF. The advent of targeted therapies is expected to further improve patient survival in the future. Efforts must nevertheless continue to find other efficient drugs, optimize treatment adherence and promote equitable access to these therapies.

Author Contributions: Writing—original draft preparation, V.S.; writing—review and editing, V.S., C.L. and C.F. All authors have read and agreed to the published version of the manuscript.

Acknowledgments: V.S. is supported by the French Institute of Health and Medical Research (Inserm). The authors are grateful to the national cystic fibrosis registries, data from which were very useful for carrying out this review.

References

1.   Welsh, M.; Ramsey, B.W.; Accurso, F.J.; Cutting, G.R. Cystic fibrosis. In *The Metabolic and Molecular Basis of Inherited Disease*, 8th ed.; Scriver, C.R., Beaudet, A.L., Sly, W.S., Valle, D., Childs, B., Vogelstein, B., Eds.; McGraw Hill: New York, NY, USA, 2001; pp. 5121–5188.
2.   Bell, S.C.; Mall, M.A.; Gutierrez, H.; Macek, M.; Madge, M.; Davies, J.C.; Burgel, P.R.; Tullis, E.; Castanos, C.; Castellani, C.; et al. The Future of Cystic Fibrosis Care: A Global Perspective. *Lancet Respir. Med.* **2020**, *8*, 65–124. [CrossRef]

3.	Dodge, J.A.; Lewis, P.A. Cystic fibrosis is no longer an important cause of childhood death in the UK. *Arch. Dis. Child.* **2005**, *90*, 547.

4.	Fajac, I.; Burgel, P.R. Demographic growth and targeted therapies: The changing face of cystic fibrosis. *Rev. Mal. Respir.* **2016**, *33*, 645–647. [CrossRef] [PubMed]

5.	Stephenson, A.L.; Stanojevic, S.; Sykes, J.; Burgel, P.R. The changing epidemiology and demography of cystic fibrosis. *Presse Med.* **2017**, *46*, e87–e95. [CrossRef]

6.	Corriveau, S.; Sykes, J.; Stephenson, A.L. Cystic fibrosis survival: The changing epidemiology. *Curr. Opin. Pulm. Med.* **2018**, *24*, 574–578. [CrossRef] [PubMed]

7.	De Boeck, K. Cystic fibrosis in the year 2020: A disease with a new face. *Acta Paediatr.* **2020**, in press. [CrossRef] [PubMed]

8.	Stephenson, A.L.; Tom, M.; Berthiaume, Y.; Singer, L.G.; Aaron, S.D.; Whitmore, G.A.; Stanojevic, S. A contemporary survival analysis of individuals with cystic fibrosis: A cohort study. *Eur. Respir. J.* **2015**, *45*, 670–679. [CrossRef] [PubMed]

9.	Anderson, D.H. Cystic fibrosis of the pancreas and its relation to celiac disease. A clinical and pathologic study. *Am. J. Dis. Child.* **1938**, *56*, 344–399. [CrossRef]

10.	Canadian Cystic Fibrosis Registry. Annual Data Report 2018. Available online: https://www.cysticfibrosis.ca /uploads/RegistryReport2018/2018RegistryAnnualDataReport.pdf (accessed on 20 April 2020).

11.	UK Cystic Fibrosis Registry (Cystic Fibrosis Trust). Annual Data Report 2018. Available online: https://www.cysticfi brosis.org.uk/~{}/media/documents/the-work-we-do/uk-cf-registry/2018-registry-annual-data-report.ashx?la=en (accessed on 20 April 2020).

12.	US Cystic Fibrosis Registry (Cystic Fibrosis Foundation). Annual Data Report 2018. Available online: https: //www.cff.org/Research/Researcher-Resources/Patient-Registry/2018-Patient-Registry-Annual-Data-Report.pdf (accessed on 20 April 2020).

13.	Rommens, J.M.; Iannuzzi, M.C.; Kerem, B.; Drumm, M.L.; Melmer, G.; Dean, M.; Rozmahel, R.; Cole, J.L.; Kennedy, D.; Hidaka, N.; et al. Identification of the cystic fibrosis gene: Chromosome walking and jumping. *Science* **1989**, *245*, 1059–1065. [CrossRef]

14.	Riordan, J.R.; Rommens, J.M.; Kerem, B.; Alon, N.; Rozmahel, R.; Grzelczak, Z.; Zielenski, J.; Lok, S.; Plavsic, N.; Chou, J.L.; et al. Identification of the cystic fibrosis gene: Cloning and characterization of complementary DNA. *Science* **1989**, *245*, 1066–1073. [CrossRef]

15.	Kerem, B.; Rommens, J.M.; Buchanan, J.A.; Markiewicz, D.; Cox, T.K.; Chakravarti, A.; Buchwald, M.; Tsui, L.C. Identification of the cystic fibrosis gene: Genetic analysis. *Science* **1989**, *245*, 1073–1080. [CrossRef] [PubMed]

16.	Farrell, P.M.; Rock, M.J.; Baker, M.W. The Impact of the CFTR Gene Discovery on Cystic Fibrosis Diagnosis, Counseling, and Preventive Therapy. *Genes* **2020**, *11*, 401. [CrossRef]

17.	Férec, C.; Scotet, V. Genetics ofcystic fibrosis: Basics. *Arch. Pediatr.* **2020**, *27* (Suppl. 1), eS4–eS7.

18.	Southern, K.W.; Munck, A.; Pollitt, R.; Travert, G.; Zanolla, L.; Dankert-Roelse, J.; Castellani, C.; ECFS CF Neonatal Screening Working Group. A survey of newborn screening for cystic fibrosis in Europe. *J. Cyst. Fibros.* **2007**, *6*, 57–65. [CrossRef] [PubMed]

19.	Scotet, V.; Gutierrez, H.; Farrell, P.M. Newborn screening for CF across the globe —Where is it worthwhile? *Int. J. Neonatal Screen.* **2020**, *6*, 18. [CrossRef]

20.	Farrell, P.M.; Joffe, S.; Foley, L.; Canny, G.J.; Mayne, P.; Rosenberg, M. Diagnosis of cystic fibrosis in the Republic of Ireland: Epidemiology and costs. *Ir. Med. J.* **2007**, *100*, 557–560.

21.	Kere, J.; Estivill, X.; Chillon, M.; Morral, N.; Nunes, V.; Norio, R.; Savilahti, E.; de la Chapelle, A. Cystic fibrosis in a low-incidence population: Two major mutations in Finland. *Hum. Genet.* **1994**, *93*, 162–166. [CrossRef]

22.	Audrézet, M.P.; Munck, A.; Scotet, V.; Claustres, M.; Roussey, M.; Delmas, D.; Férec, C.; Desgeorges, M. Comprehensive CFTR gene analysis of the French cystic fibrosis screened newborn cohort: Implications for diagnosis, genetic counseling, and mutation-specific therapy. *Genet. Med.* **2015**, *17*, 108–116. [CrossRef]

23.	Castellani, C.; Picci, L.; Tridello, G.; Casati, E.; Tamanini, A.; Bartoloni, L.; Scarpa, M.; Assael, B.M.; Veneto CF Lab Network. Cystic fibrosis carrier screening effects on birth prevalence and newborn screening. *Genet. Med.* **2016**, *18*, 145–151. [CrossRef]

24.	Dankert-Roelse, J.E.; Bouva, M.J.; Jakobs, B.S.; Janssens, H.M.; de Winter-de Groot, K.M.; Schonbeck, Y.; Gille, J.J.P.; Gulmans, V.A.M.; Verschoof-Puite, R.K.; Schielen, P.; et al. Newborn blood spot screening for cystic fibrosis with a four-step screening strategy in the Netherlands. *J. Cyst. Fibros.* **2019**, *18*, 54–63. [CrossRef]

25. Skov, M.; Baekvad-Hansen, M.; Hougaard, D.M.; Skogstrand, K.; Lund, A.M.; Pressler, T.; Olesen, H.V.; Duno, M. Cystic fibrosis newborn screening in Denmark: Experience from the first 2 years. *Pediatr. Pulmonol.* **2020**, *55*, 549–555. [CrossRef] [PubMed]

26. Soltysova, A.; Tothova Tarova, E.; Ficek, A.; Baldovic, M.; Polakova, H.; Kayserova, H.; Kadasi, L. Comprehensive genetic study of cystic fibrosis in Slovak patients in 25 years of genetic diagnostics. *Clin. Respir. J.* **2018**, *12*, 1197–1206. [CrossRef] [PubMed]

27. David, J.; Chrastina, P.; Peskova, K.; Kozich, V.; Friedecky, D.; Adam, T.; Hlidkova, E.; Vinohradska, H.; Novotna, D.; Hedelova, M.; et al. Epidemiology of rare diseases detected by newborn screening in the Czech Republic. *Cent. Eur. J. Public Health* **2019**, *27*, 153–159. [CrossRef] [PubMed]

28. Massie, R.J.; Curnow, L.; Glazner, J.; Armstrong, D.S.; Francis, I. Lessons learned from 20 years of newborn screening for cystic fibrosis. *Med. J. Aust.* **2012**, *196*, 67–70. [CrossRef]

29. Lilley, M.; Christian, S.; Hume, S.; Scott, P.; Montgomery, M.; Semple, L.; Zuberbuhler, P.; Tabak, J.; Bamforth, F.; Somerville, M.J. Newborn screening forcystic fibrosisin Alberta: Two years of experience. *Paediatr. Child. Health* **2010**, *15*, 590–594. [CrossRef]

30. Kosorok, M.R.; Wei, W.H.; Farrell, P.M. The incidence ofcystic fibrosis. *Stat. Med.* **1996**, *15*, 449–462. [CrossRef]

31. Sullivan, B.P.; Freedman, S.D. Cystic fibrosis. *Lancet* **2009**, *373*, 1891–1904. [CrossRef]

32. Klinger, K.W. Cystic fibrosisin the OhioAmish: Gene frequency and founder effect. *Hum. Genet.* **1983**, *65*, 94–98. [CrossRef]

33. Daigneault, J.; Aubin, G.; Simard, F.; De Braekeleer, M. Genetic epidemiology of cystic fibrosis in Saguenay-Lac-St-Jean (Quebec, Canada). *Clin. Genet.* **1991**, *40*, 298–303. [CrossRef]

34. Nazer, H.M. Early diagnosis of cystic fibrosis in Jordanian children. *J. Trop. Pediatr.* **1992**, *38*, 113–115. [CrossRef]

35. Yamashiro, Y.; Shimizu, T.; Oguchi, S.; Shioya, T.; Nagata, S.; Ohtsuka, Y. The estimated incidence of cystic fibrosis in Japan. *J. Pediatr. Gastroenterol. Nutr.* **1997**, *24*, 544–547. [CrossRef] [PubMed]

36. Goodchild, M.C.; Insley, J.; Rushton, D.I.; Gaze, H. Cystic fibrosisin 3 Pakistani children. *Arch. Dis. Child.* **1974**, *49*, 739–741. [CrossRef] [PubMed]

37. Kapoor, V.; Shastri, S.S.; Kabra, M.; Kabra, S.K.; Ramachandran, V.; Arora, S.; Balakrishnan, P.; Deorari, A.K.; Paul, V.K. Carrier frequency of F508del mutation of cystic fibrosis in Indian population. *J. Cyst. Fibros.* **2006**, *5*, 43–46. [CrossRef] [PubMed]

38. Kwarteng Owusu, S.; Morrow, B.M.; White, D.; Klugman, S.; Vanker, A.; Gray, D.; Zampoli, M. Cystic Fibrosis in Black African Children in South Africa: A Case Control Study. *J. Cyst. Fibros.* **2019**. [CrossRef]

39. Hale, J.E.; Parad, R.B.; Comeau, A.M. Newborn screening showing decreasing incidence of cystic fibrosis. *N. Engl. J. Med.* **2008**, *358*, 973–974. [CrossRef]

40. Castellani, C.; Picci, L.; Tamanini, A.; Girardi, P.; Rizzotti, P.; Assael, B.M. Association between carrier screening and incidence of cystic fibrosis. *JAMA* **2009**, *302*, 2573–2579. [CrossRef]

41. Massie, J.; Curnow, L.; Gaffney, L.; Carlin, J.; Francis, I. Declining prevalence of cystic fibrosis since the introduction of newborn screening. *Arch. Dis. Child.* **2010**, *95*, 531–533. [CrossRef]

42. Scotet, V.; Duguépéroux, I.; Saliou, P.; Rault, G.; Roussey, M.; Audrézet, M.P.; Férec, C. Evidence for decline in the incidence of cystic fibrosis: A 35-year observational study in Brittany, France. *Orphanet J. Rare Dis.* **2012**, *7*, 14. [CrossRef]

43. Stafler, P.; Mei-Zahav, M.; Wilschanski, M.; Mussaffi, H.; Efrati, O.; Lavie, M.; Shoseyov, D.; Cohen-Cymberknoh, M.; Gur, M.; Bentur, L.; et al. The impact of a national population carrier screening program on cystic fibrosis birth rate and age at diagnosis: Implications for newborn screening. *J. Cyst. Fibros.* **2016**, *15*, 460–466. [CrossRef]

44. Sontag, M.L.; Wagener, J.S.; Accurso, F.; Sager, S.D. Consistent incidence of cystic fibrosis in a long-term newborn screen population. In Proceedings of the 22nd AnnualNorth American Cystic Fibrosis Conference Meeting, Orlando, FL, USA, 23–26 October 2008.

45. Parker-McGill, K.; Nugent, M.; Bersie, R.; Hoffman, G.; Rock, M.; Baker, M.; Farrell, P.M.; Simpson, P.; Levy, H. Changing incidence of cystic fibrosis in Wisconsin, USA. *Pediatr. Pulmonol.* **2015**, *50*, 1065–1072. [CrossRef]

46. Scotet, V.; Audrézet, M.P.; Roussey, M.; Rault, G.; Blayau, M.; De Braekeleer, M.; Férec, C. Impact of public health strategies on the birth prevalence of cystic fibrosis in Brittany, France. *Hum. Genet.* **2003**, *113*, 280–285. [CrossRef] [PubMed]

47. Australian Cystic Fibrosis Registry. Annual Data Report 2017. Available online: https://www.cysticfibrosis.org.au/getmedia/24e94d66-29fa-4e3f-8e65-21ee24ed2e5a/ACFDR-2017-Annual-Report_highres_singles.pdf.aspx (accessed on 20 April 2020).

48. Belgian Cystic Fibrosis Registry. Annual Data Report 2016. Available online: https://www.sciensano.be/sites/www.wiv-isp.be/files/report_belgian_cf_registry_2016_en_final_1.pdf (accessed on 20 April 2020).

49. European (ECFS) Cystic Fibrosis Registry. Annual Data Report 2018. Available online: https://www.ecfs.eu/sites/default/files/general-content-images/working-groups/ecfs-patient-registry/ECFSPR_Report2017_v1.3.pdf (accessed on 20 April 2020).

50. French Cystic Fibrosis Registry. Annual Data Report 2017. Available online: http://www.vaincrelamuco.org/sites/default/files/rapport_du_registre_-_donnees_2017.pdf (accessed on 20 April 2020).

51. Irish Cystic Fibrosis Registry. Annual Data Report 2018. Available online: https://cfri.ie/annual-reports/ (accessed on 20 April 2020).

52. Burgel, P.R.; Bellis, G.; Olesen, H.V.; Viviani, L.; Zolin, A.; Blasi, F.; Elborn, J.S.; ERS/ECFS Task force on provision of care for adults withcystic fibrosisin Europe. Future trends in cystic fibrosis demography in 34 European countries. *Eur. Respir. J.* **2015**, *46*, 133–141. [CrossRef] [PubMed]

53. Coyne, I.; Sheehan, A.M.; Heery, E.; While, A.E. Improvingtransitiontoadulthealthcare for young people withcysticfibrosis: A systematic review. *J. Child. Health Care* **2017**, *21*, 312–330. [CrossRef] [PubMed]

54. Hughan, K.S.; Daley, T.; Rayas, M.S.; Kelly, A.; Roe, A. Female reproductive health in cystic fibrosis. *J. Cyst. Fibros.* **2019**, *18* (Suppl. 2), S95–S104. [CrossRef]

55. Vekaria, S.; Popowicz, N.; White, S.W.; Mulrennan, S.J. To be or not to be on CFTR modulators duringpregnancy: Risks to be considered. *J. Cyst. Fibros.* **2019**, *S1569-1993*, 30983-X.

56. Hodson, M.E.; Simmonds, N.J.; Warwick, W.J.; Tullis, E.; Castellani, C.; Assael, B.; Dodge, J.A.; Corey, M.; International study of aging in cystic fibrosis. An international/multicentre report on patients with cystic fibrosis (CF) over the age of 40 years. *J. Cyst. Fibros.* **2008**, *7*, 537–542. [CrossRef]

57. Nick, J.A.; Chacon, C.S.; Brayshaw, S.J.; Jones, M.C.; Barboa, C.M.; St Clair, C.G.; Young, R.L.; Nichols, D.P.; Janssen, J.S.; Huitt, G.A.; et al. Effects of gender and age at diagnosis on disease progression in long-term survivors of cystic fibrosis. *Am. J. Respir. Crit. Care Med.* **2010**, *182*, 614–626. [CrossRef]

58. Férec, C.; Verlingue, C.; Guillermit, H.; Quéré, I.; Raguénès, O.; Feigelson, J.; Audrézet, M.P.; Moullier, P.; Mercier, B. Genotype Analysis of Adult Cystic Fibrosis Patients. *Hum. Mol. Genet.* **1993**, *2*, 1557–1560. [CrossRef]

59. Keogh, R.H.; Stanojevic, S. A guide to interpreting estimated median age of survival in cystic fibrosispatient registry reports. *J. Cyst. Fibros.* **2018**, *17*, 213–217. [CrossRef]

60. Sykes, J.; Stanojevic, S.; Goss, C.H.; Quon, B.S.; Marshall, B.C.; Petren, K.; Ostrenga, J.; Fink, A.; Elbert, A.; Stephenson, A.L. A standardized approach to estimating survival statistics for population-basedcystic fibrosisregistry cohorts. *J. Clin. Epidemiol.* **2016**, *70*, 206–213. [CrossRef]

61. Keogh, R.H.; Szczesniak, R.; Taylor-Robinson, D.; Bilton, D. Up-to-date and projected estimates of survival for people with cystic fibrosis using baseline characteristics: A longitudinal study using UK patient registry data. *J. Cyst. Fibros.* **2018**, *17*, 218–227. [CrossRef] [PubMed]

62. Kerem, E.; Reisman, J.; Corey, M.; Canny, G.J.; Levison, H. Prediction of mortality in patients with cystic fibrosis. *N. Engl. J. Med.* **1992**, *326*, 1187–1191. [CrossRef] [PubMed]

63. Liou, T.G.; Adler, F.R.; Fitzsimmons, S.C.; Cahill, B.C.; Hibbs, J.R.; Marshall, B.C. Predictive 5-year survivorship model of cystic fibrosis. *Am. J. Epidemiol.* **2001**, *153*, 345–352. [CrossRef] [PubMed]

64. Aaron, S.D.; Stephenson, A.L.; Cameron, D.W.; Whitmore, G.A. A statistical model to predict one-year risk of death in patients with cystic fibrosis. *J. Clin. Epidemiol.* **2015**, *68*, 1336–1345. [CrossRef]

65. Nkam, L.; Lambert, J.; Latouche, A.; Bellis, G.; Burgel, P.R.; Hocine, M.N. A 3-year Prognostic Score for Adults with Cystic Fibrosis. *J. Cyst. Fibros.* **2017**, *16*, 702–708. [CrossRef]

66. Stanojevic, S.; Sykes, J.; Stephenson, A.L.; Aaron, S.D.; Whitmore, G.A. Development and External Validation of 1- And 2-year Mortality Prediction Models in Cystic Fibrosis. *Eur. Respir. J.* **2019**, *54*, 1900224. [CrossRef]

67. Keogh, R.H.; Bilton, D.; Cosgriff, R.; Kavanagh, D.; Rayner, O.; Sedgwick, P.M. Results from an online survey of adults with cystic fibrosis: Accessing and using life expectancy information. *PLoS ONE* **2019**, *14*, e0213639. [CrossRef]

68. Keogh, R.H.; Seaman, S.R.; Barrett, J.K.; Taylor-Robinson, D.; Szczesniak, R. Dynamic Prediction of Survival in Cystic Fibrosis: A Landmarking Analysis Using UK Patient Registry Data. *Epidemiology* **2019**, *30*, 29–37. [CrossRef]

69. Cystic Fibrosis Mutation Database. Available online: http://www.genet.sickkids.on.ca/app (accessed on 20 April 2020).

70. Kerem, E.; Corey, M.; Kerem, B.S.; Rommens, J.; Markiewicz, D.; Levison, H.; Tsui, L.C.; Durie, P. The relation between genotype and phenotype in cystic fibrosis – analysis of the most common mutation (delta F508). *N. Engl. J. Med.* **1990**, *323*, 1517–1522. [CrossRef]

71. The Cystic Fibrosis Genotype-Phenotype Consortium. Correlation between genotype and phenotype in patients with cystic fibrosis. *N. Engl. J. Med.* **1993**, *329*, 1308–1313. [CrossRef]

72. Welsh, M.J.; Smith, A.E. Molecular mechanisms of CFTR chloride channel dysfunction in cystic fibrosis. *Cell* **1993**, *73*, 1251–1254. [CrossRef]

73. Drumm, M.L.; Konstan, M.W.; Schluchter, M.D.; Handler, A.; Pace, R.; Zou, F.; Zariwala, M.; Fargo, D.; Xu, A.; Dunn, J.M.; et al. Genetic modifiers of lung disease in cystic fibrosis. *N. Engl. J. Med.* **2005**, *353*, 1443–1453. [CrossRef] [PubMed]

74. Corvol, H.; Blackman, S.M.; Boelle, P.Y.; Gallins, P.J.; Pace, R.G.; Stonebraker, J.R.; Accurso, F.J.; Clement, A.; Collaco, J.M.; Dang, H.; et al. Genome-wide association meta-analysis identifies five modifier loci of lung disease severity in cystic fibrosis. *Nat. Commun.* **2015**, *6*, 8382. [CrossRef] [PubMed]

75. Szczesniak, R.; Rice, J.L.; Brokamp, C.; Ryan, P.; Pestian, T.; Ni, Y.; Andrinopoulou, E.R.; Keogh, R.H.; Gecili, E.; Huang, R.; et al. Influences of environmental exposures on individuals living with cystic fibrosis. *Expert Rev. Respir. Med.* **2020**, in press. [CrossRef] [PubMed]

76. Bombieri, C.; Claustres, M.; De Boeck, K.; Derichs, N.; Dodge, J.; Girodon, E.; Sermet, I.; Schwarz, M.; Tzetis, M.; Wilschanski, M.; et al. Recommendations for the Classification of Diseases as CFTR-related Disorders. *J. Cyst. Fibros.* **2011**, *10* (Suppl. 2), S86–S102. [CrossRef]

77. Bareil, C.; Bergougnoux, A. CFTR gene variants, epidemiology and molecular pathology. *Arch. Pediatr.* **2020**, *27* (Suppl. 1), eS8–eS12. [CrossRef]

78. Farrell, P.M.; Mishler, E.H.; Fost, N.C.; Wilfond, B.S.; Tluczek, A.; Gregg, R.G.; Bruns, W.T.; Hassemer, D.J.; Laessig, R.H. Current issues in neonatal screening for cystic fibrosis and implications of the CF gene discovery. *Pediatr. Pulmonol.* **1991**, *7*, S11–S18. [CrossRef]

79. Scotet, V.; de Braekeleer, M.; Roussey, M.; Rault, G.; Parent, P.; Dagorne, M.; Journel, H.; Lemoigne, A.; Codet, J.P.; Catheline, M.; et al. Neonatal Screening for Cystic Fibrosis in Brittany, France: Assessment of 10 Years' Experience and Impact on Prenatal Diagnosis. *Lancet* **2000**, *356*, 789–794. [CrossRef]

80. Farrell, P.M.; Kosorok, M.R.; Laxova, A.; Shen, G.; Koscik, R.E.; Bruns, W.T.; Splaingard, M.; Mischler, E.H. Nutritional benefits of neonatal screening for cystic fibrosis. Wisconsin Cystic Fibrosis Neonatal Screening Study Group. *N. Engl. J. Med.* **1997**, *337*, 963–969. [CrossRef]

81. Farrell, P.M.; Lai, H.J.; Li, Z.; Kosorok, M.R.; Laxova, A.; Green, C.G.; Collins, J.; Hoffman, G.; Laessig, R.; Rock, M.J.; et al. Evidence on improved outcomes with early diagnosis of cystic fibrosis through neonatal screening: Enough is enough! *J. Pediatr.* **2005**, *147*, S30–S36. [CrossRef]

82. Mak, D.Y.; Sykes, J.; Stephenson, A.L.; Lands, L.C. The benefits of newborn screening for cystic fibrosis: The Canadian experience. *J. Cyst. Fibros.* **2016**, *15*, 302–308. [CrossRef] [PubMed]

83. Zhang, Z.; Lindstrom, M.J.; Farrell, P.M.; Lai, H.J.; Wisconsin Cystic Fibrosis Neonatal Screening Group. Pubertal Height Growth and Adult Height in Cystic Fibrosis After Newborn Screening. *Pediatrics* **2015**, *137*, e20152907. [CrossRef] [PubMed]

84. Mérelle, M.E.; Schouten, J.P.; Gerritsen, J.; Dankert-Roelse, J.E. Influence of neonatal screening and centralized treatment on long-term clinical outcome and survival of CF patients. *Eur. Respir. J.* **2001**, *18*, 306–315. [CrossRef]

85. Mastella, G.; Zanolla, L.; Castellani, C.; Altieri, S.; Furnari, M.; Giglio, L.; Lombardo, M.; Miano, A.; Sciuto, C.; Pardo, F.; et al. Neonatal screening for cystic fibrosis: Long-term clinical balance. *Pancreatology* **2001**, *1*, 531–537. [CrossRef]

86. Lai, H.J.; Cheng, Y.; Farrell, P.M. The survival advantage of patients with cystic fibrosis diagnosed through neonatal screening: Evidence from the United States Cystic Fibrosis Foundation registry data. *J. Pediatr.* **2005**, *147*, S57–S63. [CrossRef] [PubMed]

87. Tridello, G.; Castellani, C.; Meneghelli, I.; Tamanini, A.; Assael, B.M. Early Diagnosis from Newborn Screening Maximises Survival in Severe Cystic Fibrosis. *ERJ Open Res.* **2018**, *4*, 00109-2017. [CrossRef]

88. Clancy, J.P.; Cotton, C.U.; Donaldson, S.H.; Solomon, G.M.; Van Devanter, D.R.; Boyle, M.P.; Gentzsch, M.; Nick, J.A.; Illek, B.; Wallenburg, J.C.; et al. CFTR Modulator Theratyping: Current Status, Gaps and Future Directions. *J. Cyst. Fibros.* **2019**, *18*, 22–34. [CrossRef]

89. Lopes-Pacheco, M. CFTR Modulators: The Changing Face of Cystic Fibrosis in the Era of Precision Medicine. *Front. Pharmacol.* **2020**, *10*, 1662. [CrossRef]

90. Shteinberg, M.; Taylor-Cousar, J.L. Impact of CFTR modulator use on outcomes in people with severe cystic fibrosis lung disease. *Eur. Respir. Rev.* **2020**, *29*, pii: 190112. [CrossRef]

91. Accurso, F.J.; Rowe, S.M.; Clancy, J.P.; Boyle, M.P.; Dunitz, J.M.; Durie, P.R.; Sagel, S.D.; Hornick, D.B.; Konstan, M.W.; Donaldson, S.H.; et al. Effect of VX-770 in persons with cystic fibrosis and the G551D-CFTR mutation. *N. Engl. J. Med.* **2010**, *363*, 1991–2003. [CrossRef]

92. Wainwright, C.E.; Elborn, J.S.; Ramsey, B.W.; Marigowda, G.; Huang, X.; Cipolli, M.; Colombo, C.; Davies, J.C.; De Boeck, K.; Flume, P.A.; et al. Lumacaftor-Ivacaftor in Patients with Cystic Fibrosis Homozygous for Phe508del CFTR. *N. Engl. J. Med.* **2015**, *373*, 220–231. [CrossRef] [PubMed]

93. Taylor-Cousar, J.L.; Munck, A.; McKone, E.F.; van der Ent, C.K.; Moeller, A.; Simard, C.; Wang, L.T.; Ingenito, E.P.; McKee, C.; Lu, Y.; et al. Tezacaftor-Ivacaftor in Patients with Cystic Fibrosis Homozygous for Phe508del. *N. Engl. J. Med.* **2017**, *377*, 2013–2023. [CrossRef] [PubMed]

94. Keating, D.; Marigowda, G.; Burr, L.; Daines, C.; Mall, M.A.; McKone, E.F.; Ramsey, B.W.; Rowe, S.M.; Sass, L.A.; Tullis, E.; et al. VX-445-Tezacaftor-Ivacaftor in Patients with Cystic Fibrosis and One or Two Phe508del Alleles. *N. Engl. J. Med.* **2018**, *379*, 1612–1620. [CrossRef] [PubMed]

95. Rubin, J.L.; O'Callaghan, L.; Pelligra, C.; Konstan, M.W.; Ward, A.; Ishak, J.K.; Chandler, C.; Liou, T.G. Modeling long-term health outcomes of patients with cystic fibrosis homozygous for F508del-CFTR treated with lumacaftor/ivacaftor. *Ther. Adv. Respir. Dis.* **2019**, *13*, 1–23. [CrossRef]

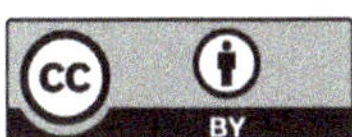

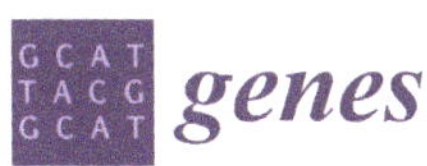 *genes*

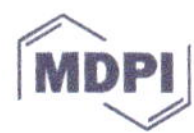

Review

Transcriptomic and Proteostasis Networks of CFTR and the Development of Small Molecule Modulators for the Treatment of Cystic Fibrosis Lung Disease

Matthew D. Strub [1,2] **and Paul B. McCray, Jr.** [1,2,*]

[1]   Interdisciplinary Graduate Program in Genetics, The University of Iowa, Iowa City, IA 52242, USA; matthew-strub@uiowa.edu

[2]   Stead Family Department of Pediatrics, The University of Iowa, Iowa City, IA 52242, USA

*   Correspondence: paul-mccray@uiowa.edu; Tel.: +1-(319)-335-6844

Received: 3 April 2020; Accepted: 8 May 2020; Published: 13 May 2020

Abstract: Cystic fibrosis (CF) is a lethal autosomal recessive disease caused by mutations in the CF transmembrane conductance regulator (*CFTR*) gene. The diversity of mutations and the multiple ways by which the protein is affected present challenges for therapeutic development. The observation that the Phe508del-CFTR mutant protein is temperature sensitive provided proof of principle that mutant CFTR could escape proteosomal degradation and retain partial function. Several specific protein interactors and quality control checkpoints encountered by CFTR during its proteostasis have been investigated for therapeutic purposes, but remain incompletely understood. Furthermore, pharmacological manipulation of many CFTR interactors has not been thoroughly investigated for the rescue of Phe508del-CFTR. However, high-throughput screening technologies helped identify several small molecule modulators that rescue CFTR from proteosomal degradation and restore partial function to the protein. Here, we discuss the current state of CFTR transcriptomic and biogenesis research and small molecule therapy development. We also review recent progress in CFTR proteostasis modulators and discuss how such treatments could complement current FDA-approved small molecules.

Keywords: Cystic fibrosis; CFTR; transcriptomics; proteostasis; small molecules; drug development

1. Cystic Fibrosis

Cystic Fibrosis (CF) is the most common lethal autosomal recessive disease in Caucasian populations, with approximately 75,000 individuals worldwide suffering from the condition [1,2]. In the United States, CF was first identified as a clinical syndrome in 1938 by Dr. Dorothy Andersen, who observed fluid-filled cysts and scars within the pancreas and similar tissue damage in the lungs of deceased children that had experienced digestive and respiratory problems [3]. Dr. Andersen termed the disease "cystic fibrosis of the pancreas". CF negatively affects multiple organ systems and can cause meconium ileus, cholestasis, biliary cirrhosis, increased sweat chloride concentrations, infertility, diabetes, and growth failure, among other symptoms [4–11]. However, the majority of morbidity and mortality associated with CF results from chronic and progressive lung dysfunction, characterized by altered airway surface liquid pH, decreased host defenses at the airway surface, impaired mucociliary transport resulting in chronic bacterial infections, bronchiectasis, irreversible tissue remodeling, and respiratory failure. Following the identification of elevated levels of chloride in the sweat of CF patients, it was hypothesized that the sweat ducts of these patients were impermeable to chloride [12]. Subsequent patch-clamp analyses of nasal and airway epithelial cells confirmed the defect in chloride permeability of the plasma membranes [13–16]. In 1989 Choi, Collins, and colleagues used linkage-based techniques to identify the gene responsible for CF, which they named the *Cystic Fibrosis Transmembrane conductance Regulator (CFTR)* [17–19].

2. CFTR Mutation Classes

The *CFTR* gene is on the long end of chromosome 7 and approximately 180,000 base pairs in length. *CFTR* is a member of the superfamily of ATP-binding cassette (ABC) genes and encodes an anion channel that conducts chloride, bicarbonate, and other substrates, thereby regulating the composition and volume of epithelial secretions [20–24]. To date, over 2,000 unique mutations have been identified in *CFTR*, resulting in an extensive range of disease severity [25]. These mutations have been grouped into six different classes based on the mechanisms by which they are believed to alter CFTR expression and function (Figure 1) [26,27]. Individual mutations may negatively affect CFTR function by more than one mechanism, and therefore, fall into multiple classes.

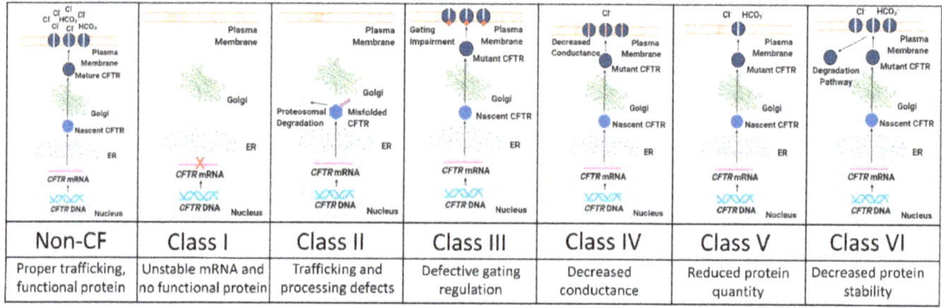

Figure 1. Schematic representation of CFTR (CF transmembrane conductance regulator) mutation classes. The top panels briefly illustrate CFTR trafficking along its proteostasis pathway and how protein maturation is disrupted by mutations. The middle panels list the mutation class, while the bottom panels briefly describe the defect(s) associated with each class. Adapted from [28].

2.1. Class I Mutations: Unstable mRNA and No Protein Production

Approximately 5–10% of *CFTR* mutations are associated with protein production, resulting from unstable mRNA and little or no CFTR protein [29]. These mutations can be caused by insertion/deletion frameshifts, abnormal splicing, or premature stop codons [30]. Examples of Class I mutations include R553X and G542X, the second most common *CFTR* mutation.

2.2. Class II Mutations: Trafficking and Processing Defects

Defective protein processing occurs in the most common class of *CFTR* mutations. Class II proteins fail to traffic through the CFTR proteostasis pathway and rarely arrive at the cell membrane [31,32]. Phe508del, the most common CF-causing mutation, is caused by a three base pair deletion (Δ) on exon 11 that results in the loss of a phenylalanine at residue 508 (Phe508del). Phe508del accounts for an estimated 70% of mutant *CFTR* alleles in the United States, and thus, roughly 90% of CF patients have one or two Phe508del alleles [33]. Class II mutant proteins often fail to reach the Golgi apparatus and are therefore never fully glycosylated [34]. Instead, these proteins are identified as misfolded by endoplasmic reticulum-associated protein degradation (ERAD) quality control mechanisms and are subsequently degraded [26]. As a result, Class II proteins rarely reach the cell surface to function [34]. Importantly, if Class II proteins do reach the cell surface, partial function can occur, although membrane stability is often impaired following rescue [31,35].

2.3. Class III Mutations: Gating Impairments

Mutations in the nucleotide binding domains (NBD) or phosphorylation sites of the regulatory domain of *CFTR* can cause reduced channel activity [26,36,37]. The third most common *CFTR* mutation,

G551D, produces a protein that, despite reaching the cell membrane, has approximately 100-fold lower open probability than that of wild-type (wt) [38]. Dimerization of the NBDs of CFTR forms two ATP binding pockets, termed ABP1 and ABP2 [39]. Whereas binding of ATP to ABP1 helps to stabilize the open channel conformation of CFTR, channel opening is dependent on ATP binding of ABP2 [40]. The G551D mutation, located in ABP2, prevents ATP binding, thus inhibiting opening of the CFTR channel [38]. The S1255P mutation, found in NBD2, also does not disrupt CFTR maturation, but instead alters the ATP-binding pocket, resulting in gating instability [41].

2.4. Class IV Mutations: Decreased Conductance

Class IV proteins achieve proper processing and gating, but mutations in their membrane spanning domains cause a misshapen protein that restricts anion transport [26]. This results in a decreased rate of ion flow through each open channel and an overall decrease in current conducted by CFTR [42]. Mutations affecting channel pore activity often arise in arginine residues (e.g., R117H, R347P, R334W). Some Class IV mutations, including R117H, also decrease the open probability of CFTR [43].

2.5. Class V Mutations: Reduced Protein Quantity

Inefficient protein maturation can be caused by alternative splicing, amino acid substitutions, or promoter mutations [26]. Class V mutations often produce incorrectly spliced versions of the *CFTR* mRNA in variable proportions, and the resultant proteins rarely transit to the cell membrane, resulting in a decreased number of functioning CFTR channels [44,45]. The most prevalent examples of Class V mutations include c.3717+12191C>T and c.3140-26A>G [46,47].

2.6. Class VI mutations: Unstable Protein

Class VI mutants can act as functional proteins at the cell surface. However, instability in the protein structure results in reduced residency at the cell surface, more rapid protein turnover, and therefore, less ion conductance [33,45]. Examples include c.120del123 and Phe508del when rescued by low temperature or correctors (rPhe508del) [48].

3. CFTR Structure and Function

CFTR is a 1,480 amino acid transmembrane glycoprotein containing two homologous halves, each consisting of six transmembrane alpha helices (termed TMD or transmembrane domain) that form an anion conduction pore, and a nucleotide-binding domain that serves as the binding site for ATP hydrolysis (Figure 2). These halves are connected by a regulatory (R) domain that contains multiple phosphorylation sites and regulates channel activity. The R domain is intrinsically unstructured and adapts its conformation upon binding to the NBDs and the CFTR N-terminus [49,50]. Recently, the cryo-EM structure of full length human CFTR was published, highlighting several key structural elements required for a fully functional protein [51,52]. First, an unphosphorylated R domain prevents the dimerization of NBD1 and NBD2, resulting in a closed channel. Secondly, a small inhibitory helix exists in the R domain that is docked inside the intracellular vestibule between the nucleotide binding domains, which precludes channel opening. It is believed that the disruption of the interaction between this inhibitory helix and the nucleotide binding domains would allow for protein kinase A (PKA)-mediated phosphorylation of the R domain, resulting in NBD dimerization and subsequent opening of the ion channel. Third, the authors sought to explain why CFTR acts as an ion channel, whereas other ABC transporters function as pumps that move ions against electrochemical gradients. When comparing the structures of CFTR and other ABC proteins, differences in two transmembrane helices (TM7 and TM8) were identified, leading to the hypothesis that these helices affect ion conduction and gating.

CFTR is neither isolated from neighboring proteins nor does it act alone. Instead, CFTR is part of a multiprotein assembly at the apical membrane surface, and is anchored via PDZ domains commonly found in plasma membrane proteins and other intracellular signaling proteins [53,54]. When at the apical membrane, CFTR is spatially located near other ion channels, membrane receptors, and cytoskeletal proteins. Additionally, transcriptomic studies in human CF cells suggest that significant changes in gene expression may result from the absence of functional CFTR [55]. Affected genes include members of the protein processing and inflammatory response functional families, among others. Likewise, proteomic analyses of the wt and Phe508del-CFTR interactomes by Pankow et al. identified novel effectors belonging to mRNA decay, co-translational control, endocytic recycling, ER quality control and folding, and protein degradation networks [56]. Such relationships between *CFTR* and other genes suggest that CFTR does not act solely as an ion channel, but instead, may have various roles throughout its biogenesis. Interactions between *CFTR* and genes that influence its processing or maturation could help to explain the wide range of phenotypes and severities in CF patients with identical mutations [33]. A better understanding of such interactions could also lead to the development of small molecule modulators for CF lung disease.

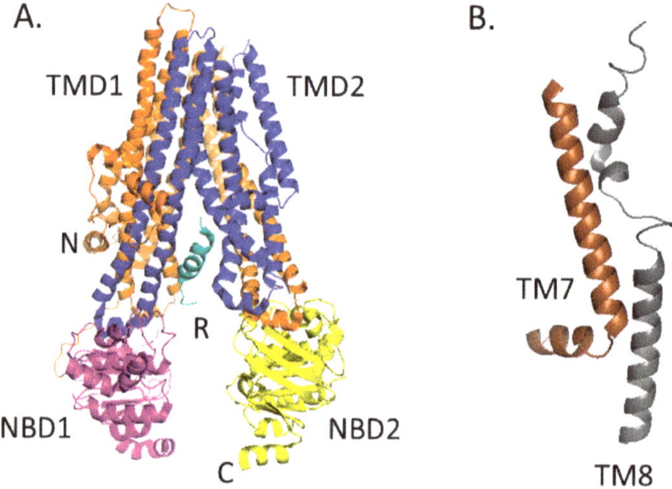

Figure 2. Cryo-EM structure of dephosphorylated, ATP-free CFTR. **A.** CFTR contains two transmembrane domains (TMD1 in orange, TMD2 in blue), two nucleotide binding domains (NBD1 in purple, NBD2 in yellow), and a regulatory (R) domain (cyan). CFTR is activated by phosphorylation of the R domain and ATP hydrolysis by the NBDs. Note that the structural flexibility of the R domain limits its visibility by Cryo-EM. Instead, 19 alanines are shown that correspond to the C-terminal region of the R domain. **B.** Magnified view of transmembrane helices (TM) 7 (brown) and 8 (gray). CFTR differs from other ABC transporters in that TM7 is displaced from its usual position and TM8 breaks into three short helices, rather than being a continuous helix as seen in other ABC transporters. TM7 and TM8 are found in TMD2. PBD ID: 5UAK.

4. Cystic Fibrosis Transcriptome

4.1. mRNA Profiling

The first transcriptomic profiling of well-differentiated primary cultures of human airway epithelia from Phe508del/Phe508del donors was performed by Zabner et al. in 2005 [57]. Of the approximately 22,000 genes represented on the Affymetrix U133A GeneChip, 18 were observed to be significantly upregulated in CF, while 6 were downregulated. The KCl cotransporter *KCC4* was identified as elevated in CF and was deemed a candidate for further studies. Interestingly, this profiling concluded that the level of *CFTR* mRNA was not significantly different in Phe508del/Phe508del cells compared to non-CF. Differences were also not observed when comparing cells from male and female donors. Figure 3 shows a general workflow of transcriptomic profiling for CF.

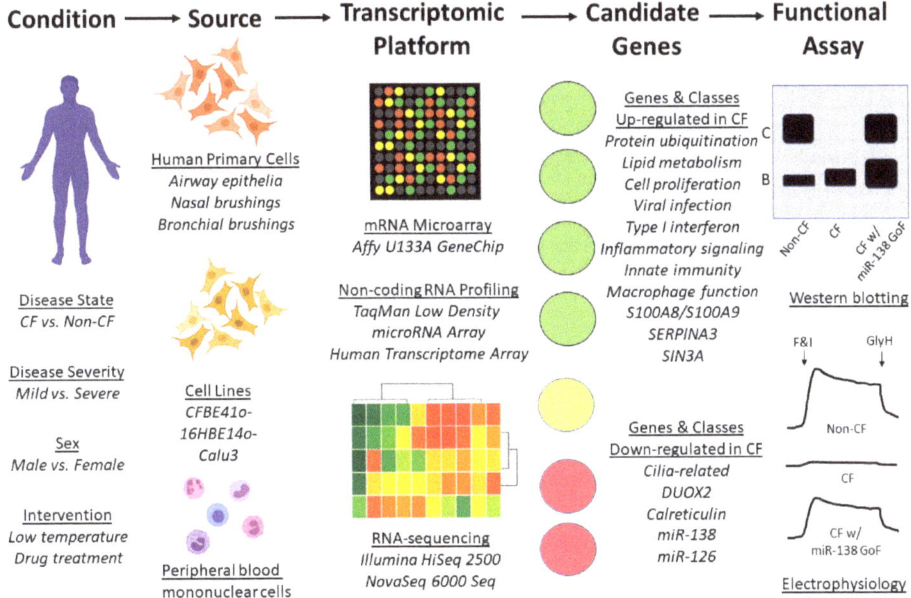

Figure 3. Workflow of transcriptomic profiling. To identify transcriptomic changes resulting from cystic fibrosis (e.g., disease presence or severity), multiple primary and immortalized cell sources are available, as are several profiling platforms. Analysis of profiling output reveals differentially expressed genes (DEGs) and gene classes; findings highlighted in the text are shown under "Candidate Genes". The effects of manipulating DEGs (e.g., gain of function (GoF) can be assessed using multiple assays. Examples of CFTR western blotting and electrophysiology as endpoints are presented with hypothetical data representing overexpression of miR-138 [58]. F&I represent the cyclic AMP agonists forskolin and IBMX. GlyH represents CFTR inhibitor GlyH-101.

One of the earliest transcriptomic studies using nasal epithelium of CF subjects was performed by Wright et al., in which they compared Phe508del homozygotes in the most severe 20th percentile of lung disease (as measured by forced expiratory volume; FEV_1) to those in the mildest 20th percentile [59]. Phe508del homozygotes and age-matched non-CF controls were also compared. Significant upregulation of 569 genes was observed in severe CF lung disease, while genes involved in protein ubiquitination (discussed later in Phe508del-CFTR Proteostasis and Quality Control), mitochondrial oxidoreductase activity, and lipid metabolism were significantly enriched. Among genes downregulated in CF were *DUOX2*, a key producer of hydrogen peroxide for airway mucosal defense, and calreticulin, an ER chaperone involved in protein metabolism (also discussed later in Phe508del-CFTR Proteostasis and Quality Control). Genes upregulated in mild CF lung disease compared to severe CF and non-CF included statherin, which is known to be produced in the submucosal cavities of the upper airways and to have antibacterial properties, and *ADIPOQ*, an anti-inflammatory cytokine and inducer of IL-10. RT-PCR revealed no significant differences in the transcriptomic levels of *CFTR* between Phe508del homozygotes and non-CF controls, in agreement with the findings by Zabner et al. [57].

Clarke and colleagues carried out a whole genome microarray study of primary nasal epithelial cells from Phe508del homozygotes and non-CF controls, and compared their results with several other relevant microarray datasets [60]. In their expression profile, genes involved in cell proliferation were significantly upregulated in CF, while cilia-related genes were downregulated. Due to great variability in the gene expression profiles across the independent studies, the meta-analysis comparing this study to five other microarray experiments (including the Zabner, Wright, and Ogilvie studies described in this section) yielded few common dysregulated genes across at least three experiments. However, when the authors compared their microarray results with the Ogilvie microarray, a molecular signature of native CF airway epithelial cells was observed, consisting of 21 common upregulated genes and 9 common downregulated genes [61]. A significant number of these genes were involved in inflammation and defense, including the upregulated *CXCR4, FOS, S100A8, S100A9,* and *SERPINA3* transcripts.

Although several gene expression studies have used nasal epithelial brushings from CF donors, Ogilvie et al. concluded that transcriptomics of the CF nasal epithelium is not representative of gene expression in the lung respiratory epithelium. Following bead array profiling of CF and non-CF nasal and bronchial epithelium, 863 genes were found to be significantly dysregulated in the bronchial cells, whereas only 15 genes were identified as dysregulated in nasal cells [61].

Polineni et al. performed RNA-sequencing of nasal mucosal cells from 134 CF subjects with varying genotypes and disease severities, as assessed by cytokine levels in nasal lavages [62]. Pathway analysis of the gene expression data highlighted the positive correlation between CF disease severity and viral infection, inflammatory signaling, lipid metabolism, macrophage function, and innate immunity. Multiple human leukocyte antigen (HLA) genes robustly contributed to the enriched pathways and several were also observed at the intersection of the gene expression profiling and previously identified CF GWAS risk alleles. The authors concluded that HLA genes may serve as targets for interventions aiming to improve CF lung health.

A meta-analysis of 13 microarray experiments was performed by Clarke and colleagues, comparing CF with similar disorders (e.g., chronic obstructive pulmonary disease, asthma, and idiopathic pulmonary fibrosis), environmental factors (e.g., smoking), relevant cellular processes (e.g., epithelial regeneration), and non-respiratory controls (e.g., schizophrenia) [63]. Genes whose expression was inversely related with *CFTR* across samples expressing Phe508del were subjected to an siRNA knockdown assay to identify potential negative regulators of CFTR. Nine genes, including *SNX6, PSEN1,* and *RCN2,* produced an appreciable increase in CFTR trafficking to the cell membrane. While the siRNA knockdown experiments were considered preliminary by the authors, these genes may serve as intriguing leads for therapeutic targets.

An additional transcriptomic study comparing the peripheral blood leukocytes of CF subjects with mild and severe lung disease was performed by Kormann et al. [64] Enrichment analyses identified genes of the type I interferon response, as well as ribosomal stalk proteins, as upregulated in mild disease. Such modifiers of CF lung disease may have implications as new biomarkers or targets for intervention.

4.2. Non-coding RNA Profiling

While most CF-related transcriptomic studies have focused on mRNA profiling, McCray and colleagues profiled global microRNA expression in well-differentiated primary cultures of human airway epithelia by qPCR and identified 31 highly expressed microRNAs in CF [58]. Further analyses of these microRNAs identified *SIN3A* as a highly conserved target of miR-138. As *SIN3A* has conserved motifs that bind to the transcriptional repressor CTCF and the *CFTR* locus contains functional CTCF-binding sites, the authors hypothesized that miR-138 and *SIN3A* regulate *CFTR*. Functional assays determined that overexpression of miR-138 or knockdown of *SIN3A* partially restored the maturation, trafficking, and function of Phe508del-CFTR. Oglesby et al. also identified miR-126 as downregulated in CF airway epithelial cells [65]. Overexpression of miR-126 resulted in downregulated TOM1 protein production. Furthermore, knockdown of *TOM1* mRNA significantly increased NF-κB regulated IL-8 secretion, linking miR-126 to innate immune responses in CF. Additionally, miR-145 has been shown to mediate TGF-β inhibition of CFTR function and knockdown of miR-145 restored Phe508del function in human primary epithelial cells [66]. Likewise, miR-200b reduces CFTR during prolonged hypoxia, although inhibition of miR-200b also rescues *CFTR* mRNA levels in primary bronchial epithelial cells [67]. These studies lend further support to the strategy of manipulating microRNAs or their target genes to enhance CFTR expression or alleviate symptoms associated with CF.

Likewise, Kamei and colleagues analyzed the expression of non-coding genes, or functional RNAs with no protein-coding capacity [68]. Using the Human Transcriptome Array, 91 dysregulated non-coding RNAs were identified in the CFBE41o- cell line. Linc-SUMF1-2, an intergenic non-coding RNA with no known function, was found to be inversely correlated with wild-type CFTR. Further analyses identified eight dysregulated genes, including *CXCL10*, *MYC*, and *LAMB3*, as both CFTR- and linc-SUMF-1-2-dependent in CF airway epithelial cells, uncovering a novel regulatory pathway of CF-associated gene regulation.

5. Phe508del-CFTR Proteostasis and Quality Control

CFTR was among the first membrane proteins identified as being regulated by the ERAD pathway [69]. Wild-type CFTR undergoes co-translation and N-glycosylation in the ER before being packed into COPII vesicles at ER exit sites and trafficked to the Golgi apparatus. Upon reaching the Golgi, glycan processing and modification occurs, rendering a complex, mature form of the protein. CFTR is then trafficked to the cell surface, where its stability is tightly regulated by protein interactors. Upon removal from the plasma membrane, CFTR can undergo endocytosis or be recycled back to the cell surface [70]. Despite its proteostasis pathway being incompletely understood, CFTR interacts with several classes of proteins and must pass multiple quality control checkpoints during trafficking from the ER to the cell surface (Figure 4).

5.1. Chaperones and Protein Folding

Heat shock proteins (Hsps) serve as the first quality control constituents of CFTR biogenesis, as these molecular chaperones co-translationally interact directly with CFTR. Hsp90, the constitutively expressed isoform of Hsp70 (often referred to as Hsc70), and the stress-induced isoform of Hsp70 bind CFTR during translation and assist in proper folding via ATP hydrolysis [71–75]. Small molecule-induced inhibition of Hsp90 in cultured human cells prevents proper CFTR folding, leading to protein degradation [71]. However, both Hsp90 and Hsp70 can recruit channel folding and maturation antagonizers, such as the Hsp70/Hsp90 organizing protein (HOP) [76,77]. HOP directs CFTR towards the degradation pathway by recruiting the E3 ubiquitin ligase CHIP (sometimes referred to as STUB1) to the CFTR-Hsp70/90 complex [78,79]. CHIP tags CFTR with ubiquitin (discussed in *E3 Ubiquitin Ligases*) and the CFTR protein is ushered toward the proteasome for degradation. The pro-degradation effects of CHIP can be reversed, however, by the Hsp/Hsc70 nucleotide exchange factor HspBP1, which inhibits CHIP and results in the continuation of CFTR along the pro-folding pathway [78,79]. The Hsp90 co-chaperone Aha1 is believed to prevent Hsp90 from properly interacting with CFTR, resulting in degradation of nascent protein [80,81]. An additional nucleotide exchange factor for Hsc70, Hsp105, has been observed to both promote the post-translational maturation of CFTR, while also at times assisting in the co-translational degradation of CFTR [82,83].

Hsp40 co-chaperones, often referred to as J proteins, have also been shown to interact with CFTR during its initial translation stages. DNAJA1 (Hsp40/Hdj2) and DNAJB1 (Hsp40/Hdj1) interact with Hsc70 to promote folding of the NBD1 of CFTR and assist in rescuing wtCFTR from endoplasmic reticulum retention [73,84,85]. However, these DNAJ proteins have been unable to rescue Phe508del-CFTR from being degraded and sometimes actually serve as pro-degradation components of the quality control machinery [86]. DNAJA1 has been shown to promote CHIP ubiquitin ligase activity and DNAJC5 (Hsp40 cysteine string protein; sometimes referred to as Csp) independently recruits CHIP to the CFTR-Hsp90 complex [87–89]. Similarly, DNAJB12 recruits the E3 ubiquitin ligase RMA1 to the CFTR-Hsc70 complex, promoting degradation of both Phe508del-CFTR and immature wtCFTR [90,91].

An additional subclass of Hsps, termed small heat shock proteins (sHsps), have also been shown to affect CFTR biogenesis through holdase activity of misfolded proteins [92]. HSPB1 (sHsp Hsp27) recruits Ubc9 to the immature NBD1 domain, where it catalyzes the attachment of small ubiquitin-like modifier (SUMO), leading to ubiquitination [93,94]. Likewise, HSPB4 (sHsp αA-crystallin) can also assist with CFTR degradation [93].

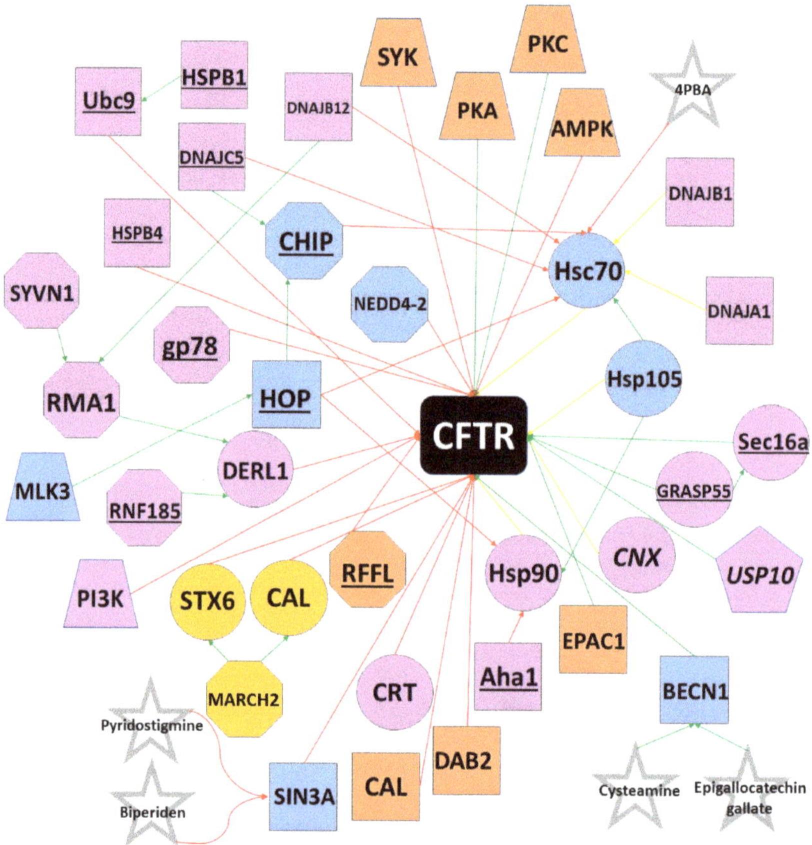

Figure 4. CFTR Proteostasis Interactors. Selected proteins active in the CFTR proteostasis pathway are shown. Octagons represent E3 ubiquitin ligases; trapezoids indicate kinases; circles represent chaperones; pentagons indicate deubiquitinases; co-chaperones and all other proteins are represented as squares; proteostasis modulators are represented as stars. Red arrows indicate degradation interactions; green arrows represent activation or maturation interactions; yellow arrows indicate that the protein can have degradative or activation interactions. In most cases, these proteins degrade Phe508del, while promoting wtCFTR maturation. Proteins shaded in purple primarily interact with co-factors or CFTR at the ER; orange at the cell surface; yellow at the Golgi apparatus. Proteins shaded in blue can interact with co-factors or CFTR at the ER or cell surface. Underlined proteins are primarily only found in the Phe508del proteostasis pathway, whereas italicized proteins are usually found in the wtCFTR pathway. Curved lines indicate that pyridostigmine and biperiden are believed to act by mimicking the transcriptional changes resulting from downregulation of SIN3A. Please note that the most common interactions and locations for each protein are shown. Some proteins are active at multiple locations.

Calnexin (CNX) is a membrane chaperone found in the ER that affects the folding of CFTR transmembrane domains [95]. While the binding of CNX to CFTR can prevent pro-degradation quality control proteins from binding immaturely folded CFTR, studies also suggest that CNX can obstruct channel maturation [96,97]. In fact, inhibition of CNX improves trafficking of wtCFTR from the ER to the cell membrane [96]. However, such inhibition has little effect on Phe508del-CFTR, perhaps indicating that Phe508del is targeted for degradation prior to the role of CNX in the quality control pathway. Calreticulin (CRT), found in the ER lumen, does not contribute to CFTR folding, but instead increases the length of time that CFTR remains in the ER, resulting in increased CFTR turnover [98].

5.2. E3 Ubiquitin Ligases and Protein Degradation

The complex quality control mechanisms responsible for CFTR folding, maturation, and processing result in a high rate of protein turnover, even for wtCFTR. In fact, current estimates indicate that only one fourth of wtCFTR is folded correctly and trafficked from the ER, whereas virtually no Phe508del-CFTR manages to escape [99]. Proteins unreleased from the ER enter the ubiquitin-proteasome ERAD pathway [34]. Proteins targeted for ERAD by chaperones like CHIP and RMA1 (discussed in *Heat-shock proteins*) are tagged with ubiquitin, a 76-amino acid polypeptide that signals the release of CFTR from the ER membrane. However, rather than trafficking to the cell membrane, ubiquitin-tagged CFTR is hydrolyzed by the proteolytic chymotrypsin-like activity of the proteasome [100].

The first step of the ubiquitin-proteasome ERAD pathway requires the ATP-dependent binding of ubiquitin to an E1 ubiquitin activating enzyme. The E1 enzyme catalyzes the C-terminus of ubiquitin and then transfers ubiquitin to an E1 active site cysteine residue. UBA1 and UBA6 are the only known E1 ubiquitin activating enzymes in humans [101]. Next, E2 ubiquitin-conjugating enzymes are recruited to E1-ubiquitin complex and catalyze the transfer of ubiquitin to the active site cysteine of E2. Currently, 35 unique E2 conjugating enzymes have been identified in the human genome [102]. Lastly, E3 ubiquitin ligases function as substrate identification molecules and bind both E2 enzymes and substrates while transferring ubiquitin from the E2 to the substrate. E3 ubiquitin ligases often transfer multiple ubiquitin polypeptides to a substrate, creating a polyubiquitin chain. Ubiquitinated proteins are then trafficked to the proteasome for degradation. E3 ubiquitin ligases have been sorted into multiple classes, including HECT and RING, depending on their active domains. Over 600 unique E3 ubiquitin ligases have been identified thus far, and most E3s can target multiple substrates. Likewise, individual substrates may be ubiquitinated by multiple E3s [103,104].

To date, several E3 ubiquitin ligases have been shown to ubiquitinate CFTR. RMA1 (sometimes called RNF5) and RNF185, a highly conserved homologue of RMA1, ubiquitinate misfolded CFTR following NBD1 translation [90,105,106]. An additional E3 ubiquitin ligase, gp78, acts by elongating the polyubiquitin chains initiated by RMA1 and RNF185 [107]. Unlike RMA1 and RNF185, the E3 ubiquitin ligase CHIP only acts on fully translated CFTR [78,79,86]. As RMA1, RNF185, and CHIP are unable to directly bind to CFTR, these proteins ubiquitinate misfolded CFTR through adaptor proteins. Specifically, RMA1 and RNF185 require Derlin-1, whereas CHIP binds Hsc70 or Hsp70 [108–110]. Interestingly, whereas Hsc70/Hsp70 often promote CFTR folding, CHIP is able to "hijack" these chaperones to trigger ERAD [111]. CHIP and E3 ubiquitin ligase RFFL can ubiquitinate CFTR at the cell periphery. Unlike CHIP, RFFL binds directly to CFTR and is independent of molecular chaperones. RFFL does not affect turnover of wtCFTR, but instead targets only misfolded protein on the cell surface [112].

Additional E3 ubiquitin enzymes that target CFTR include MARCH2, NEDD4-2, SYVN1, and FBXO2. MARCH2 ubiquitinates CFTR through adaptor proteins CAL and STX6 [113]. NEDD4-2 is a HECT E3 ubiquitin ligase that binds both wtCFTR and Phe508del-CFTR [114]. SYVN1 regulates CFTR ubiquitination through the RNF5/AMFR pathway, whereas FBX02 binds directly to CFTR via the SCF complex [115]. Knockdown of MARCH2, NEDD4-2, and SYVN1 has been demonstrated to improve Phe508del-CFTR maturation and trafficking and restore partial function to the mutant protein.

Lastly, the deubiquitinase USP10 has been shown to interact with wtCFTR in endosomes, reducing polyubiquitination and improving rates of endocytic recycling of wtCFTR [116,117].

5.3. ER Stress and Anterograde Trafficking

Whereas properly folded CFTR usually enters COPII-coated vesicles budding from the ER and subsequently traffics to the Golgi en route to the cell surface, mutant CFTR can also undergo unconventional anterograde trafficking. Such trafficking is commonly induced by ER stress and involves the bypassing of the ER-to-Golgi transport, resulting in CFTR trafficking from the ER straight to the cell periphery [118,119]. During ER stress, IRE1 initiates the unfolded protein response (UPR), which increases both the expression of Sec16a and the number of possible exit sites in the ER. Sec16a acts as a secretory protein at such exit sites and facilitates scaffolding of COPII-coated vesicles. ER stress also causes GRASP55, usually found in the Golgi, to traffic to the ER, where it interacts with Sec16a. Although the mechanism by which GRASP55/Sec16a aids in the trafficking of CFTR to the cell surface is not currently understood, the resultant membrane bound CFTR lacks complex glycosylation, indicating that the protein bypassed the Golgi [119–121]. Despite being misfolded and incompletely glycosylated, Phe508del-CFTR protein that reaches the cell surface through unconventional anterograde trafficking retains partial function, suggesting that the GRASP55 pathway may serve as an interesting therapeutic target.

5.4. Protein Kinases and Membrane Stability

Membrane stability of CFTR is partially regulated by protein kinases. PKA and protein kinase C (PKC) have been shown to phosphorylate CFTR predominately at the R domain, although NBD1 and C-terminal residues can also be phosphorylated [122–124]. While phosphorylation generally suppresses endocytosis, AMP-activated protein kinase (AMPK) and spleen tyrosine kinase (SYK) have been shown to decrease CFTR plasma membrane stability [124,125]. In the ER, mixed-lineage kinase 3 (MLK3) is believed to promote degradation by interacting with HOP [126]. Additionally, inhibition of the phosphatidylinositol 3-kinase (PI3K) pathway can increase CFTR stability and expression [127,128].

5.5. Tethering Factors and Endocytosis Adaptors

Also contributing to CFTR's plasma membrane stability are endocytosis adaptors and tethering factors. Knockdown of the endocytosis factor DAB2 has been shown to stabilize Phe508del-CFTR at the cell surface by inhibiting endocytosis [129,130]. CFTR has a PDZ binding motif at the C-terminus that tethers to the PDZ domain of NHERF1, supporting channel activation and CFTR membrane stability for both wild-type and mutant proteins [131]. The exchange protein EPAC1 strengthens this interaction and further suppresses endocytosis [132]. However, the CFTR-associated ligand (CAL) decreases the stability of CFTR at the cell membrane through its PDZ domain. Knockdown of CAL has been shown to improve function and stability of Phe508del-CFTR, suggesting that inhibition of the protein may be a therapeutic option [113,133,134].

6. Small Molecule Modulators

The observation by Welsh and colleagues that Phe508del-CFTR could be rescued and traffic to the cell surface via low temperature (27° C) incubation was transformative because it demonstrated that if Phe508del (and potentially other mutations) could escape the ERAD pathway and traffic to the cell membrane, they retained partial function [31]. While low temperature treatment is not a therapeutically viable option for CF patients, this observation encouraged researchers to target genes affecting the processing and maturation of CFTR [135]. Furthermore, through the use of high-throughput screening technology, several small molecules that interact directly with CFTR and positively affect processing or function have been identified. Following lead optimization and clinical trials, four small molecules are now FDA-approved for CF, providing potentially 90% of patients with at least one modulator option. Several other small molecules are currently being investigated in clinical trials (Table 1).

Table 1. Selected clinical trials using small molecule modulators for cystic fibrosis.

Small molecule(s)	Trade Name	Company	Phase	Modulator Type	Mutations	Clinical Trial
Ivacaftor	Kalydeco	Vertex Pharmaceuticals	Approved	Potentiator	G551D, 37 others *	NCT02725567
Lumacaftor + Ivacaftor	Orkambi	Vertex Pharmaceuticals	Approved	Lumacaftor = Corrector; Ivacaftor = Potentiator	Phe508del/Phe508del	NCT03601637
Tezacaftor + Ivacaftor	Symdeko	Vertex Pharmaceuticals	Approved	Tezacaftor = Corrector; Ivacaftor = Potentiator	Phe508del/Phe508del,26 others **	NCT02412111
Elexacaftor + Tezacaftor + Ivacaftor	Trikafta	Vertex Pharmaceuticals	Approved	Elexacaftor, Tezacaftor = Correctors; Ivacaftor = Potentiator	Phe508del + any other mutation	NCT04183790
PTC124 + Ivacaftor	Ataluren	PTC Therapeutics	Phase 4	Premature stop codon readthrough	Class I mutations	NCT03256968
VX-561	—	Vertex Pharmaceuticals	Phase 2	Potentiator	G551D, 8 others ***	NCT03911713
ABBV-2222	—	AbbVie	Phase 2	Corrector	Phe508del/Phe508del	NCT03969888
ABBV-3067	—	AbbVie	Phase 2	Potentiator	Phe508del/Phe508del	NCT03969888
ELX-02	—	Eloxx Pharmaceuticals	Phase 2	Nonsense mutation readthrough agent	G542X	NCT04135495
FDL169	—	Flatley Discovery Lab	Phase 2	Corrector	Phe508del/Phe508del	NCT02767297
PTI-428 + Ivacaftor	—	Proteostasis Therapeutics	Phase 2	Amplifier	Same as Ivacaftor	NCT03258424
PTI-801	—	Proteostasis Therapeutics	Phase 2	Corrector	Phe508del/Phe508del	NCT03140527
PTI-808	—	Proteostasis Therapeutics	Phase 2	Potentiator	Phe508del/Phe508del	NCT03251092
VX-121	—	Vertex Pharmaceuticals	Phase 2	Corrector	Phe508del + minimal function (MF) mutation	NCT03912233
MRT5005	—	Translate Bio	Phase 1	mRNA delivery	Class I or II mutations	NCT03375047

* Mutations *A455E, A1067T, D100E, D110H, D579G, D1152H, D1270N, E56K, E193K, E831X, F1052V, F1074L, G178R, G551S, G1069R, G1244E, G1349D, K1060T, L206W, P67L, R74W, R117C, R347H, R352Q, R1070Q, R1070W, S549N, S549R, S945L, S977F, S1251N, S1255P, R117H, c.579+3A>G, c.2657+5G>A, c.3140-26A>G, c.3717+12191C>T.* ** Mutations *A455E, A1067T, D100E, D110H, D579G, D1152H, D1270N, E56K, E193K, E831X, F1052V, F1074L, K1060T, L206W, P67L, R74W, R117C, R347H, R352Q, R1070W, S945L, S977F, c.579+3A>G, c.2657+5G>A, c.3140-26A>G, c.3717+12191C>T.* *** *G178R, G551S, G1244E, G1349D, S549N, S549R, S1251N, S1255P.*

6.1. CFTR Potentiators

Potentiators are a class of small molecules that increase anion transport via CFTR at the cell membrane by increasing the channel open probability. As discussed previously, Class III CFTR mutations have gating defects, whereas Class IV CFTR mutations exhibit abnormal conductance. However, in both mutation classes, CFTR is trafficked to the cell membrane and partial function can be restored with the use of potentiators. Furthermore, clinical benefits have been observed in patients with G551D and related mutations when receiving monotherapy with a single potentiator [136–141]. As will be discussed later, potentiators can also help to restore function in Class II mutations, including Phe508del-CFTR, when coupled with one or more correctors.

Vertex Pharmaceuticals (Boston, MA, USA) identified the first FDA-approved CFTR potentiator. Ivacaftor (trade name Kalydeco) was approved in 2012 for CF patients with the G551D mutation and was later approved for additional Class III mutations, including G1244E, G1349D, S549R, among others [140,142–146]. Kalydeco has also been approved for the Class IV mutation R117H and related mutations [141,147,148]. Ivacaftor was identified through a high throughput screen using NIH-3T3 mouse fibroblast cells expressing Phe508del-CFTR [149]. These cells were first incubated at 27 °C to rescue the mutant protein to the cell surface and then treated with small molecule candidates, with a fluorescent signal being detected when CFTR-mediated chloride transport occurred. Vertex screened approximately 300,000 compounds using the NIH-3T3 fluorescence assay and identified four scaffolds that had significant potentiating activity. Following medicinal chemistry to optimize these scaffolds, investigators concluded that a singular scaffold was the most efficacious and lead optimization of the scaffold resulted in the testing of an additional 70 small molecules. Of these, VX-770, which would later be named ivacaftor, showed superior function. In human bronchial epithelial (HBE) cells derived from G551D/Phe508del subjects, ivacaftor increased chloride secretion 10-fold, reaching 50% of wtCFTR levels [136]. In vivo studies in G551D patients followed, and two randomized, double-blind, placebo-controlled studies demonstrated a 10.5% increase in FEV_1 compared to placebo and markedly reduced sweat chloride levels [143]. These groundbreaking results were the first in which a small molecule acted as a clinical modulator of CFTR. Patch clamp studies of ivacaftor-treated cells expressing G551D concluded that ivacaftor increased the open probability of G551D-CFTR six-fold [136]. Additionally, ivacaftor increased the open probability of Phe508del-CFTR five-fold and even wtCFTR two-fold [136,139,150]. Further clinical trials of ivacaftor in Phe508del patients did not yield efficacious results [151].

The flavonoids genistein and curcumin have also been shown to have potentiating effects, especially when combined with lumacaftor (see CFTR Correctors), as these compounds enhance forskolin-induced swelling in rectal organoids with Phe508del and G551D mutations [152]. Rattlesnake phospholipase A_2 and several aminoarylthiazoles are also being investigated as potentiators in CFBE41o- and Phe508del-A549 cells [153–155]. Furthermore, several pharmaceutical companies and research groups have small molecule potentiators in clinical trials, including Vertex, AbbVie, and Proteostasis Therapeutics (Table 1).

6.2. CFTR Correctors

While potentiators like ivacaftor have had significant clinical benefits for patients with Class III and Class IV mutations, little effect was seen in patients with Class II mutations, including those with Phe508del. As approximately 90% of CF patients have at least one Phe508del allele, there is substantial interest in identifying small molecule correctors that can restore function to misfolded proteins with processing defects.

Corr-4a was the first corrector discovered that restored function to Phe508del-CFTR-transfected epithelial cells at 37 °C to the same level as low temperature incubation [156]. High throughput screening has aided researchers in the quest to discover small molecule correctors and such experiments led Vertex Pharmaceuticals to discover VRT-422 and VRT-325 [137]. These compounds restored CFTR-mediated chloride conductance to 10% of wtCFTR levels in HBE cells. Despite this modest restoration of conductance, these compounds served as an important proof-of-concept for small molecule correction at a clinically relevant level. Further medicinal chemistry and lead optimization by Vertex led to the discovery of VX-809, which reportedly rescued up to 30% of Phe508del-CFTR from degradation and restored chloride conductance to approximately 15% of wtCFTR levels [157]. VX-809 was later named lumacaftor. Interestingly, lumacaftor shows added efficacy when combined with low temperature, Corr-4a, and VRT-325, indicating that the misfolding defect(s) caused by the Phe508del-CFTR mutation is not entirely corrected by the individual compound [158–160]. This strongly supports a therapeutic strategy of combining more than one corrector compound.

Following the identification of lumacaftor and ivacaftor, the corrector-potentiator combination entered clinical trials. Once approved for Phe508del homozygous patients, the combination, marketed as Orkambi, gave up to 45% of CF patients a small molecule modulator option [161]. However, the clinical effect seen in Phe508del patients treated with Orkambi was modest, as homozygous patients experienced an average increase in FEV_1 of only 4% [162]. Additionally, an antagonistic effect between ivacaftor and lumacaftor was seen in several studies, leaving many patients without clinical improvement [163,164]. An estimated 15% of patients discontinued Orkambi within three months of use [165].

Recognizing the need for improved correctors, as well as the potential benefits of multi-corrector treatments, Vertex developed VX-661, later named tezacaftor, and VX-445, renamed elexacaftor. While tezacaftor is structurally related to and shares a mechanism with lumacaftor, elexacaftor is thought to act at a second site on CFTR, making it a corrector 2 (or C2) molecule [166]. Clinical trials with a triple-combination of tezacaftor, elexacaftor, and ivacaftor in patients with at least one Phe508del allele resulted in an average increase in FEV_1 of approximately 10%, as well as reduced sweat chloride and frequency of pulmonary exacerbations [167,168]. This triple-combination therapy was subsequently FDA-approved in 2019 for patients with at least one Phe508del allele and marketed as Trikafta.

Vertex has also completed clinical trials of VX-440 and VX-152 in combination with tezacaftor/ivacaftor, but pursued elexacaftor as the third element of their triple-combination strategy [169]. Additional correctors in clinical trials have been reported by Vertex, AbbVie, Flatley Discovery Lab, and Proteostasis Therapeutics (Table 1) [170,171].

6.3. Premature Stop Codon Readthrough Agents

Although Kalydeco and Trikafta provide up to 90% of CF patients with modulator treatments, such small molecules are not therapeutic for patients with Class I mutations, which cause unstable mRNA and often no protein production. An estimated 9% of CF-causing mutations fall in Class I and approximately half of all Israeli CF patients have such mutations [172,173]. As most Class I mutations are caused by a premature stop codon, "readthrough" of these stop codons would theoretically allow for proper translation to the normal transcript termination site. This effect has been seen in R553X- and G542X-CFTR-expressing HeLa cells treated with aminoglycoside antibiotics, such as gentamicin [174,175]. However, preclinical studies of gentamicin treatment in patients with Class I mutations showed no clinical benefit [176,177].

High-throughput screens identified ataluren as a potentially efficacious readthrough agent. In subsequent experiments in transgenic mice harboring the G542X mutation, CFTR expression at the plasma membrane was partially restored by ataluren treatment [178–180]. However, while ataluren progressed to phase III clinical trials, little benefit was observed [181]. Currently, synthetic aminoglycosides, ataluren derivatives, and escin, the FDA-approved active component of horse chestnut seed, are being investigated as readthrough agents in W1282X/Phe508del-CFBE and human primary epithelial cells [182–185]. It is important to note that such agents may cause the insertion of non-native amino acids at the site of readthrough, which may reduce channel function [186]. Currently, ELX-02, a eukaryotic ribosomal selective glycoside developed by Eloxx Pharmaceuticals (Waltham, MA, USA), is in Phase 2 clinical trials as a premature stop codon readthrough agent (NCT04135495).

6.4. CFTR Stabilizers

While CFTR correctors can rescue mutant protein to the cell surface, long-term stability of Phe508del-CFTR at the plasma membrane has not been observed following solo corrector treatment [187]. Likewise, while low temperature treatment rescues CFTR to the cell surface, the protein's half-life is still reduced and it experiences increased endocytosis and decreased recycling [188,189]. Class VI CFTR mutations result in unstable protein configurations that lead to reduced residency of CFTR at the cell surface and, therefore, less anion conductance. As correctors are currently unable to address this class of mutations, researchers have searched for small molecules to stabilize the mutant CFTR protein at the plasma membrane for longer periods.

To date, several CFTR stabilizers have been identified. Although not a small molecule, hepatocyte growth factor (HGF) has been shown to activate Rac1 signaling and resultingly stabilize CFTR through its interaction with NHERF-1 [190]. While lumacaftor can increase CFTR plasma membrane stability to a modest degree, co-treatment of lumacaftor with HGF further enhanced the anchoring of CFTR to NHERF-1 in mouse small intestine organoids [131,191]. Treatment with vasoactive intestinal peptide also stabilized interactions between CFTR and NHERF-1 by decreasing the rate of endocytosis [192]. Lastly, cavosonstat, an inhibitor of S-nitrosoglutathione reductase, helps to stabilize CFTR by preventing its interaction with HOP [76,77]. Interestingly, cavosonstat is the only CFTR stabilizer to be tested in clinical trials (NCT02589236). It is currently being administered to Phe508del/Phe508del patients using Orkambi and patients with Class III mutations using Kalydeco.

6.5. Splicing Correctors

Approximately 10% of CFTR mutations are caused by aberrant mRNA splicing that often results in immature protein that rarely trafficks to the cell membrane. Such mutations can be found across multiple classes but are particularly common in Class V. Modulators able to correct splicing and restore full-length CFTR mRNA could rescue CFTR protein function. Currently, antisense oligonucleotides are being investigated as therapeutic options for splicing mutations [193].

6.6. CFTR Amplifiers

Amplifiers increase the amount of *CFTR* mRNA production and subsequent protein production [194]. As the mRNA still contains a mutation, amplifiers do not directly correct processing or restore function to the protein. Instead, an increased amount of protein substrate is available for modulators to act upon. Therefore, amplifiers are always investigated as a component of a multi-drug therapy. Phase 2 clinical trials were recently completed for the amplifier PTI-428, or nesolifcaftor, in patients using tezacaftor/ivacaftor (NTC03591094).

6.7. mRNA Delivery Agents

Delivery of *CFTR*-encoding mRNA to the lungs would allow epithelial cells to create wtCFTR protein in a mutation-agnostic manner. Robinson and colleagues used lipid-based nanoparticles (LNPs) for delivery of chemically modified *CFTR* mRNA (cmCFTR) to CFTR knockout mice [195]. Approximately 55% of net chloride efflux of normal mice was observed 3 days post-transfection. Translate Bio is currently testing MRT5005, an agent designed to deliver *CFTR* mRNA, in Phase I clinical trials (NCT03375047).

6.8. Proteostasis Modulators

Glycerol and trimethylamine N-oxide (TMAO), when added to NIH 3T3 cells expressing Phe508del, were found to restore partial processing and function to Phe508del-CFTR [196–198]. High concentrations of 4-phenylbutrate (4PBA) emerged as a candidate CFTR modulator, as it restored function to Phe508del-CFTR by interfering with Hsc70 in HEK293 cells expressing Phe508del. However, clinical trials of 4PBA showed little improvement in respiratory function [199–202]. Balch and colleagues tested

HDAC inhibitors for the rescue of Phe508del-CFTR and identified suberoylanilide hydroxamic acid (SAHA) as efficacious in primary human bronchial epithelial cells [203,204]. The combination treatment of cysteamine and epigallocatechin gallate has been shown to rescue CFTR trafficking, function, and plasma membrane stability through the correction of Beclin-1 autophagy flux in primary nasal epithelial cells [205,206]. A phase II clinical trial of the cysteamine-epigallocatechin gallate combination reported decreased sweat chloride levels and modest increases in FEV_1 in Phe508del/Phe508del patients [207].

McCray and colleagues used a transcriptomic-based strategy to identify candidate correctors of CFTR. By querying the genomic signature of miR-138-mediated CFTR rescue in the Connectivity Map, a catalogue of gene expression profiles of various cell lines treated with bioactive small molecules, the group was able to identify molecules whose genomic signatures closely resembled that of miR-138 overexpression or *SIN3A* knockdown. After testing 27 small molecules, four were identified that partially rescued maturation and function of Phe508del-CFTR in primary human airway epithelia (HAE), including biperiden, pizotifen, pyridostigmine, and valproic acid. Of these, pyridostigmine showed cooperativity with corrector compound C18 (an analogue of lumacaftor) in improving Phe508del-CFTR function [208].

Likewise, Galietta and colleagues used connectivity mapping to identify drugs having a similar mode of action at the gene expression level as CFBE41o- and primary bronchial epithelial cells treated at 27 °C for 24 h [209]. Several anti-inflammatory glucocorticoids were found to increase Phe508del-CFTR function in the cell line, but the activity could not be confirmed in primary cells. Sondo et al. also identified 9-aminoacridine and ciclopirox as proteostasis regulators able to restore partial function to Phe508del-CFTR in cell lines [210]. However, these small molecules did not increase chloride secretion in primary bronchial epithelial cells from CF patients and subsequent microarray profiling revealed different gene expression signatures generated by the treatments in cell lines and primary cells.

Additional investigations of the repurposing of drugs currently FDA-approved for non-CF disorders yielded compounds that are efficacious in vitro. Miglustat (marketed under the trade name Zavesca and used to treat Gaucher disease) and sildenafil (marketed under the trade name Viagara and used to treat erectile dysfunction and pulmonary hypertension) treatments partially restored function to Phe508del-CFTR in human nasal epithelial cells [211,212].

7. Conclusions

A golden age of CFTR small molecule modulators has arrived, as approximately 90% of CF patients could receive clinical benefits from the use of one or more FDA-approved drugs. Clinical studies have reported improved lung function, reduced pulmonary exacerbations, increased weight, and improved quality of life measures. However, despite the profound impact that these drugs are having on patients, there are major areas that must be considered in the future of CF drug development. First, it is crucial that therapies be identified for all CFTR mutation classes. Currently, there are no approved treatments for mutations causing premature stop codons, frameshifts, or nonsense mutations. Fortunately, small molecules to address some of these mutations are currently progressing through clinical trials. However, it is possible that small molecule therapeutics will not provide clinical benefits to all mutations. For such situations, the development of gene therapy or gene editing approaches may be crucial [213,214]. Secondly, there are still patients in age ranges that are not approved to receive the FDA-approved small molecules. CFTR modulators are likely to have their greatest benefit if patients are treated before irreversible tissue remodeling of the lung occurs, presumably shortly after birth, or even *in utero*. Orkambi is currently being tested in patients 12-24 months old, whereas Trikafta is under investigation in patients 6-11 years of age. Lastly, the long-term effects of the current treatments are unknown, as the drugs only recently became available. Additionally, they are currently quite expensive, which limits their widespread availability worldwide, and places burdens on healthcare systems. It will be important for healthcare professionals to continually monitor the efficacy and any potential side effects of these compounds.

While the advancements in small molecule treatments for CF in the last decade have been monumental and are acknowledged, it is imperative that improved treatments continue to be developed. As seen with Trikafta, the co-treatment of two or more small molecules may present opportunities to improve the efficacy of pharmacological therapies. Tezacaftor and elexacaftor act synergistically, likely due to the fact that elexacator acts on a different site in CFTR than tezacaftor. An alternative strategy is to pair a corrector that interacts directly with CFTR, such as tezacaftor, which a small molecule that manipulates the CFTR proteostasis pathway. Significant additive effects have been observed in human primary airway epithelial co-treated with pyridostigmine and corrector compound C18, as well as in SAHA paired with corrector compound C3. While these small molecules have not yet advanced to clinical trials, they lend support to the strategy of targeting proteostasis interactors. Furthermore, although several modulators of CFTR proteostasis have not shown significant efficacy in clinical trials, it would be unwise to abandon investigations of such therapies. Some failed candidates, such as glycerol and 9-aminoacridine, have incompletely understood mechanisms, making lead optimization difficult. Others, such as 4PBA, target proteins that can act in both degradation and maturation pathways, further complicating the already delicate process of rescuing Phe508del. However, as seen in Figure 4, many proteins involved in the CFTR proteostasis pathway have not been targeted pharmaceutically for correction of Phe508del and may be therapeutic targets. Lastly, as transcriptomic and proteomic studies of CFTR proteostasis continue to uncover new interactors, it is important for researchers to investigate whether such interactors can be targeted therapeutically. Modulators of the CFTR proteostasis pathway could serve as pharmaceutical leads and complement the already existing drugs discovered via high throughput screening.

Author Contributions: M.D.S., P.B.M.J. writing, review, figure creation, and editing. All authors have read and agreed to the published version of the manuscript.

Funding: This work was supported by National Institutes of Health Predoctoral Training Grant T32GM008629 (PI Daniel Eberl). We also acknowledge support from the NIH (UG3 HL-147366, P01 HL51670, P01 HL091842), the Cystic Fibrosis Foundation, the University of Iowa Center for Gene Therapy (DK54759), and the Roy J. Carver Chair in Pulmonary Research (PBM).

Acknowledgments: We thank Jennifer A. Bartlett and Ashley L. Cooney for their critical review of the manuscript.

Conflicts of Interest: The authors have no conflicts of interest to declare.

References

1. Ratjen, F.; Doring, G. Cystic fibrosis. *Lancet* **2003**, *361*, 681–689. [CrossRef]
2. Brown, S.D.; White, R.; Tobin, P. Keep them breathing: Cystic fibrosis pathophysiology, diagnosis, and treatment. *JAAPA* **2017**, *30*, 23–27. [CrossRef] [PubMed]
3. Clague, S. Dorothy Hansine Andersen. *Lancet Respir. Med.* **2014**, *2*, 184–185. [CrossRef]
4. Fakhoury, K.; Durie, P.R.; Levison, H.; Canny, G.J. Meconium ileus in the absence of cystic fibrosis. *Arch. Dis. Child.* **1992**, *67*, 1204–1206. [CrossRef] [PubMed]
5. Kelly, A.; Moran, A. Update on cystic fibrosis-related diabetes. *J. Cyst. Fibros.* **2013**, *12*, 318–331. [CrossRef] [PubMed]
6. Kobelska-Dubiel, N.; Klincewicz, B.; Cichy, W. Liver disease in cystic fibrosis. *Prz. Gastroenterol.* **2014**, *9*, 136–141. [CrossRef]
7. Quinton, P.M. Missing Cl conductance in cystic fibrosis. *Am. J. Physiol.* **1986**, *251*, C649–C652. [CrossRef]
8. Sokol, R.Z. Infertility in men with cystic fibrosis. *Curr. Opin. Pulm. Med.* **2001**, *7*, 421–426. [CrossRef]
9. Thalhammer, G.H.; Eber, E.; Uranus, S.; Pfeifer, J.; Zach, M.S. Partial splenectomy in cystic fibrosis patients with hypersplenism. *Arch. Dis. Child.* **2003**, *88*, 143–146. [CrossRef]
10. Chesdachai, S.; Tangpricha, V. Treatment of vitamin D deficiency in cystic fibrosis. *J. Steroid Biochem. Mol. Biol.* **2016**, *164*, 36–39. [CrossRef]
11. Scaparrotta, A.; Di Pillo, S.; Attanasi, M.; Consilvio, N.P.; Cingolani, A.; Rapino, D.; Mohn, A.; Chiarelli, F. Growth failure in children with cystic fibrosis. *J. Pediatr. Endocrinol. Metab.* **2012**, *25*, 393–405. [CrossRef] [PubMed]

12. Quinton, P.M. Chloride impermeability in cystic fibrosis. *Nature* **1983**, *301*, 421–422. [CrossRef]

13. Knowles, M.; Gatzy, J.; Boucher, R. Relative ion permeability of normal and cystic fibrosis nasal epithelium. *J. Clin. Investig.* **1983**, *71*, 1410–1417. [CrossRef] [PubMed]

14. Welsh, M.J. An apical-membrane chloride channel in human tracheal epithelium. *Science* **1986**, *232*, 1648–1650. [CrossRef] [PubMed]

15. Welsh, M.J.; Liedtke, C.M. Chloride and potassium channels in cystic fibrosis airway epithelia. *Nature* **1986**, *322*, 467–470. [CrossRef] [PubMed]

16. Schoumacher, R.A.; Shoemaker, R.L.; Halm, D.R.; Tallant, E.A.; Wallace, R.W.; Frizzell, R.A. Phosphorylation fails to activate chloride channels from cystic fibrosis airway cells. *Nature* **1987**, *330*, 752–754. [CrossRef]

17. Riordan, J.R.; Rommens, J.M.; Kerem, B.; Alon, N.; Rozmahel, R.; Grzelczak, Z.; Zielenski, J.; Lok, S.; Plavsic, N.; Chou, J.L.; et al. Identification of the cystic fibrosis gene: Cloning and characterization of complementary DNA. *Science* **1989**, *245*, 1066–1073. [CrossRef]

18. Kerem, B.; Rommens, J.M.; Buchanan, J.A.; Markiewicz, D.; Cox, T.K.; Chakravarti, A.; Buchwald, M.; Tsui, L.C. Identification of the cystic fibrosis gene: Genetic analysis. *Science* **1989**, *245*, 1073–1080. [CrossRef]

19. Rommens, J.M.; Iannuzzi, M.C.; Kerem, B.; Drumm, M.L.; Melmer, G.; Dean, M.; Rozmahel, R.; Cole, J.L.; Kennedy, D.; Hidaka, N.; et al. Identification of the cystic fibrosis gene: Chromosome walking and jumping. *Science* **1989**, *245*, 1059–1065. [CrossRef]

20. Anderson, M.P.; Gregory, R.J.; Thompson, S.; Souza, D.W.; Paul, S.; Mulligan, R.C.; Smith, A.E.; Welsh, M.J. Demonstration that CFTR is a chloride channel by alteration of its anion selectivity. *Science* **1991**, *253*, 202–205. [CrossRef]

21. Anderson, M.P.; Rich, D.P.; Gregory, R.J.; Smith, A.E.; Welsh, M.J. Generation of cAMP-activated chloride currents by expression of CFTR. *Science* **1991**, *251*, 679–682. [CrossRef] [PubMed]

22. Bear, C.E.; Li, C.H.; Kartner, N.; Bridges, R.J.; Jensen, T.J.; Ramjeesingh, M.; Riordan, J.R. Purification and functional reconstitution of the cystic fibrosis transmembrane conductance regulator (CFTR). *Cell* **1992**, *68*, 809–818. [CrossRef]

23. Kunzelmann, K.; Schreiber, R.; Nitschke, R.; Mall, M. Control of epithelial Na+ conductance by the cystic fibrosis transmembrane conductance regulator. *Pflugers Arch.* **2000**, *440*, 193–201. [CrossRef]

24. Rich, D.P.; Anderson, M.P.; Gregory, R.J.; Cheng, S.H.; Paul, S.; Jefferson, D.M.; McCann, J.D.; Klinger, K.W.; Smith, A.E.; Welsh, M.J. Expression of cystic fibrosis transmembrane conductance regulator corrects defective chloride channel regulation in cystic fibrosis airway epithelial cells. *Nature* **1990**, *347*, 358–363. [CrossRef] [PubMed]

25. Castellani, C.; CFTR2 team. CFTR2: How will it help care? *Paediatr. Respir. Rev.* **2013**, *14* (Suppl. 1), 2–5. [CrossRef] [PubMed]

26. Welsh, M.J.; Smith, A.E. Molecular mechanisms of CFTR chloride channel dysfunction in cystic fibrosis. *Cell* **1993**, *73*, 1251–1254. [CrossRef]

27. Veit, G.; Avramescu, R.G.; Chiang, A.N.; Houck, S.A.; Cai, Z.; Peters, K.W.; Hong, J.S.; Pollard, H.B.; Guggino, W.B.; Balch, W.E.; et al. From CFTR biology toward combinatorial pharmacotherapy: Expanded classification of cystic fibrosis mutations. *Mol. Biol. Cell* **2016**, *27*, 424–433. [CrossRef] [PubMed]

28. Boyle, M.P.; De Boeck, K. A new era in the treatment of cystic fibrosis: Correction of the underlying CFTR defect. *Lancet Respir. Med.* **2013**, *1*, 158–163. [CrossRef]

29. Hamosh, A.; Trapnell, B.C.; Zeitlin, P.L.; Montrose-Rafizadeh, C.; Rosenstein, B.J.; Crystal, R.G.; Cutting, G.R. Severe deficiency of cystic fibrosis transmembrane conductance regulator messenger RNA carrying nonsense mutations R553X and W1316X in respiratory epithelial cells of patients with cystic fibrosis. *J. Clin. Investig.* **1991**, *88*, 1880–1885. [CrossRef] [PubMed]

30. Tsui, L.C. Mutations and sequence variations detected in the cystic fibrosis transmembrane conductance regulator (CFTR) gene: A report from the Cystic Fibrosis Genetic Analysis Consortium. *Hum. Mutat.* **1992**, *1*, 197–203. [CrossRef] [PubMed]

31. Denning, G.M.; Ostedgaard, L.S.; Welsh, M.J. Abnormal localization of cystic fibrosis transmembrane conductance regulator in primary cultures of cystic fibrosis airway epithelia. *J. Cell Biol.* **1992**, *118*, 551–559. [CrossRef] [PubMed]

32. Kartner, N.; Augustinas, O.; Jensen, T.J.; Naismith, A.L.; Riordan, J.R. Mislocalization of delta F508 CFTR in cystic fibrosis sweat gland. *Nat. Genet.* **1992**, *1*, 321–327. [CrossRef] [PubMed]

33. Rowe, S.M.; Miller, S.; Sorscher, E.J. Cystic fibrosis. *N. Engl. J. Med.* **2005**, *352*, 1992–2001. [CrossRef] [PubMed]
34. Cheng, S.H.; Gregory, R.J.; Marshall, J.; Paul, S.; Souza, D.W.; White, G.A.; O'Riordan, C.R.; Smith, A.E. Defective intracellular transport and processing of CFTR is the molecular basis of most cystic fibrosis. *Cell* **1990**, *63*, 827–834. [CrossRef]
35. Lukacs, G.L.; Chang, X.B.; Bear, C.; Kartner, N.; Mohamed, A.; Riordan, J.R.; Grinstein, S. The delta F508 mutation decreases the stability of cystic fibrosis transmembrane conductance regulator in the plasma membrane. Determination of functional half-lives on transfected cells. *J. Biol. Chem.* **1993**, *268*, 21592–21598.
36. Drumm, M.L.; Wilkinson, D.J.; Smit, L.S.; Worrell, R.T.; Strong, T.V.; Frizzell, R.A.; Dawson, D.C.; Collins, F.S. Chloride conductance expressed by delta F508 and other mutant CFTRs in Xenopus oocytes. *Science* **1991**, *254*, 1797–1799. [CrossRef]
37. Anderson, M.P.; Welsh, M.J. Regulation by ATP and ADP of CFTR chloride channels that contain mutant nucleotide-binding domains. *Science* **1992**, *257*, 1701–1704. [CrossRef]
38. Bompadre, S.G.; Li, M.; Hwang, T.C. Mechanism of G551D-CFTR (cystic fibrosis transmembrane conductance regulator) potentiation by a high affinity ATP analog. *J. Biol. Chem.* **2008**, *283*, 5364–5369. [CrossRef]
39. Zhou, Z.; Wang, X.; Liu, H.Y.; Zou, X.; Li, M.; Hwang, T.C. The two ATP binding sites of cystic fibrosis transmembrane conductance regulator (CFTR) play distinct roles in gating kinetics and energetics. *J. Gen. Physiol.* **2006**, *128*, 413–422. [CrossRef]
40. Bompadre, S.G.; Sohma, Y.; Li, M.; Hwang, T.C. G551D and G1349D, two CF-associated mutations in the signature sequences of CFTR, exhibit distinct gating defects. *J. Gen. Physiol.* **2007**, *129*, 285–298. [CrossRef]
41. Zeitlin, P.L. Novel pharmacologic therapies for cystic fibrosis. *J. Clin. Investig.* **1999**, *103*, 447–452. [CrossRef]
42. Sheppard, D.N.; Rich, D.P.; Ostedgaard, L.S.; Gregory, R.J.; Smith, A.E.; Welsh, M.J. Mutations in CFTR associated with mild-disease-form Cl- channels with altered pore properties. *Nature* **1993**, *362*, 160–164. [CrossRef] [PubMed]
43. Yu, Y.C.; Sohma, Y.; Hwang, T.C. On the mechanism of gating defects caused by the R117H mutation in cystic fibrosis transmembrane conductance regulator. *J. Physiol.* **2016**, *594*, 3227–3244. [CrossRef] [PubMed]
44. Zielenski, J.; Tsui, L.C. Cystic fibrosis: Genotypic and phenotypic variations. *Annu. Rev. Genet.* **1995**, *29*, 777–807. [CrossRef] [PubMed]
45. Haardt, M.; Benharouga, M.; Lechardeur, D.; Kartner, N.; Lukacs, G.L. C-terminal truncations destabilize the cystic fibrosis transmembrane conductance regulator without impairing its biogenesis. A novel class of mutation. *J. Biol. Chem.* **1999**, *274*, 21873–21877. [CrossRef] [PubMed]
46. Stern, R.C.; Doershuk, C.F.; Drumm, M.L. 3849+10 kb C–>T mutation and disease severity in cystic fibrosis. *Lancet* **1995**, *346*, 274–276. [CrossRef]
47. Beck, S.; Penque, D.; Garcia, S.; Gomes, A.; Farinha, C.; Mata, L.; Gulbenkian, S.; Gil-Ferreira, K.; Duarte, A.; Pacheco, P.; et al. Cystic fibrosis patients with the 3272-26A–>G mutation have mild disease, leaky alternative mRNA splicing, and CFTR protein at the cell membrane. *Hum. Mutat.* **1999**, *14*, 133–144. [CrossRef]
48. Marson, F.A.L.; Bertuzzo, C.S.; Ribeiro, J.D. Classification of CFTR mutation classes. *Lancet Respir. Med.* **2016**, *4*, e37–e38. [CrossRef]
49. Ma, J.; Zhao, J.; Drumm, M.L.; Xie, J.; Davis, P.B. Function of the R domain in the cystic fibrosis transmembrane conductance regulator chloride channel. *J. Biol. Chem.* **1997**, *272*, 28133–28141. [CrossRef]
50. Ostedgaard, L.S.; Baldursson, O.; Vermeer, D.W.; Welsh, M.J.; Robertson, A.D. A functional R domain from cystic fibrosis transmembrane conductance regulator is predominantly unstructured in solution. *Proc. Natl. Acad. Sci. USA* **2000**, *97*, 5657–5662. [CrossRef]
51. Zhang, Z.; Liu, F.; Chen, J. Conformational changes of CFTR upon phosphorylation and ATP binding. *Cell* **2017**, *170*, 483–491. [CrossRef] [PubMed]
52. Liu, F.; Zhang, Z.; Csanady, L.; Gadsby, D.C.; Chen, J. Molecular structure of the human CFTR ion channel. *Cell* **2017**, *169*, 85–95. [CrossRef] [PubMed]
53. Short, D.B.; Trotter, K.W.; Reczek, D.; Kreda, S.M.; Bretscher, A.; Boucher, R.C.; Stutts, M.J.; Milgram, S.L. An apical PDZ protein anchors the cystic fibrosis transmembrane conductance regulator to the cytoskeleton. *J. Biol. Chem.* **1998**, *273*, 19797–19801. [CrossRef] [PubMed]

54. Moyer, B.D.; Duhaime, M.; Shaw, C.; Denton, J.; Reynolds, D.; Karlson, K.H.; Pfeiffer, J.; Wang, S.; Mickle, J.E.; Milewski, M.; et al. The PDZ-interacting domain of cystic fibrosis transmembrane conductance regulator is required for functional expression in the apical plasma membrane. *J. Biol. Chem.* **2000**, *275*, 27069–27074. [CrossRef]

55. Xu, Y.; Clark, J.C.; Aronow, B.J.; Dey, C.R.; Liu, C.; Wooldridge, J.L.; Whitsett, J.A. Transcriptional adaptation to cystic fibrosis transmembrane conductance regulator deficiency. *J. Biol. Chem.* **2003**, *278*, 7674–7682. [CrossRef]

56. Pankow, S.; Bamberger, C.; Calzolari, D.; Martinez-Bartolome, S.; Lavallee-Adam, M.; Balch, W.E.; Yates, J.R., 3rd. F508 CFTR interactome remodelling promotes rescue of cystic fibrosis. *Nature* **2015**, *528*, 510–516. [CrossRef]

57. Zabner, J.; Scheetz, T.E.; Almabrazi, H.G.; Casavant, T.L.; Huang, J.; Keshavjee, S.; McCray, P.B., Jr. CFTR DeltaF508 mutation has minimal effect on the gene expression profile of differentiated human airway epithelia. *Am. J. Physiol. Lung Cell Mol. Physiol.* **2005**, *289*, L545–L553. [CrossRef]

58. Ramachandran, S.; Karp, P.H.; Jiang, P.; Ostedgaard, L.S.; Walz, A.E.; Fisher, J.T.; Keshavjee, S.; Lennox, K.A.; Jacobi, A.M.; Rose, S.D.; et al. A microRNA network regulates expression and biosynthesis of wild-type and DeltaF508 mutant cystic fibrosis transmembrane conductance regulator. *Proc. Natl. Acad. Sci. USA* **2012**, *109*, 13362–13367. [CrossRef]

59. Wright, J.M.; Merlo, C.A.; Reynolds, J.B.; Zeitlin, P.L.; Garcia, J.G.; Guggino, W.B.; Boyle, M.P. Respiratory epithelial gene expression in patients with mild and severe cystic fibrosis lung disease. *Am. J. Respir. Cell Mol. Biol.* **2006**, *35*, 327–336. [CrossRef]

60. Clarke, L.A.; Sousa, L.; Barreto, C.; Amaral, M.D. Changes in transcriptome of native nasal epithelium expressing F508del-CFTR and intersecting data from comparable studies. *Respir. Res.* **2013**, *14*, 38. [CrossRef]

61. Ogilvie, V.; Passmore, M.; Hyndman, L.; Jones, L.; Stevenson, B.; Wilson, A.; Davidson, H.; Kitchen, R.R.; Gray, R.D.; Shah, P.; et al. Differential global gene expression in cystic fibrosis nasal and bronchial epithelium. *Genomics* **2011**, *98*, 327–336. [CrossRef]

62. Polineni, D.; Dang, H.; Gallins, P.J.; Jones, L.C.; Pace, R.G.; Stonebraker, J.R.; Commander, L.A.; Krenicky, J.E.; Zhou, Y.H.; Corvol, H.; et al. Airway mucosal host defense is key to genomic regulation of cystic fibrosis lung disease severity. *Am. J. Respir. Crit. Care Med.* **2018**, *197*, 79–93. [CrossRef] [PubMed]

63. Clarke, L.A.; Botelho, H.M.; Sousa, L.; Falcao, A.O.; Amaral, M.D. Transcriptome meta-analysis reveals common differential and global gene expression profiles in cystic fibrosis and other respiratory disorders and identifies CFTR regulators. *Genomics* **2015**, *106*, 268–277. [CrossRef] [PubMed]

64. Kormann, M.S.D.; Dewerth, A.; Eichner, F.; Baskaran, P.; Hector, A.; Regamey, N.; Hartl, D.; Handgretinger, R.; Antony, J.S. Transcriptomic profile of cystic fibrosis patients identifies type I interferon response and ribosomal stalk proteins as potential modifiers of disease severity. *PLoS ONE* **2017**, *12*, e0183526. [CrossRef] [PubMed]

65. Oglesby, I.K.; Bray, I.M.; Chotirmall, S.H.; Stallings, R.L.; O'Neill, S.J.; McElvaney, N.G.; Greene, C.M. miR-126 is downregulated in cystic fibrosis airway epithelial cells and regulates TOM1 expression. *J. Immunol.* **2010**, *184*, 1702–1709. [CrossRef]

66. Lutful Kabir, F.; Ambalavanan, N.; Liu, G.; Li, P.; Solomon, G.M.; Lal, C.V.; Mazur, M.; Halloran, B.; Szul, T.; Gerthoffer, W.T.; et al. MicroRNA-145 antagonism reverses TGF-beta inhibition of F508del CFTR correction in airway epithelia. *Am. J. Respir. Crit. Care Med.* **2018**, *197*, 632–643. [CrossRef]

67. Bartoszewska, S.; Kamysz, W.; Jakiela, B.; Sanak, M.; Kroliczewski, J.; Bebok, Z.; Bartoszewski, R.; Collawn, J.F. miR-200b downregulates CFTR during hypoxia in human lung epithelial cells. *Cell Mol. Biol. Lett.* **2017**, *22*, 23. [CrossRef]

68. Kamei, S.; Maruta, K.; Fujikawa, H.; Nohara, H.; Ueno-Shuto, K.; Tasaki, Y.; Nakashima, R.; Kawakami, T.; Eto, Y.; Suico, M.A.; et al. Integrative expression analysis identifies a novel interplay between CFTR and linc-SUMF1-2 that involves CF-associated gene dysregulation. *Biochem. Biophys. Res. Commun.* **2019**, *509*, 521–528. [CrossRef]

69. Jensen, T.J.; Loo, M.A.; Pind, S.; Williams, D.B.; Goldberg, A.L.; Riordan, J.R. Multiple proteolytic systems, including the proteasome, contribute to CFTR processing. *Cell* **1995**, *83*, 129–135. [CrossRef]

70. Farinha, C.M.; Matos, P.; Amaral, M.D. Control of cystic fibrosis transmembrane conductance regulator membrane trafficking: Not just from the endoplasmic reticulum to the Golgi. *FEBS J.* **2013**, *280*, 4396–4406. [CrossRef]

71. Loo, M.A.; Jensen, T.J.; Cui, L.; Hou, Y.; Chang, X.B.; Riordan, J.R. Perturbation of Hsp90 interaction with nascent CFTR prevents its maturation and accelerates its degradation by the proteasome. *EMBO J.* **1998**, *17*, 6879–6887. [CrossRef] [PubMed]

72. Scott-Ward, T.S.; Amaral, M.D. Deletion of Phe508 in the first nucleotide-binding domain of the cystic fibrosis transmembrane conductance regulator increases its affinity for the heat shock cognate 70 chaperone. *FEBS J.* **2009**, *276*, 7097–7109. [CrossRef] [PubMed]

73. Meacham, G.C.; Lu, Z.; King, S.; Sorscher, E.; Tousson, A.; Cyr, D.M. The Hdj-2/Hsc70 chaperone pair facilitates early steps in CFTR biogenesis. *EMBO J.* **1999**, *18*, 1492–1505. [CrossRef]

74. Bagdany, M.; Veit, G.; Fukuda, R.; Avramescu, R.G.; Okiyoneda, T.; Baaklini, I.; Singh, J.; Sovak, G.; Xu, H.; Apaja, P.M.; et al. Chaperones rescue the energetic landscape of mutant CFTR at single molecule and in cell. *Nat. Commun.* **2017**, *8*, 398. [CrossRef] [PubMed]

75. Matsumura, Y.; David, L.L.; Skach, W.R. Role of Hsc70 binding cycle in CFTR folding and endoplasmic reticulum-associated degradation. *Mol. Biol. Cell* **2011**, *22*, 2797–2809. [CrossRef]

76. Marozkina, N.V.; Yemen, S.; Borowitz, M.; Liu, L.; Plapp, M.; Sun, F.; Islam, R.; Erdmann-Gilmore, P.; Townsend, R.R.; Lichti, C.F.; et al. Hsp 70/Hsp 90 organizing protein as a nitrosylation target in cystic fibrosis therapy. *Proc. Natl. Acad. Sci. USA* **2010**, *107*, 11393–11398. [CrossRef]

77. Zaman, K.; Sawczak, V.; Zaidi, A.; Butler, M.; Bennett, D.; Getsy, P.; Zeinomar, M.; Greenberg, Z.; Forbes, M.; Rehman, S.; et al. Augmentation of CFTR maturation by S-nitrosoglutathione reductase. *Am. J. Physiol. Lung Cell Mol. Physiol.* **2016**, *310*, L263–L270. [CrossRef] [PubMed]

78. Kabani, M.; McLellan, C.; Raynes, D.A.; Guerriero, V.; Brodsky, J.L. HspBP1, a homologue of the yeast Fes1 and Sls1 proteins, is an Hsc70 nucleotide exchange factor. *FEBS Lett.* **2002**, *531*, 339–342. [CrossRef]

79. Alberti, S.; Bohse, K.; Arndt, V.; Schmitz, A.; Hohfeld, J. The cochaperone HspBP1 inhibits the CHIP ubiquitin ligase and stimulates the maturation of the cystic fibrosis transmembrane conductance regulator. *Mol. Biol. Cell* **2004**, *15*, 4003–4010. [CrossRef]

80. Koulov, A.V.; LaPointe, P.; Lu, B.; Razvi, A.; Coppinger, J.; Dong, M.Q.; Matteson, J.; Laister, R.; Arrowsmith, C.; Yates, J.R., 3rd; et al. Biological and structural basis for Aha1 regulation of Hsp90 ATPase activity in maintaining proteostasis in the human disease cystic fibrosis. *Mol. Biol. Cell* **2010**, *21*, 871–884. [CrossRef]

81. Wang, X.; Venable, J.; LaPointe, P.; Hutt, D.M.; Koulov, A.V.; Coppinger, J.; Gurkan, C.; Kellner, W.; Matteson, J.; Plutner, H.; et al. Hsp90 cochaperone Aha1 downregulation rescues misfolding of CFTR in cystic fibrosis. *Cell* **2006**, *127*, 803–815. [CrossRef] [PubMed]

82. Saxena, A.; Banasavadi-Siddegowda, Y.K.; Fan, Y.; Bhattacharya, S.; Roy, G.; Giovannucci, D.R.; Frizzell, R.A.; Wang, X. Human heat shock protein 105/110 kDa (Hsp105/110) regulates biogenesis and quality control of misfolded cystic fibrosis transmembrane conductance regulator at multiple levels. *J. Biol. Chem.* **2012**, *287*, 19158–19170. [CrossRef] [PubMed]

83. Bracher, A.; Verghese, J. The nucleotide exchange factors of Hsp70 molecular chaperones. *Front. Mol. Biosci.* **2015**, *2*, 10. [CrossRef] [PubMed]

84. Strickland, E.; Qu, B.H.; Millen, L.; Thomas, P.J. The molecular chaperone Hsc70 assists the in vitro folding of the N-terminal nucleotide-binding domain of the cystic fibrosis transmembrane conductance regulator. *J. Biol. Chem.* **1997**, *272*, 25421–25424. [CrossRef] [PubMed]

85. Farinha, C.M.; Nogueira, P.; Mendes, F.; Penque, D.; Amaral, M.D. The human DnaJ homologue (Hdj)-1/heat-shock protein (Hsp) 40 co-chaperone is required for the in vivo stabilization of the cystic fibrosis transmembrane conductance regulator by Hsp70. *Biochem. J.* **2002**, *366*, 797–806. [CrossRef]

86. Younger, J.M.; Ren, H.Y.; Chen, L.; Fan, C.Y.; Fields, A.; Patterson, C.; Cyr, D.M. A foldable CFTR{Delta}F508 biogenic intermediate accumulates upon inhibition of the Hsc70-CHIP E3 ubiquitin ligase. *J. Cell Biol.* **2004**, *167*, 1075–1085. [CrossRef]

87. Schmidt, B.Z.; Watts, R.J.; Aridor, M.; Frizzell, R.A. Cysteine string protein promotes proteasomal degradation of the cystic fibrosis transmembrane conductance regulator (CFTR) by increasing its interaction with the C terminus of Hsp70-interacting protein and promoting CFTR ubiquitylation. *J. Biol. Chem.* **2009**, *284*, 4168–4178. [CrossRef]

88. Zhang, H.; Peters, K.W.; Sun, F.; Marino, C.R.; Lang, J.; Burgoyne, R.D.; Frizzell, R.A. Cysteine string protein interacts with and modulates the maturation of the cystic fibrosis transmembrane conductance regulator. *J. Biol. Chem.* **2002**, *277*, 28948–28958. [CrossRef]

89. Zhang, H.; Schmidt, B.Z.; Sun, F.; Condliffe, S.B.; Butterworth, M.B.; Youker, R.T.; Brodsky, J.L.; Aridor, M.; Frizzell, R.A. Cysteine string protein monitors late steps in cystic fibrosis transmembrane conductance regulator biogenesis. *J. Biol. Chem.* **2006**, *281*, 11312–11321. [CrossRef]

90. Grove, D.E.; Fan, C.Y.; Ren, H.Y.; Cyr, D.M. The endoplasmic reticulum-associated Hsp40 DNAJB12 and Hsc70 cooperate to facilitate RMA1 E3-dependent degradation of nascent CFTRDeltaF508. *Mol. Biol. Cell* **2011**, *22*, 301–314. [CrossRef]

91. Yamamoto, Y.H.; Kimura, T.; Momohara, S.; Takeuchi, M.; Tani, T.; Kimata, Y.; Kadokura, H.; Kohno, K. A novel ER J-protein DNAJB12 accelerates ER-associated degradation of membrane proteins including CFTR. *Cell Struct. Funct.* **2010**, *35*, 107–116. [CrossRef] [PubMed]

92. Mogk, A.; Ruger-Herreros, C.; Bukau, B. Cellular functions and mechanisms of action of small heat shock proteins. *Annu. Rev. Microbiol.* **2019**, *73*, 89–110. [CrossRef] [PubMed]

93. Ahner, A.; Gong, X.; Schmidt, B.Z.; Peters, K.W.; Rabeh, W.M.; Thibodeau, P.H.; Lukacs, G.L.; Frizzell, R.A. Small heat shock proteins target mutant cystic fibrosis transmembrane conductance regulator for degradation via a small ubiquitin-like modifier-dependent pathway. *Mol. Biol. Cell* **2013**, *24*, 74–84. [CrossRef] [PubMed]

94. Gong, X.; Ahner, A.; Roldan, A.; Lukacs, G.L.; Thibodeau, P.H.; Frizzell, R.A. Non-native conformers of cystic fibrosis transmembrane conductance regulator NBD1 are recognized by Hsp27 and conjugated to SUMO-2 for degradation. *J. Biol. Chem.* **2016**, *291*, 2004–2017. [CrossRef] [PubMed]

95. Rosser, M.F.; Grove, D.E.; Chen, L.; Cyr, D.M. Assembly and misassembly of cystic fibrosis transmembrane conductance regulator: Folding defects caused by deletion of F508 occur before and after the calnexin-dependent association of membrane spanning domain (MSD) 1 and MSD2. *Mol. Biol. Cell* **2008**, *19*, 4570–4579. [CrossRef]

96. Farinha, C.M.; Amaral, M.D. Most F508del-CFTR is targeted to degradation at an early folding checkpoint and independently of calnexin. *Mol. Cell Biol.* **2005**, *25*, 5242–5252. [CrossRef]

97. Okiyoneda, T.; Niibori, A.; Harada, K.; Kohno, T.; Michalak, M.; Duszyk, M.; Wada, I.; Ikawa, M.; Shuto, T.; Suico, M.A.; et al. Role of calnexin in the ER quality control and productive folding of CFTR; differential effect of calnexin knockout on wild-type and DeltaF508 CFTR. *Biochim. Biophys. Acta* **2008**, *1783*, 1585–1594. [CrossRef]

98. Harada, K.; Okiyoneda, T.; Hashimoto, Y.; Ueno, K.; Nakamura, K.; Yamahira, K.; Sugahara, T.; Shuto, T.; Wada, I.; Suico, M.A.; et al. Calreticulin negatively regulates the cell surface expression of cystic fibrosis transmembrane conductance regulator. *J. Biol. Chem.* **2006**, *281*, 12841–12848. [CrossRef]

99. Ward, C.L.; Kopito, R.R. Intracellular turnover of cystic fibrosis transmembrane conductance regulator. Inefficient processing and rapid degradation of wild-type and mutant proteins. *J. Biol. Chem.* **1994**, *269*, 25710–25718.

100. Oberdorf, J.; Carlson, E.J.; Skach, W.R. Redundancy of mammalian proteasome beta subunit function during endoplasmic reticulum associated degradation. *Biochemistry* **2001**, *40*, 13397–13405. [CrossRef]

101. Mulder, M.P.; Witting, K.; Berlin, I.; Pruneda, J.N.; Wu, K.P.; Chang, J.G.; Merkx, R.; Bialas, J.; Groettrup, M.; Vertegaal, A.C.; et al. A cascading activity-based probe sequentially targets E1-E2-E3 ubiquitin enzymes. *Nat. Chem. Biol.* **2016**, *12*, 523–530. [CrossRef] [PubMed]

102. Ardley, H.C.; Robinson, P.A. E3 ubiquitin ligases. *Essays Biochem.* **2005**, *41*, 15–30. [CrossRef] [PubMed]

103. Nakayama, K.I.; Nakayama, K. Ubiquitin ligases: Cell-cycle control and cancer. *Nat. Rev. Cancer* **2006**, *6*, 369–381. [CrossRef]

104. Li, W.; Bengtson, M.H.; Ulbrich, A.; Matsuda, A.; Reddy, V.A.; Orth, A.; Chanda, S.K.; Batalov, S.; Joazeiro, C.A. Genome-wide and functional annotation of human E3 ubiquitin ligases identifies MULAN, a mitochondrial E3 that regulates the organelle's dynamics and signaling. *PLoS ONE* **2008**, *3*, e1487. [CrossRef]

105. Younger, J.M.; Chen, L.; Ren, H.Y.; Rosser, M.F.; Turnbull, E.L.; Fan, C.Y.; Patterson, C.; Cyr, D.M. Sequential quality-control checkpoints triage misfolded cystic fibrosis transmembrane conductance regulator. *Cell* **2006**, *126*, 571–582. [CrossRef] [PubMed]

106. El Khouri, E.; Le Pavec, G.; Toledano, M.B.; Delaunay-Moisan, A. RNF185 is a novel E3 ligase of endoplasmic reticulum-associated degradation (ERAD) that targets cystic fibrosis transmembrane conductance regulator (CFTR). *J. Biol. Chem.* **2013**, *288*, 31177–31191. [CrossRef]

107. Morito, D.; Hirao, K.; Oda, Y.; Hosokawa, N.; Tokunaga, F.; Cyr, D.M.; Tanaka, K.; Iwai, K.; Nagata, K. Gp78 cooperates with RMA1 in endoplasmic reticulum-associated degradation of CFTRDeltaF508. *Mol. Biol. Cell* **2008**, *19*, 1328–1336. [CrossRef]

108. Mehnert, M.; Sommer, T.; Jarosch, E. Der1 promotes movement of misfolded proteins through the endoplasmic reticulum membrane. *Nat. Cell Biol.* **2014**, *16*, 77–86. [CrossRef]

109. Mehnert, M.; Sommermeyer, F.; Berger, M.; Kumar Lakshmipathy, S.; Gauss, R.; Aebi, M.; Jarosch, E.; Sommer, T. The interplay of Hrd3 and the molecular chaperone system ensures efficient degradation of malfolded secretory proteins. *Mol. Biol. Cell* **2015**, *26*, 185–194. [CrossRef]

110. Carvalho, P.; Stanley, A.M.; Rapoport, T.A. Retrotranslocation of a misfolded luminal ER protein by the ubiquitin-ligase Hrd1p. *Cell* **2010**, *143*, 579–591. [CrossRef]

111. Meacham, G.C.; Patterson, C.; Zhang, W.; Younger, J.M.; Cyr, D.M. The Hsc70 co-chaperone CHIP targets immature CFTR for proteasomal degradation. *Nat. Cell Biol.* **2001**, *3*, 100–105. [CrossRef] [PubMed]

112. Okiyoneda, T.; Veit, G.; Sakai, R.; Aki, M.; Fujihara, T.; Higashi, M.; Susuki-Miyata, S.; Miyata, M.; Fukuda, N.; Yoshida, A.; et al. Chaperone-independent peripheral quality control of CFTR by RFFL E3 ligase. *Dev. Cell* **2018**, *44*, 694–708. [CrossRef] [PubMed]

113. Cheng, J.; Guggino, W. Ubiquitination and degradation of CFTR by the E3 ubiquitin ligase MARCH2 through its association with adaptor proteins CAL and STX6. *PLoS ONE* **2013**, *8*, e68001. [CrossRef] [PubMed]

114. Caohuy, H.; Jozwik, C.; Pollard, H.B. Rescue of DeltaF508-CFTR by the SGK1/Nedd4-2 signaling pathway. *J. Biol. Chem.* **2009**, *284*, 25241–25253. [CrossRef] [PubMed]

115. Ramachandran, S.; Osterhaus, S.R.; Parekh, K.R.; Jacobi, A.M.; Behlke, M.A.; McCray, P.B., Jr. SYVN1, NEDD8, and FBXO2 proteins regulate DeltaF508 cystic fibrosis transmembrane conductance regulator (CFTR) ubiquitin-mediated proteasomal degradation. *J. Biol. Chem.* **2016**, *291*, 25489–25504. [CrossRef]

116. Bomberger, J.M.; Barnaby, R.L.; Stanton, B.A. The deubiquitinating enzyme USP10 regulates the post-endocytic sorting of cystic fibrosis transmembrane conductance regulator in airway epithelial cells. *J. Biol. Chem.* **2009**, *284*, 18778–18789. [CrossRef] [PubMed]

117. Bomberger, J.M.; Barnaby, R.L.; Stanton, B.A. The deubiquitinating enzyme USP10 regulates the endocytic recycling of CFTR in airway epithelial cells. *Channels (Austin)* **2010**, *4*, 150–154. [CrossRef]

118. Farhan, H.; Weiss, M.; Tani, K.; Kaufman, R.J.; Hauri, H.P. Adaptation of endoplasmic reticulum exit sites to acute and chronic increases in cargo load. *EMBO J.* **2008**, *27*, 2043–2054. [CrossRef]

119. Piao, H.; Kim, J.; Noh, S.H.; Kweon, H.S.; Kim, J.Y.; Lee, M.G. Sec16A is critical for both conventional and unconventional secretion of CFTR. *Sci. Rep.* **2017**, *7*, 39887. [CrossRef]

120. Gee, H.Y.; Noh, S.H.; Tang, B.L.; Kim, K.H.; Lee, M.G. Rescue of DeltaF508-CFTR trafficking via a GRASP-dependent unconventional secretion pathway. *Cell* **2011**, *146*, 746–760. [CrossRef]

121. Kim, J.; Noh, S.H.; Piao, H.; Kim, D.H.; Kim, K.; Cha, J.S.; Chung, W.Y.; Cho, H.S.; Kim, J.Y.; Lee, M.G. Monomerization and ER Relocalization of GRASP Is a Requisite for Unconventional Secretion of CFTR. *Traffic* **2016**, *17*, 733–753. [CrossRef] [PubMed]

122. Chappe, V.; Irvine, T.; Liao, J.; Evagelidis, A.; Hanrahan, J.W. Phosphorylation of CFTR by PKA promotes binding of the regulatory domain. *EMBO J.* **2005**, *24*, 2730–2740. [CrossRef] [PubMed]

123. Jia, Y.; Mathews, C.J.; Hanrahan, J.W. Phosphorylation by protein kinase C is required for acute activation of cystic fibrosis transmembrane conductance regulator by protein kinase A. *J. Biol. Chem.* **1997**, *272*, 4978–4984. [CrossRef] [PubMed]

124. Hallows, K.R.; Raghuram, V.; Kemp, B.E.; Witters, L.A.; Foskett, J.K. Inhibition of cystic fibrosis transmembrane conductance regulator by novel interaction with the metabolic sensor AMP-activated protein kinase. *J. Clin. Investig.* **2000**, *105*, 1711–1721. [CrossRef] [PubMed]

125. Farinha, C.M.; Swiatecka-Urban, A.; Brautigan, D.L.; Jordan, P. Regulatory crosstalk by protein kinases on CFTR trafficking and activity. *Front. Chem.* **2016**, *4*, 1. [CrossRef]

126. Hegde, R.N.; Parashuraman, S.; Iorio, F.; Ciciriello, F.; Capuani, F.; Carissimo, A.; Carrella, D.; Belcastro, V.; Subramanian, A.; Bounti, L.; et al. Unravelling druggable signalling networks that control F508del-CFTR proteostasis. *eLife* **2015**, *4*. [CrossRef]

127. Tuo, B.; Wen, G.; Zhang, Y.; Liu, X.; Wang, X.; Liu, X.; Dong, H. Involvement of phosphatidylinositol 3-kinase in cAMP- and cGMP-induced duodenal epithelial CFTR activation in mice. *Am. J. Physiol. Cell Physiol.* **2009**, *297*, C503–C515. [CrossRef]

128. Reilly, R.; Mroz, M.S.; Dempsey, E.; Wynne, K.; Keely, S.J.; McKone, E.F.; Hiebel, C.; Behl, C.; Coppinger, J.A. Targeting the PI3K/Akt/mTOR signalling pathway in cystic fibrosis. *Sci. Rep.* **2017**, *7*, 7642. [CrossRef]

129. Fu, L.; Rab, A.; Tang, L.P.; Rowe, S.M.; Bebok, Z.; Collawn, J.F. Dab2 is a key regulator of endocytosis and post-endocytic trafficking of the cystic fibrosis transmembrane conductance regulator. *Biochem. J.* **2012**, *441*, 633–643. [CrossRef]

130. Madden, D.R.; Swiatecka-Urban, A. Tissue-specific control of CFTR endocytosis by Dab2: Cargo recruitment as a therapeutic target. *Commun. Integr. Biol.* **2012**, *5*, 473–476. [CrossRef]

131. Loureiro, C.A.; Matos, A.M.; Dias-Alves, A.; Pereira, J.F.; Uliyakina, I.; Barros, P.; Amaral, M.D.; Matos, P. A molecular switch in the scaffold NHERF1 enables misfolded CFTR to evade the peripheral quality control checkpoint. *Sci. Signal.* **2015**, *8*, ra48. [CrossRef]

132. Lobo, M.J.; Amaral, M.D.; Zaccolo, M.; Farinha, C.M. EPAC1 activation by cAMP stabilizes CFTR at the membrane by promoting its interaction with NHERF1. *J. Cell Sci.* **2016**, *129*, 2599–2612. [CrossRef] [PubMed]

133. Cheng, J.; Cebotaru, V.; Cebotaru, L.; Guggino, W.B. Syntaxin 6 and CAL mediate the degradation of the cystic fibrosis transmembrane conductance regulator. *Mol. Biol. Cell* **2010**, *21*, 1178–1187. [CrossRef]

134. Cheng, J.; Wang, H.; Guggino, W.B. Modulation of mature cystic fibrosis transmembrane regulator protein by the PDZ domain protein CAL. *J. Biol. Chem.* **2004**, *279*, 1892–1898. [CrossRef] [PubMed]

135. Lopes-Pacheco, M.; Boinot, C.; Sabirzhanova, I.; Rapino, D.; Cebotaru, L. Combination of correctors rescues CFTR transmembrane-domain mutants by mitigating their interactions with proteostasis. *Cell Physiol. Biochem.* **2017**, *41*, 2194–2210. [CrossRef] [PubMed]

136. Van Goor, F.; Hadida, S.; Grootenhuis, P.D.; Burton, B.; Cao, D.; Neuberger, T.; Turnbull, A.; Singh, A.; Joubran, J.; Hazlewood, A.; et al. Rescue of CF airway epithelial cell function in vitro by a CFTR potentiator, VX-770. *Proc. Natl. Acad. Sci. USA* **2009**, *106*, 18825–18830. [CrossRef]

137. Van Goor, F.; Straley, K.S.; Cao, D.; Gonzalez, J.; Hadida, S.; Hazlewood, A.; Joubran, J.; Knapp, T.; Makings, L.R.; Miller, M.; et al. Rescue of DeltaF508-CFTR trafficking and gating in human cystic fibrosis airway primary cultures by small molecules. *Am. J. Physiol. Lung Cell Mol. Physiol.* **2006**, *290*, L1117–L1130. [CrossRef]

138. Van Goor, F.; Yu, H.; Burton, B.; Hoffman, B.J. Effect of ivacaftor on CFTR forms with missense mutations associated with defects in protein processing or function. *J. Cyst. Fibros.* **2014**, *13*, 29–36. [CrossRef]

139. Eckford, P.D.; Li, C.; Ramjeesingh, M.; Bear, C.E. Cystic fibrosis transmembrane conductance regulator (CFTR) potentiator VX-770 (ivacaftor) opens the defective channel gate of mutant CFTR in a phosphorylation-dependent but ATP-independent manner. *J. Biol. Chem.* **2012**, *287*, 36639–36649. [CrossRef]

140. De Boeck, K.; Munck, A.; Walker, S.; Faro, A.; Hiatt, P.; Gilmartin, G.; Higgins, M. Efficacy and safety of ivacaftor in patients with cystic fibrosis and a non-G551D gating mutation. *J. Cyst. Fibros* **2014**, *13*, 674–680. [CrossRef]

141. Moss, R.B.; Flume, P.A.; Elborn, J.S.; Cooke, J.; Rowe, S.M.; McColley, S.A.; Rubenstein, R.C.; Higgins, M.; Group, V.X.S. Efficacy and safety of ivacaftor in patients with cystic fibrosis who have an Arg117His-CFTR mutation: A double-blind, randomised controlled trial. *Lancet Respir. Med.* **2015**, *3*, 524–533. [CrossRef]

142. Accurso, F.J.; Rowe, S.M.; Clancy, J.P.; Boyle, M.P.; Dunitz, J.M.; Durie, P.R.; Sagel, S.D.; Hornick, D.B.; Konstan, M.W.; Donaldson, S.H.; et al. Effect of VX-770 in persons with cystic fibrosis and the G551D-CFTR mutation. *N. Engl. J. Med.* **2010**, *363*, 1991–2003. [CrossRef] [PubMed]

143. Ramsey, B.W.; Davies, J.; McElvaney, N.G.; Tullis, E.; Bell, S.C.; Drevinek, P.; Griese, M.; McKone, E.F.; Wainwright, C.E.; Konstan, M.W.; et al. A CFTR potentiator in patients with cystic fibrosis and the G551D mutation. *N. Engl. J. Med.* **2011**, *365*, 1663–1672. [CrossRef] [PubMed]

144. Davies, J.; Sheridan, H.; Bell, N.; Cunningham, S.; Davis, S.D.; Elborn, J.S.; Milla, C.E.; Starner, T.D.; Weiner, D.J.; Lee, P.S.; et al. Assessment of clinical response to ivacaftor with lung clearance index in cystic fibrosis patients with a G551D-CFTR mutation and preserved spirometry: A randomised controlled trial. *Lancet Respir. Med.* **2013**, *1*, 630–638. [CrossRef]

145. Davies, J.C.; Wainwright, C.E.; Canny, G.J.; Chilvers, M.A.; Howenstine, M.S.; Munck, A.; Mainz, J.G.; Rodriguez, S.; Li, H.; Yen, K.; et al. Efficacy and safety of ivacaftor in patients aged 6 to 11 years with cystic fibrosis with a G551D mutation. *Am. J. Respir. Crit. Care Med.* **2013**, *187*, 1219–1225. [CrossRef]

146. McKone, E.F.; Borowitz, D.; Drevinek, P.; Griese, M.; Konstan, M.W.; Wainwright, C.; Ratjen, F.; Sermet-Gaudelus, I.; Plant, B.; Munck, A.; et al. Long-term safety and efficacy of ivacaftor in patients with cystic fibrosis who have the Gly551Asp-CFTR mutation: A phase 3, open-label extension study (PERSIST). *Lancet Respir. Med.* **2014**, *2*, 902–910. [CrossRef]

147. Carter, S.; Kelly, S.; Caples, E.; Grogan, B.; Doyle, J.; Gallagher, C.G.; McKone, E.F. Ivacaftor as salvage therapy in a patient with cystic fibrosis genotype F508del/R117H/IVS8-5T. *J. Cyst. Fibros.* **2015**, *14*, e4–e5. [CrossRef]

148. Ronan, N.J.; Fleming, C.; O'Callaghan, G.; Maher, M.M.; Murphy, D.M.; Plant, B.J. The role of Ivacaftor in severe cystic fibrosis in a patient with the R117H mutation. *Chest* **2015**, *148*, e72–e75. [CrossRef]

149. Hadida, S.; Van Goor, F.; Zhou, J.; Arumugam, V.; McCartney, J.; Hazlewood, A.; Decker, C.; Negulescu, P.; Grootenhuis, P.D. Discovery of N-(2,4-di-tert-butyl-5-hydroxyphenyl)-4-oxo-1,4-dihydroquinoline-3-carboxamide (VX-770, ivacaftor), a potent and orally bioavailable CFTR potentiator. *J. Med. Chem.* **2014**, *57*, 9776–9795. [CrossRef]

150. Jih, K.Y.; Hwang, T.C. Vx-770 potentiates CFTR function by promoting decoupling between the gating cycle and ATP hydrolysis cycle. *Proc. Natl. Acad. Sci. USA* **2013**, *110*, 4404–4409. [CrossRef]

151. Flume, P.A.; Liou, T.G.; Borowitz, D.S.; Li, H.; Yen, K.; Ordonez, C.L.; Geller, D.E.; Group, V.X.S. Ivacaftor in subjects with cystic fibrosis who are homozygous for the F508del-CFTR mutation. *Chest* **2012**, *142*, 718–724. [CrossRef] [PubMed]

152. Dekkers, J.F.; Van Mourik, P.; Vonk, A.M.; Kruisselbrink, E.; Berkers, G.; de Winter-de Groot, K.M.; Janssens, H.M.; Bronsveld, I.; van der Ent, C.K.; de Jonge, H.R.; et al. Potentiator synergy in rectal organoids carrying S1251N, G551D, or F508del CFTR mutations. *J. Cyst. Fibros.* **2016**, *15*, 568–578. [CrossRef] [PubMed]

153. Pedemonte, N.; Tomati, V.; Sondo, E.; Caci, E.; Millo, E.; Armirotti, A.; Damonte, G.; Zegarra-Moran, O.; Galietta, L.J. Dual activity of aminoarylthiazoles on the trafficking and gating defects of the cystic fibrosis transmembrane conductance regulator chloride channel caused by cystic fibrosis mutations. *J. Biol. Chem.* **2011**, *286*, 15215–15226. [CrossRef] [PubMed]

154. Pesce, E.; Bellotti, M.; Liessi, N.; Guariento, S.; Damonte, G.; Cichero, E.; Galatini, A.; Salis, A.; Gianotti, A.; Pedemonte, N.; et al. Synthesis and structure-activity relationship of aminoarylthiazole derivatives as correctors of the chloride transport defect in cystic fibrosis. *Eur. J. Med. Chem.* **2015**, *99*, 14–35. [CrossRef] [PubMed]

155. Faure, G.; Bakouh, N.; Lourdel, S.; Odolczyk, N.; Premchandar, A.; Servel, N.; Hatton, A.; Ostrowski, M.K.; Xu, H.; Saul, F.A.; et al. Rattlesnake phospholipase A2 increases CFTR-chloride channel current and corrects F508CFTR dysfunction: Impact in cystic fibrosis. *J. Mol. Biol.* **2016**, *428*, 2898–2915. [CrossRef]

156. Pedemonte, N.; Lukacs, G.L.; Du, K.; Caci, E.; Zegarra-Moran, O.; Galietta, L.J.; Verkman, A.S. Small-molecule correctors of defective DeltaF508-CFTR cellular processing identified by high-throughput screening. *J. Clin. Investig.* **2005**, *115*, 2564–2571. [CrossRef]

157. Van Goor, F.; Hadida, S.; Grootenhuis, P.D.; Burton, B.; Stack, J.H.; Straley, K.S.; Decker, C.J.; Miller, M.; McCartney, J.; Olson, E.R.; et al. Correction of the F508del-CFTR protein processing defect in vitro by the investigational drug VX-809. *Proc. Natl. Acad. Sci. USA* **2011**, *108*, 18843–18848. [CrossRef]

158. Loo, T.W.; Bartlett, M.C.; Clarke, D.M. Corrector VX-809 stabilizes the first transmembrane domain of CFTR. *Biochem. Pharmacol.* **2013**, *86*, 612–619. [CrossRef]

159. Ren, H.Y.; Grove, D.E.; De La Rosa, O.; Houck, S.A.; Sopha, P.; Van Goor, F.; Hoffman, B.J.; Cyr, D.M. VX-809 corrects folding defects in cystic fibrosis transmembrane conductance regulator protein through action on membrane-spanning domain 1. *Mol. Biol. Cell* **2013**, *24*, 3016–3024. [CrossRef]

160. Farinha, C.M.; King-Underwood, J.; Sousa, M.; Correia, A.R.; Henriques, B.J.; Roxo-Rosa, M.; Da Paula, A.C.; Williams, J.; Hirst, S.; Gomes, C.M.; et al. Revertants, low temperature, and correctors reveal the mechanism of F508del-CFTR rescue by VX-809 and suggest multiple agents for full correction. *Chem. Biol.* **2013**, *20*, 943–955. [CrossRef]

161. Cholon, D.M.; Esther, C.R., Jr.; Gentzsch, M. Efficacy of lumacaftor-ivacaftor for the treatment of cystic fibrosis patients homozygous for the F508del-CFTR mutation. *Expert Rev. Precis. Med. Drug Dev.* **2016**, *1*, 235–243. [CrossRef] [PubMed]

162. Wainwright, C.E.; Elborn, J.S.; Ramsey, B.W. Lumacaftor-Ivacaftor in patients with cystic fibrosis homozygous for Phe508del CFTR. *N. Engl. J. Med.* **2015**, *373*, 1783–1784. [CrossRef] [PubMed]

163. Veit, G.; Avramescu, R.G.; Perdomo, D.; Phuan, P.W.; Bagdany, M.; Apaja, P.M.; Borot, F.; Szollosi, D.; Wu, Y.S.; Finkbeiner, W.E.; et al. Some gating potentiators, including VX-770, diminish DeltaF508-CFTR functional expression. *Sci. Transl. Med.* **2014**, *6*, 246ra297. [CrossRef]

164. Cholon, D.M.; Quinney, N.L.; Fulcher, M.L.; Esther, C.R., Jr.; Das, J.; Dokholyan, N.V.; Randell, S.H.; Boucher, R.C.; Gentzsch, M. Potentiator ivacaftor abrogates pharmacological correction of DeltaF508 CFTR in cystic fibrosis. *Sci. Transl. Med.* **2014**, *6*, 246ra296. [CrossRef]

165. Walker, J. Vertex Pharmaceuticals' Cystic Fibrosis Drug Disappoints. *Wall Street J.* 2016. Available online: https://www.wsj.com/articles/vertex-pharmaceuticals-loss-narrows-as-sales-surge-1461792448 (accessed on 12 May 2020).

166. Keating, D.; Marigowda, G.; Burr, L.; Daines, C.; Mall, M.A.; McKone, E.F.; Ramsey, B.W.; Rowe, S.M.; Sass, L.A.; Tullis, E.; et al. VX-445-Tezacaftor-Ivacaftor in patients with cystic fibrosis and one or two Phe508del alleles. *N. Engl. J. Med.* **2018**, *379*, 1612–1620. [CrossRef] [PubMed]

167. Heijerman, H.G.M.; McKone, E.F.; Downey, D.G.; Van Braeckel, E.; Rowe, S.M.; Tullis, E.; Mall, M.A.; Welter, J.J.; Ramsey, B.W.; McKee, C.M.; et al. Efficacy and safety of the elexacaftor plus tezacaftor plus ivacaftor combination regimen in people with cystic fibrosis homozygous for the F508del mutation: A double-blind, randomised, phase 3 trial. *Lancet* **2019**, *394*, 1940–1948. [CrossRef]

168. Middleton, P.G.; Mall, M.A.; Drevinek, P.; Lands, L.C.; McKone, E.F.; Polineni, D.; Ramsey, B.W.; Taylor-Cousar, J.L.; Tullis, E.; Vermeulen, F.; et al. Elexacaftor-Tezacaftor-Ivacaftor for cystic fibrosis with a single Phe508del allele. *N. Engl. J. Med.* **2019**, *381*, 1809–1819. [CrossRef]

169. Vertex. Vertex Announces Positive Phase 1 & Phase 2 Data from Three Different Triple Combination Regimens in People with Cystic Fibrosis Who Have One F508del Mutation and One Minimal Function Mutation (F508del/Min). 2017. Available online: investors.vrtx.com (accessed on 12 May 2020).

170. Wang, X.; Liu, B.; Searle, X.; Yeung, C.; Bogdan, A.; Greszler, S.; Singh, A.; Fan, Y.; Swensen, A.M.; Vortherms, T.; et al. Discovery of 4-[(2R,4R)-4-({[1-(2,2-Difluoro-1,3-benzodioxol-5-yl)cyclopropyl]carbonyl}amino)-7-(difluoromethoxy)-3,4-dihydro-2H-chromen-2-yl]benzoic Acid (ABBV/GLPG-2222), a potent cystic fibrosis transmembrane conductance regulator (CFTR) corrector for the treatment of cystic fibrosis. *J. Med. Chem.* **2018**, *61*, 1436–1449. [CrossRef]

171. Kym, P.R.; Wang, X.; Pizzonero, M.; Van der Plas, S.E. Recent progress in the discovery and development of small-molecule modulators of CFTR. *Prog. Med. Chem.* **2018**, *57*, 235–276. [CrossRef]

172. Kerem, B.; Chiba-Falek, O.; Kerem, E. Cystic fibrosis in Jews: Frequency and mutation distribution. *Genet. Test.* **1997**, *1*, 35–39. [CrossRef]

173. Bobadilla, J.L.; Macek, M., Jr.; Fine, J.P.; Farrell, P.M. Cystic fibrosis: A worldwide analysis of CFTR mutations–correlation with incidence data and application to screening. *Hum. Mutat* **2002**, *19*, 575–606. [CrossRef]

174. Howard, M.; Frizzell, R.A.; Bedwell, D.M. Aminoglycoside antibiotics restore CFTR function by overcoming premature stop mutations. *Nat. Med.* **1996**, *2*, 467–469. [CrossRef]

175. Wilschanski, M.; Yahav, Y.; Yaacov, Y.; Blau, H.; Bentur, L.; Rivlin, J.; Aviram, M.; Bdolah-Abram, T.; Bebok, Z.; Shushi, L.; et al. Gentamicin-induced correction of CFTR function in patients with cystic fibrosis and CFTR stop mutations. *N. Engl. J. Med.* **2003**, *349*, 1433–1441. [CrossRef]

176. Clancy, J.P.; Rowe, S.M.; Bebok, Z.; Aitken, M.L.; Gibson, R.; Zeitlin, P.; Berclaz, P.; Moss, R.; Knowles, M.R.; Oster, R.A.; et al. No detectable improvements in cystic fibrosis transmembrane conductance regulator by nasal aminoglycosides in patients with cystic fibrosis with stop mutations. *Am. J. Respir. Cell Mol. Biol.* **2007**, *37*, 57–66. [CrossRef] [PubMed]

177. Prayle, A.; Watson, A.; Fortnum, H.; Smyth, A. Side effects of aminoglycosides on the kidney, ear and balance in cystic fibrosis. *Thorax* **2010**, *65*, 654–658. [CrossRef] [PubMed]

178. Du, M.; Liu, X.; Welch, E.M.; Hirawat, S.; Peltz, S.W.; Bedwell, D.M. PTC124 is an orally bioavailable compound that promotes suppression of the human CFTR-G542X nonsense allele in a CF mouse model. *Proc. Natl. Acad. Sci. USA* **2008**, *105*, 2064–2069. [CrossRef] [PubMed]

179. Kerem, E.; Hirawat, S.; Armoni, S.; Yaakov, Y.; Shoseyov, D.; Cohen, M.; Nissim-Rafinia, M.; Blau, H.; Rivlin, J.; Aviram, M.; et al. Effectiveness of PTC124 treatment of cystic fibrosis caused by nonsense mutations: A prospective phase II trial. *Lancet* **2008**, *372*, 719–727. [CrossRef]

180. Wilschanski, M.; Miller, L.L.; Shoseyov, D.; Blau, H.; Rivlin, J.; Aviram, M.; Cohen, M.; Armoni, S.; Yaakov, Y.; Pugatsch, T.; et al. Chronic ataluren (PTC124) treatment of nonsense mutation cystic fibrosis. *Eur. Respir. J.* **2011**, *38*, 59–69. [CrossRef]

181. Kerem, E.; Konstan, M.W.; De Boeck, K.; Accurso, F.J.; Sermet-Gaudelus, I.; Wilschanski, M.; Elborn, J.S.; Melotti, P.; Bronsveld, I.; Fajac, I.; et al. Ataluren for the treatment of nonsense-mutation cystic fibrosis: A randomised, double-blind, placebo-controlled phase 3 trial. *Lancet Respir. Med.* **2014**, *2*, 539–547. [CrossRef]

182. Rowe, S.M.; Sloane, P.; Tang, L.P.; Backer, K.; Mazur, M.; Buckley-Lanier, J.; Nudelman, I.; Belakhov, V.; Bebok, Z.; Schwiebert, E.; et al. Suppression of CFTR premature termination codons and rescue of CFTR protein and function by the synthetic aminoglycoside NB54. *J. Mol. Med.* **2011**, *89*, 1149–1161. [CrossRef]

183. Pibiri, I.; Lentini, L.; Melfi, R.; Gallucci, G.; Pace, A.; Spinello, A.; Barone, G.; Di Leonardo, A. Enhancement of premature stop codon readthrough in the CFTR gene by Ataluren (PTC124) derivatives. *Eur. J. Med. Chem.* **2015**, *101*, 236–244. [CrossRef]

184. Pibiri, I.; Lentini, L.; Tutone, M.; Melfi, R.; Pace, A.; Di Leonardo, A. Exploring the readthrough of nonsense mutations by non-acidic Ataluren analogues selected by ligand-based virtual screening. *Eur. J. Med. Chem.* **2016**, *122*, 429–435. [CrossRef]

185. Mutyam, V.; Du, M.; Xue, X.; Keeling, K.M.; White, E.L.; Bostwick, J.R.; Rasmussen, L.; Liu, B.; Mazur, M.; Hong, J.S.; et al. Discovery of clinically approved agents that promote suppression of cystic fibrosis transmembrane conductance regulator nonsense mutations. *Am. J. Respir. Crit. Care Med.* **2016**, *194*, 1092–1103. [CrossRef] [PubMed]

186. Lueck, J.D.; Yoon, J.S.; Perales-Puchalt, A.; Mackey, A.L.; Infield, D.T.; Behlke, M.A.; Pope, M.R.; Weiner, D.B.; Skach, W.R.; McCray, P.B., Jr.; et al. Engineered transfer RNAs for suppression of premature termination codons. *Nat. Commun.* **2019**, *10*, 822. [CrossRef] [PubMed]

187. He, L.; Kota, P.; Aleksandrov, A.A.; Cui, L.; Jensen, T.; Dokholyan, N.V.; Riordan, J.R. Correctors of DeltaF508 CFTR restore global conformational maturation without thermally stabilizing the mutant protein. *FASEB J.* **2013**, *27*, 536–545. [CrossRef] [PubMed]

188. Sharma, M.; Pampinella, F.; Nemes, C.; Benharouga, M.; So, J.; Du, K.; Bache, K.G.; Papsin, B.; Zerangue, N.; Stenmark, H.; et al. Misfolding diverts CFTR from recycling to degradation: Quality control at early endosomes. *J. Cell Biol.* **2004**, *164*, 923–933. [CrossRef]

189. Swiatecka-Urban, A.; Brown, A.; Moreau-Marquis, S.; Renuka, J.; Coutermarsh, B.; Barnaby, R.; Karlson, K.H.; Flotte, T.R.; Fukuda, M.; Langford, G.M.; et al. The short apical membrane half-life of rescued {Delta}F508-cystic fibrosis transmembrane conductance regulator (CFTR) results from accelerated endocytosis of {Delta}F508-CFTR in polarized human airway epithelial cells. *J. Biol. Chem.* **2005**, *280*, 36762–36772. [CrossRef] [PubMed]

190. Moniz, S.; Sousa, M.; Moraes, B.J.; Mendes, A.I.; Palma, M.; Barreto, C.; Fragata, J.I.; Amaral, M.D.; Matos, P. HGF stimulation of Rac1 signaling enhances pharmacological correction of the most prevalent cystic fibrosis mutant F508del-CFTR. *ACS Chem. Biol.* **2013**, *8*, 432–442. [CrossRef]

191. Arora, K.; Moon, C.; Zhang, W.; Yarlagadda, S.; Penmatsa, H.; Ren, A.; Sinha, C.; Naren, A.P. Stabilizing rescued surface-localized deltaf508 CFTR by potentiation of its interaction with Na(+)/H(+) exchanger regulatory factor 1. *Biochemistry* **2014**, *53*, 4169–4179. [CrossRef]

192. Rafferty, S.; Alcolado, N.; Norez, C.; Chappe, F.; Pelzer, S.; Becq, F.; Chappe, V. Rescue of functional F508del cystic fibrosis transmembrane conductance regulator by vasoactive intestinal peptide in the human nasal epithelial cell line JME/CF15. *J. Pharmacol. Exp. Ther.* **2009**, *331*, 2–13. [CrossRef]

193. Igreja, S.; Clarke, L.A.; Botelho, H.M.; Marques, L.; Amaral, M.D. Correction of a cystic fibrosis splicing mutation by antisense oligonucleotides. *Hum. Mutat.* **2016**, *37*, 209–215. [CrossRef] [PubMed]

194. Molinski, S.V.; Ahmadi, S.; Ip, W.; Ouyang, H.; Villella, A.; Miller, J.P.; Lee, P.S.; Kulleperuma, K.; Du, K.; Di Paola, M.; et al. Orkambi(R) and amplifier co-therapy improves function from a rare CFTR mutation in gene-edited cells and patient tissue. *EMBO Mol. Med.* **2017**, *9*, 1224–1243. [CrossRef] [PubMed]

195. Robinson, E.; MacDonald, K.D.; Slaughter, K.; McKinney, M.; Patel, S.; Sun, C.; Sahay, G. Lipid nanoparticle-delivered chemically modified mRNA restores chloride secretion in cystic fibrosis. *Mol. Ther.* **2018**, *26*, 2034–2046. [CrossRef]

196. Brown, C.R.; Hong-Brown, L.Q.; Biwersi, J.; Verkman, A.S.; Welch, W.J. Chemical chaperones correct the mutant phenotype of the delta F508 cystic fibrosis transmembrane conductance regulator protein. *Cell Stress Chaperones* **1996**, *1*, 117–125. [CrossRef]

197. Brown, C.R.; Hong-Brown, L.Q.; Welch, W.J. Correcting temperature-sensitive protein folding defects. *J. Clin. Investig.* **1997**, *99*, 1432–1444. [CrossRef] [PubMed]

198. Sato, S.; Ward, C.L.; Krouse, M.E.; Wine, J.J.; Kopito, R.R. Glycerol reverses the misfolding phenotype of the most common cystic fibrosis mutation. *J. Biol. Chem.* **1996**, *271*, 635–638. [CrossRef] [PubMed]

199. Rubenstein, R.C.; Egan, M.E.; Zeitlin, P.L. In vitro pharmacologic restoration of CFTR-mediated chloride transport with sodium 4-phenylbutyrate in cystic fibrosis epithelial cells containing delta F508-CFTR. *J. Clin. Investig.* **1997**, *100*, 2457–2465. [CrossRef]

200. Rubenstein, R.C.; Zeitlin, P.L. Sodium 4-phenylbutyrate downregulates Hsc70: Implications for intracellular trafficking of DeltaF508-CFTR. *Am. J. Physiol. Cell Physiol.* **2000**, *278*, C259–C267. [CrossRef]

201. Rubenstein, R.C.; Zeitlin, P.L. A pilot clinical trial of oral sodium 4-phenylbutyrate (Buphenyl) in deltaF508-homozygous cystic fibrosis patients: Partial restoration of nasal epithelial CFTR function. *Am. J. Respir. Crit. Care Med.* **1998**, *157*, 484–490. [CrossRef]

202. Zeitlin, P.L.; Diener-West, M.; Rubenstein, R.C.; Boyle, M.P.; Lee, C.K.; Brass-Ernst, L. Evidence of CFTR function in cystic fibrosis after systemic administration of 4-phenylbutyrate. *Mol. Ther.* **2002**, *6*, 119–126. [CrossRef] [PubMed]

203. Bouchecareilh, M.; Hutt, D.M.; Szajner, P.; Flotte, T.R.; Balch, W.E. Histone deacetylase inhibitor (HDACi) suberoylanilide hydroxamic acid (SAHA)-mediated correction of alpha1-antitrypsin deficiency. *J. Biol. Chem.* **2012**, *287*, 38265–38278. [CrossRef] [PubMed]

204. Hutt, D.M.; Herman, D.; Rodrigues, A.P.; Noel, S.; Pilewski, J.M.; Matteson, J.; Hoch, B.; Kellner, W.; Kelly, J.W.; Schmidt, A.; et al. Reduced histone deacetylase 7 activity restores function to misfolded CFTR in cystic fibrosis. *Nat. Chem. Biol.* **2010**, *6*, 25–33. [CrossRef] [PubMed]

205. De Stefano, D.; Villella, V.R.; Esposito, S.; Tosco, A.; Sepe, A.; De Gregorio, F.; Salvadori, L.; Grassia, R.; Leone, C.A.; De Rosa, G.; et al. Restoration of CFTR function in patients with cystic fibrosis carrying the F508del-CFTR mutation. *Autophagy* **2014**, *10*, 2053–2074. [CrossRef] [PubMed]

206. Tosco, A.; De Gregorio, F.; Esposito, S.; De Stefano, D.; Sana, I.; Ferrari, E.; Sepe, A.; Salvadori, L.; Buonpensiero, P.; Di Pasqua, A.; et al. A novel treatment of cystic fibrosis acting on-target: Cysteamine plus epigallocatechin gallate for the autophagy-dependent rescue of class II-mutated CFTR. *Cell Death Differ.* **2017**, *24*, 1305. [CrossRef] [PubMed]

207. Izzo, V.; Pietrocola, F.; Sica, V.; Durand, S.; Lachkar, S.; Enot, D.; Bravo-San Pedro, J.M.; Chery, A.; Esposito, S.; Raia, V.; et al. Metabolic interactions between cysteamine and epigallocatechin gallate. *Cell Cycle* **2017**, *16*, 271–279. [CrossRef]

208. Ramachandran, S.; Osterhaus, S.R.; Karp, P.H.; Welsh, M.J.; McCray, P.B., Jr. A genomic signature approach to rescue DeltaF508-cystic fibrosis transmembrane conductance regulator biosynthesis and function. *Am. J. Respir. Cell Mol. Biol.* **2014**, *51*, 354–362. [CrossRef]

209. Pesce, E.; Gorrieri, G.; Sirci, F.; Napolitano, F.; Carrella, D.; Caci, E.; Tomati, V.; Zegarra-Moran, O.; di Bernardo, D.; Galietta, L.J. Evaluation of a systems biology approach to identify pharmacological correctors of the mutant CFTR chloride channel. *J. Cyst. Fibros.* **2016**, *15*, 425–435. [CrossRef]

210. Sondo, E.; Tomati, V.; Caci, E.; Esposito, A.I.; Pfeffer, U.; Pedemonte, N.; Galietta, L.J. Rescue of the mutant CFTR chloride channel by pharmacological correctors and low temperature analyzed by gene expression profiling. *Am. J. Physiol. Cell Physiol.* **2011**, *301*, C872–C885. [CrossRef]

211. Dormer, R.L.; Harris, C.M.; Clark, Z.; Pereira, M.M.; Doull, I.J.; Norez, C.; Becq, F.; McPherson, M.A. Sildenafil (Viagra) corrects DeltaF508-CFTR location in nasal epithelial cells from patients with cystic fibrosis. *Thorax* **2005**, *60*, 55–59. [CrossRef]

212. Norez, C.; Antigny, F.; Noel, S.; Vandebrouck, C.; Becq, F. A cystic fibrosis respiratory epithelial cell chronically treated by miglustat acquires a non-cystic fibrosis-like phenotype. *Am. J. Respir. Cell Mol. Biol.* **2009**, *41*, 217–225. [CrossRef]

213. Krishnamurthy, S.; Wohlford-Lenane, C.; Kandimalla, S.; Sartre, G.; Meyerholz, D.K.; Theberge, V.; Hallee, S.; Duperre, A.M.; Del'Guidice, T.; Lepetit-Stoffaes, J.P.; et al. Engineered amphiphilic peptides enable delivery of proteins and CRISPR-associated nucleases to airway epithelia. *Nat. Commun.* **2019**, *10*, 4906. [CrossRef] [PubMed]

214. Yan, Z.; McCray, P.B., Jr.; Engelhardt, J.F. Advances in gene therapy for cystic fibrosis lung disease. *Hum. Mol. Genet.* **2019**, *28*, R88–R94. [CrossRef] [PubMed]

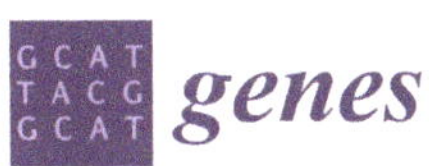 *genes*

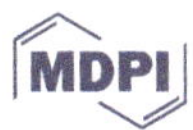

Review

The Microbiome in Cystic Fibrosis Pulmonary Disease

Alice Françoise [1] and Geneviève Héry-Arnaud [1,2,*]

[1]   UMR 1078 GGB, University of Brest, Inserm, EFS, F-29200 Brest, France; alice1francoise.af@gmail.com
[2]   Unité de Bactériologie, Pôle de Biologie-Pathologie, Centre Hospitalier Régional et Universitaire de Brest, Hôpital de la Cavale Blanche, Boulevard Tanguy Prigent, 29200 Brest, France
*   Correspondence: hery@univ-brest.fr; Tel.: +33-298145102; Fax: +33-298145149

Received: 30 March 2020; Accepted: 8 May 2020; Published: 11 May 2020

Abstract: Cystic fibrosis (CF) is a genetic disease with mutational changes leading to profound dysbiosis, both pulmonary and intestinal, from a very young age. This dysbiosis plays an important role in clinical manifestations, particularly in the lungs, affected by chronic infection. The range of microbiological tools has recently been enriched by metagenomics based on next-generation sequencing (NGS). Currently applied essentially in a gene-targeted manner, metagenomics has enabled very exhaustive description of bacterial communities in the CF lung niche and, to a lesser extent, the fungi. Aided by progress in bioinformatics, this now makes it possible to envisage shotgun sequencing and opens the door to other areas of the microbial world, the virome, and the archaeome, for which almost everything remains to be described in cystic fibrosis. Paradoxically, applying NGS in microbiology has seen a rebirth of bacterial culture, but in an extended manner (culturomics), which has proved to be a perfectly complementary approach to NGS. Animal models have also proved indispensable for validating microbiome pathophysiological hypotheses. Description of pathological microbiomes and correlation with clinical status and therapeutics (antibiotic therapy, cystic fibrosis transmembrane conductance regulator (CFTR) modulators) revealed the richness of microbiome data, enabling description of predictive and follow-up biomarkers. Although monogenic, CF is a multifactorial disease, and both genotype and microbiome profiles are crucial interconnected factors in disease progression. Microbiome-genome interactions are thus important to decipher.

Keywords: cystic fibrosis; lung microbiome; metagenomics; gut–lung axis

---

1. Introduction

Gene discovery and progress in genetics and genomics have dramatically modified our view of precision medicine [1,2]. Cystic fibrosis (CF) is a monogenic disease implicating mutations of both copies of the gene coding the cystic fibrosis transmembrane conductance regulator (CFTR) protein, thus inherited in an autosomal recessive manner. The *cftr* gene has been known for more than 30 years and mutation screening for CF is now routine [3]. However, CF shows great and incompletely understood clinical heterogeneity, which wide allelic heterogeneity and functional classification of clinical mutations fail to explain. Several studies over the last five years explored *cftr* genotype–phenotype relationships [4,5], establishing that the disease depends on a balance between *cftr* mutations and the combined influence of modifier genes and other poorly characterized factors [6,7].

CF is thus a multifactorial monogenic disease, whose pathophysiology remains to be explained, particularly concerning infectious pulmonary disease. Chronic lung infections are the primary cause of morbidity-mortality in CF. The CF respiratory tract is colonized by numerous bacteria from an early age [8]. Despite tremendous progress, CF patients still die from lung infection. Discovering factors for airway infection could help identify mechanisms for increased susceptibility to infection, with subpopulations for aggressive screening and therapy. Many studies explored the link between cftr genotype and respiratory phenotype [9–12]. While p.F508del mutation was associated with *Pseudomonas aeruginosa* colonization [12], the most threatening microbial pathogen in CF [13], the correlations that can be established between *cftr* mutations and the progression of lung disease do not fully explain the lung phenotypes of CF patients. For example, patients with the same *cftr* genotype may have a clinical discordance, including siblings with CF [14].

Until recently, CF-related lung disease research focused on major pathogens such as *P. aeruginosa*. However, just as genetics has been interested in genes other than *cftr* [4,15], microbiology is also undergoing a paradigm shift, considering the whole microbial environment and not just one pathogen. In both fields, this shift was enabled by new technology: next-generation sequencing (NGS).

This review aims to describe the modalities and value of microbiome exploration in CF pulmonary disease, complementing genetic data. The development of metagenomics tools and of "-omics" in general provides decisive new knowledge about microbial communities associated with humans and their interactions with host and environmental factors. This review will focus mainly on describing the airways microbiome, but it will also address the gut microbiome through the gut–lung axis, which is very important to decipher the respiratory disease.

2. Deciphering the Microbiome

2.1. New Technology, New Vocabulary

The term "microbiota" refers to all the microorganisms (bacteria, viruses, fungi, archaea, protists) present in an ecosystem [16]. It can be explored by genomic mapping of all microorganisms in the studied environment, leading to the description of the microbiome (microbi-*ome*, i.e., "-*ome*" part of the microbes) [16,17]. In microbial ecology, the term "microbiome" also refers to the entire habitat: microorganisms, their genomes, and microscopic environmental conditions (micro-*biome*) [16,17]. Complete microbiome study further includes intracellular mechanisms and interactions between microorganisms or between microorganisms and their host and environment; this is the aim of complementary approaches such as transcriptomics or metabolomics [18,19]. Disease-associated microbiome alterations are often referred to as a "dysbiosis", a term that is widely used in the microbiome field but remains vaguely defined and is often misused. However, in chronic conditions such as CF, the term is relevant. Dysbiosis can be analyzed at different levels (taxonomic, functional), but most often it is assessed at the taxonomic level; dysbiosis is defined as the loss or gain of bacteria that promotes health or disease, respectively [18,19].

Most microbiome studies actually concern only a fraction of it: bacterial communities, but the microbiome also comprises all the genetic material provided by viruses, fungi and archaea: virome, mycobiome, and archaeome; however, data remain scant, and "microbiome" implicitly still refers to bacteria. All microbiome data are based on taxonomy enabling predictions and hypotheses based on knowledge of identical microorganisms. The most commonly used ranks, in ascending order, are species, genera, families, orders, classes, phyla, and domains (Table 1) [20–23]. With the emergence of genomics, other dimensions have been added. Operational taxonomic units (OTUs) are clusters of similar sequence variants recovered from high-throughput marker gene analysis (usually *rrs* gene that encodes bacterial 16S rRNA). Each cluster represents a taxonomic unit (species or genus depending on sequence similarity threshold and type of bacterium). Typically, a 97% 16S gene sequence identity threshold defines OTUs. Amplicon sequence variant (ASV) is a new term referring to individual DNA sequences recovered after removing spurious sequences generated during amplification and sequencing [24]. ASVs use a method resolving individual sequences without clustering. ASVs are thus inferred sequences of true biological origin. Given the high diversity of human microbiomes, simplifying methods are proposed, classifying the microbiome into clusters based on OTU abundance, first applied to the gut microbiome: three human enterotypes were described worldwide, independent of age, gender, body weight, or ethnic group, but diet-dependent in the long-term [25]. This method was then applied to other niches (pulmotypes, vaginotypes, etc.).

NGS boosted analysis of human microbial communities, but without making traditional bacterial culture redundant if throughput is high. The era of metagenomics is also the era of high-throughput culture-based approach. We will see how these two complementary approaches are practiced.

2.2. Molecular-Based Strategies

2.2.1. Sampling and Pre-Analytical Consideration

In CF, the two main microbiomes are gut and lung, being the most affected [26]. For the gut microbiome, most studies use stool samples, easy to collect non-invasively. In addition, feces show less eukaryotic contamination, facilitating pre-analytical processing, especially since bacterial load is high (10^{11} colony forming unit (CFU)/gram feces). Conversely, lung microbiome samples must be retrieved from the lower respiratory tract and bacterial load is lower [17]. However, pulmonary colonization density is much higher. This allows pulmonary microbiome study in sputum, where contamination is minimal in CF patients expectorating spontaneously [27–29]. Bronchoalveolar lavage (BAL) used to be the only method for non-expectorating patients, but induced sputum has been validated as reflecting CF bronchopulmonary bacterial communities, and is far less invasive, allowing iterative sampling for close monitoring [30,31].

For molecular methods, there are many points of vigilance; two must be monitored as they greatly influence outcome [26]: nucleic acid extraction, because many species are difficult to lyse, and contamination risk, as bacteria are ubiquitous, including in the DNA extraction or amplification kits ("contaminome" or "kitome") [32].

2.2.2. Targeted or Shotgun Metagenomics

The study of microbial communities in clinical niches focuses on two key questions:

Who is there? This is addressed by ribosomal RNA gene profiling (targeted metagenomics or metagenetics) [2], resolving the richness (number of OTUs per sample), evenness (similarity of proportions of the different OTUs in a sample) and diversity (number of OTUs per sample and their abundance) of the community (bacteria, fungi) up to OTU or ASV level. For bacteria, the target is the 16S rRNA gene, common to all bacteria, with nine variable regions (V1–9) enabling taxonomic affiliation interspaced by constant regions, allowing primer hybridization. For fungi, the target is ITS1, ITS2, or 18S rRNA genes [33], and for archaea, selected 16S rRNA gene domains; however, this last domain has not been extensively studied yet [34]. Viruses lack any universal gene, precluding a targeted-metagenomic approach [35]. Choice of library preparation and sequencing method largely depends on local facilities. Illumina technology is the most widely applied worldwide in metagenomics. The MiSeq Illumina platform has short reading lengths (50–300 nt), that can be extended to 2×300 nt by reading amplified DNA in two directions. This technology provides only a partial view of genes, preventing taxonomic affiliation down to species level for all reads, and describing ecosystems at best at genus level. Conversely, long-read sequencing (e.g., real-time sequencing, Pacific Biosciences; nanopore sequencing, Oxford Nanopore Technologies) can determine genes' full-length, allowing fine microbiome resolution and use of bioinformatic tools such as Picrust software, designed to predict metagenome functional content from marker genes [36].

Table 1. Principal taxa in gut and lung cystic fibrosis (CF) microbiomes, presented according to bacterial taxonomy [20–23].

	Domain	Phylum	Class	Order	Family	Genus	Species
CF lung microbiome	Bacteria	Bacteroidetes	Bacteroidia	Bacteroidales	*Prevotellaceae*	*Prevotella* *Porphyromonas*	*P. denticola* *P. catoniae*
		Firmicutes	Bacilli	Lactobacillales	*Streptococcaceae*	*Streptococcus* *Granulicatella* *Gemella* *Staphylococcus* *Veillonella*	*S. oralis* *G.adiacens* *G. haemolysans* *S. aureus* *V. parvula*
		Proteobacteria	Gammaproteobacteria	Pseudomonales	*Pseudomonadaceae*	*Pseudomonas* *Burkholderia* *Achromobacter* *Stenotrophomonas* *Neisseria* *Haemophilus*	*P. aeruginosa* *S. maltophilia* *B. cenocepacia* *A. xylosoxidans* *N. mucosa* *H. influenzae*
		Actinobacteria	Actinobacteria	Actinomycetales	*Actinomycetaceae*	*Actinomyces* *Rothia* *Atopobium*	*A. odontolyticus* *R. mucilaginosa* *A. parvulum*
		Fusobacteria	Fusobacteriia	Fusobacteriales	*Fusobacteriaceae*	*Fusobacterium*	*F. nucleatum*
CF gut microbiome	Bacteria	Bacteroidetes	Bacteroidia	Bacteroidales	*Tannerellaceae*	*Parabacteroides* *Prevotella* *Veillonella* *Bacteroides*	*P. distasonis* *P. coprii* *V. parvula* *B. fragilis*
		Firmicutes	Clostridia	Clostridiales	*Ruminococcaceae*	*Faecalibacterium* *Blautia*	*F. prausnitzii* *B. faecis*
		Actinobacteria	Actinobacteria	Bifidobacteriales	*Bifidobacteriaceae*	*Bifidobacterium*	*B. longum*

Class, order, and family are mentioned only for the first species listed for each phylum.

What are they doing? This is addressed by whole metagenome shotgun sequencing, facilitated as high-throughput technologies become more affordable, and consisting of untargeted sequencing of all microbial genomes directly after extraction, without amplification, limiting bias induced by primers. It provides complete information whatever the microorganism (bacteria, phages, archaea, eukaryotic parasites): taxonomic composition, microbial community functional potential, and epidemiology [37]. As whole genome sequences may be reconstructed, metagenomics may elucidate community composition up to clonal complex level, reconstructing metabolic pathways [38,39]. In CF, shotgun metagenomics generated unbiased quantitative diversity data in lung, discerning more species than targeted metagenomics [35,37]. It is essential for virome study. Multiplex PCR kits detect most airway-invading viruses but do not provide quantification data or detect the entire virus population. Metagenomics offers a precious alternative for exploring the lung virome, and also the CF archaeome in years to come [35,37].

Other "-omics" approaches complete community analysis. Transcriptomics and proteomics estimate the degree of expression of previously identified genomes [26,40]. As several bacterial metabolic pathways influence many ecosystem parameters, metabolomics may extend our understanding of microbial functions in CF lung [19,41,42].

2.3. Culture-Based Strategy

Studies have shown the quantitative and qualitative importance of non-cultivable or hard-to-cultivate bacteria such as anaerobes, unable to grow or even killed by oxygen. Thus, species important in the pathophysiology of bowel disease, like *Faecalibacterium prausnitzii*, were revealed by NGS [43]. Anaerobes were expected in the gut microbiome, but their level in the lungs was surprising [44]. These NGS data encouraged a return to culture, but with high throughput by multiplying culture conditions (enriched media, strict anaerobic atmosphere, extended incubation time, etc.) and systematic identification of each colony morphotype on MALDI-TOF mass spectrometry. Many improvements in culture media broaden the spectrum of cultivable bacteria. Artificial media mimic natural conditions, recreating macromolecular composition and abiotic conditions (pH, electrolytes concentration, etc.): artificial sputum mimicking bronchopulmonary mucus [45]; or creating new culture facilities: fermenters mimicking the gastrointestinal tract [46] or artificial mucus-clogged bronchiole [47]. The "culturomics" extended-culture approach can culture bacteria previously considered "uncultivable" [48]. It also explores potential microbial interactions identified in meta-genetic studies and characterizes bacterial metabolites of interest [49–51]. In CF, extensive culture-enriched airway microbiome profiling identified bacterial families, such as *Ruminococcaceae* or *Bacteriovoracaceae*, in CF sputa not detected by 16S rDNA sequencing alone [52].

2.4. Animal Models

The microbiome is very sensitive to environmental factors such as diet, antibiotics, age, sex, etc. In animal models, these confounding factors can be better controlled (although cage effects were reported) [53,54]. In CF, there are several models, with CF mouse models being the most common, although not optimal for studying pulmonary disease [55]. As previously reviewed [55,56], CF ferret [57], rabbit [58], pig [59], sheep [60], or rat [61] models could be future alternatives for the study of microbiome as they show closer anatomy or pulmonary phenotype with humans than mice. Metagenomic studies have yet to be done. Analysis of CF mouse intestinal microbiota highlighted bacterial overgrowth as well as a decrease in microbiome richness and diversity [62–64]. This was replicated, but dysbiosis intensity seems model-dependent [64].

Different conditions can be chosen for animal microbiome experiments. Antibiotics can be used to study the effect of microbiome disruption on a function of interest, for example, to test how CF patients may react to the cocktails they receive. Lynch et al. demonstrated that changes in CF and non-CF mouse microbiome under antibiotics were greater than the pre-treatment difference between the two types of mice [65]. Germ-free animals [66] or animals under different diets [67] are other ways to explore microbiome function. Finally, animal models can explore the gut–lung axis or specific microbial interactions identified as pathophysiologically critical by -omics studies [68]. A major issue is that animal and human microbiomes are of different composition; indeed, results in mice are often not seen in humans. Humanized microbiome mouse models might overcome this [56], but have not yet been applied in CF.

3. CF Microbiome Landscape

3.1. Airway Microbiome

The respiratory tract measures approximately 50–75 m^2 and is an open door to our environment. Its anatomical diversity (trachea, bronchi, bronchioles, alveolar sacs) corresponds to pulmonary geography (biogeography) [17,19]. The main pulmonary bacterial phyla are Bacteroidetes and Firmicutes and to a lesser extent Proteobacteria and Actinobacteria [17,69]. High-throughput 16S rRNA gene sequencing highlighted a "core microbiome" of taxa present in most individuals [17,69]. In healthy subjects, it mainly comprises *Streptococcus, Prevotella, Fusobacterium, Veillonella, Porphyromonas, Haemophilus* and *Neisseria* [69]. Interestingly, this organ dedicated to oxygenation hosts abundant strictly anaerobic bacteria, such as *Prevotella, Fusobacterium, Veillonella,* and *Porphyromonas.*

3.1.1. CF Airways Microbiome Ecology

In CF, the absence or dysfunction of CFTR protein significantly impacts mucus rheology [70], particularly at the respiratory level, conferring hyperviscosity and promoting polymicrobial proliferation and microbial imbalance (dysbiosis) along the respiratory tract. More than 1000 species were identified in CF airways by shotgun metagenome sequencing of induced sputum [71,72]. On nasal microbiota analysis [71], while healthy subjects displayed a continuum in upper and lower airway microbiomes [73], graduated sample analysis of the CF respiratory tract (nasal, nasopharyngeal, oral, and lung samples) demonstrated dissimilarities between the two [71,74,75]. The more advanced the disease, the more pronounced the difference [74]. Analysis of CF sputum and BAL samples revealed complex microbial communities where all parts of the living microscopic domains could be described: bacterial microbiome, virome, and archaeome.

Bacterial microbiome: The complexity of the CF pulmonary microbiome is such that classical culture cannot provide an exhaustive bacterial inventory. NGS has greatly advanced understanding of CF pathophysiology. Actinobacteria, Bacteroidetes, Firmicutes, Fusobacteria, and Proteobacteria constitute >99% of the CF airway community. The CF pulmonary microbiome shows overrepresentation of Proteobacteria and Actinobacteria [72]. The core microbiome comprises *Streptococcus, Prevotella, Veillonella, Rothia, Actinomyces, Gemella, Granulicatella, Fusobacterium, Neisseria, Atopobium,* and *Porphyromonas* [23,76–78], with variations in other taxa [22]. Notably, anaerobics are fewer than in non-CF lung microbiomes, which may be significant for CF pulmonary physiopathology [44]. The microbiome perspective also better deciphers the multidrug-resistance gene determinants by predicting the ecosystem "resistome" (i.e., all antibiotic-resistance genes in both pathogenic and non-pathogenic bacteria) [79].

Virome: The CF lung virome is strongly affected by the mucosal environment and impaired immunity [35]. Common respiratory viruses are found in 60% of CF patients (more than in the general population) and cause greater morbidity than in non-CF subjects [80]. Presence correlates with inflammation, as they interfere with IFN and NF-kappaB pathways, and with bacterial co-infection (including *P. aeruginosa*), inducing exacerbation and impaired lung function [35,80]. In addition to eukaryotic viruses, the CF lung microbiome contains phages adapted to this particular environment [35, 72,81], and known to impact the microbiome, driving pathogen adaptation and antibiotic resistance [81].

Mycobiome: Fungi such as *Aspergillus fumigatus* are long-known opportunistic pathogens for CF patients, detected in sputum [82]. However, most CF airway fungi belong to the *Candida* or *Malassezia* families and are mostly transient [33]. Fungal species may interact with the bacteriome and/or virome and be a cofactor in inflammation and immune response [83]. Deciphering the inter-kingdom network may elucidate CF pulmonary disease [84].

Archaeome: Archaea are a group of single-cell prokaryotic organisms, previously classified as bacteria but now distinguished in a specific domain, beside bacteria and eukaryotes. They are found in anaerobic environments, including human. Exploration of human-associated archaea is still very new but has demonstrated diversity between anatomical niches [85]. In the CF lung, all archaeal phyla show <0.1% abundance [72,85].

3.1.2. CF Airway Microbiome Dynamics Throughout Disease Course

Disease course can be seen through the prism of the lung microbiome. Microbiome progression is individual-specific, requiring personalized medical follow-up [20]; nevertheless, trends emerge. The intestinal microenvironment predisposes young CF children to intestinal and respiratory dysbiosis, possibly from birth [8]. Up to 11 years of age, microbial diversity is high [86], then, as *P. aeruginosa* colonization becomes chronic, richness and diversity is lost with age, disease progression, and dominance of pathogens [29,87]. Diversity is a marker of lung function. In long-term follow-up (10 years), diversity was maintained in patients with stable respiratory function, and decreased in patients with impaired function on FEV1 [87]. This decrease correlates with the establishment of a dominant pathogen [88], usually *P. aeruginosa*, whose prevalence increases with age [20,22]. Other taxa associated with CF pathogenicity (*Staphylococcus*, *Haemophilus*, *Burkholderia*) are also more prevalent in older patients [20,74]. Other pathogens of increasing concern (non-fermentative Gram-negative bacilli: *Achromobacter*, *Stenotrophomonas*) show similar colonization patterns, leading to persistent infection [89].

Variations in microbiome profile were also described in patients with pulmonary exacerbations (PEx). *P. aeruginosa* or other pathogens are systematic in sputum of CF PEx patients [90], but anaerobes are key components in PEx [91]. Variations in several anaerobic genera (e.g., *Prevotella*) account more for variability in respiratory function after treatment and in the metabolic environmental shift during PEx than the dominant opportunistic genera *Pseudomonas* [40,90]; thus, anaerobes may be better PEx biomarkers than the commonly used diversity, which shows no difference or diminution [20,92]. Long-course antibiotics also impact microbiome maturation and evolution. During exacerbations, antibiotherapy modulates the microbiome, decreasing diversity and richness; long-term effects include reduced commensal bacterial population not corrected after wash-out [92].

3.2. Gut–Lung Connection

CF gut–lung dialogue is interesting, as gut and lung microbiomes are disrupted by the same etiology (loss of CFTR function), making their interactions more complex. Dysbiosis of the two sites is partially independent. Altered microbial communities in gut and lung is governed by organ-specific micro-environmental conditions (viscous mucus, hyperinflammation, etc.). However, the two microbiomes also interact. The intestinal microbiome especially impacts pulmonary microbiome constitution via microbial metabolite exchange [69]. In CF, the gut–lung axis is disrupted by decreased abundance of bacteria producing short-chain fatty acids (SCFAs) [93,94], which have immunomodulatory properties, so that the gut dysbiosis correlates with pulmonary immune homeostasis defects [93,94]. Close interaction between intestinal and pulmonary microbiotes was shown in a murine CF model; Bazett et al. [63] revealed pulmonary hyper-reactivity in response to antibiotic-induced intestinal dysbiosis. Therefore, loss of gut microbiome diversity and functional potential under repeated antibiotic treatment (often started at an early age) may exacerbate pulmonary disease in CF patients [95].

4. Deciphering Genome–Microbiome Interactions

4.1. Influence of Cftr Mutation on Pulmotypes and Enterotypes

Human genetic variation is a factor in interpersonal differences in microbiomes. Genes directly influence health by promoting a beneficial microbiome [96]. Studies of intestinal microbiome heritability revealed a subset of microbes whose abundance is partly genetically determined by the host [97]. Microbiomes are more similar for monozygotic twins than for dizygotic twins [97]. One of the most hereditary taxa is the *Christensenellaceae*, a family of bacteria that has been shown to promote a lean host phenotype. It is estimated that the host genotype influences 30–60% of the variation in the relative abundance of *Christensenellaceae* [97]. However, genome-wide association studies to identify human genetic variants associated with microbiome phenotypes is proving difficult. What about cystic fibrosis?

In mice, loss of *cftr* gene function causes intestinal dysbiosis. A close relationship was demonstrated between *cftr* genotype and microbiome constitution [66]. CF mice initially germ-free and transplanted with fecal microbiota from non-CF mice had a different microbiological profile than non-CF controls [66]. However, the exact mechanisms of microorganism selection by genotype are unknown. In humans too, CFTR protein functional impairment alters the gut microbiome [98]. Studies of the link between the type of *cftr* mutation and effect on the microbiome showed conflicting results. Microbiomes differed depending on whether the patient had one or two alleles with p.F508del mutation or else two alleles with other mutations [11,95], but further analyses found no such significant differences [99,100]. This may be explained by two factors. The first is the possible involvement of many modulator genes, in addition to the *cftr* gene, in microbial community selection [9,101]. In CF gut samples, abundance of Actinobacteria depends on the number of p.F508del alleles, but the *cftr* mutation profile does not explain the modulated bacterial metabolic pathways whereas more than 1000 genes can be otherwise over- or under-expressed [9]. The second factor is the mutual influence of genotypes and microbiome patterns (e.g., enterotypes for the gut microbiome and pulmotypes for the lung microbiome). Microbiome disruption, by antibiotics [101] or diet [67], also affects the level of expression of essential intestinal genes and even CF modifier genes such as *Slc6a14* [101].

4.2. Effects of CFTR-Modulating Therapies on the Microbiome

CFTR modulators, including ivacaftor, have CFTR-dependent and CFTR-independent effects on the microbiome [102]. In the intestinal microbiome [103], ivacaftor increases *Akkermansia*, a beneficial bacterium involved in mucosal protection, and decreases *Enterobacteriaceae*, which correlates with decreased fecal calprotectin, an inflammation marker. In the lung microbiome, significant positive changes occurred within 48 h of initiation of ivacaftor and lasted for the first year; it reduced relative abundance of *Pseudomonas* [104,105], and increased relative abundance of endogenous species (*Streptococcus*, anaerobes) [76]. This shift to a more diverse microbiome is the hallmark of a "healthier" CF microbiome. Studies showed a negative association between microbial diversity and respiratory tract inflammation [20], and positive correlation between increased taxa count and FEV1 [64]. However, neither gut nor lung microbiome changes were sustained in the second year [76,105–107].

5. Toward A New Microbiome-Based Medicine

5.1. A Source of New Prognosis and Diagnosis Biomarkers

Global microbiome parameters such as diversity, richness, or dominant populations are potential prognostic factors to be monitored [108–110]. Microbiome diversity in particular is a major predictive marker of disease progression in young adults, correlating with risk of subsequent lung transplantation and death [109]. In a decade-long study of the CF lung microbiome, community diversity decreased significantly over time in patients with typically progressive lung disease but remained relatively stable in mild lung disease phenotypes [87]. This rethinking of CF-associated airway infection in the light of microbiome analysis may be useful for clinicians making the often complicated decision about what antibiotic(s) to use in these complex infections [111]. That is the goal of the CF-MATTERS study, the first randomized controlled trial to compare microbiome-directed versus standard antibiotic therapy for CF patients with respiratory infections (https://www.cfmatters.eu/).

Similarly, clinical trial designs may need a baseline microbiome study to stratify patients according to dominant microbe. The efficacy of inhaled aztreonam, an antibiotic targeting *P. aeruginosa* in the CF airway, was evaluated using alternative outcomes according to microbiome effect [112]; benefit depended essentially on impact on species other than *P. aeruginosa*.

In the era of predictive medicine, the microbiome may be a source of new biomarkers for follow-up and early intervention. Risk of *P. aeruginosa* early colonization may be assessed on predictive biomarkers within the microbiome. *Porphyromonas* is a candidate biomarker in the lungs (BEACH study; ClinicalTrials.gov Identifier: NCT03947957) [78], and *Parabacteroides* in the gut [8]. The predictive potential of the microbiome for exacerbation was studied to adapt antibiotic therapeutic strategies. Three genera (*Streptococcus*, *Haemophilus*, *Staphylococcus*) emerged as predictive markers of antibiotic response [112].

5.2. A Source of Innovative Therapies

5.2.1. Identification of Beneficial Microbes

Identifying potentially beneficial bacteria in CF consists first in comparing patients' microbiomes versus healthy subjects to detect significant differences in abundance of well-known beneficial microbes such as *Bifidobacterium* or *Lactobacillus*, or new-generation probiotics such as *F. prausnitzii* [98]. For the lung microbiome, larger genetic screening is needed, as the concept of lung probiotics is new, and beneficial microbes maybe different from those in the gut [78,113,114]. Candidate probiotic properties must then be confirmed in vitro and in vivo. The immuno-modulatory potential of *Bacteroides* from CF patients has been assessed in vitro [115], which should be followed by in vivo safety and efficacy experiments [116–118].

5.2.2. Other Innovative Therapies for the Gut Microbiota

In the gut–lung axis, dietary involvement offers a microbiome-based therapeutic perspective for preventing lung disease by manipulating the gut microbiome. Diet fortification with certain fatty acids [119] or carbohydrates is of interest, as these regulate production of SCFAs, which have a positive impact on lung function in CF patients [93,120]. Vitamin D supplementation, essential for the development of a healthy intestinal microbiota, could also be beneficial for patients who are generally deficient due to malabsorption and dysbiosis [121]. Ultimately, knowledge acquired on the "gut–lung" axis may guide fecal microbiota transplantation in respiratory pathologies; only randomized controlled trials can enable progress on this therapeutic track.

6. Conclusions

In conclusion, in the era of NGS, it seems just as fundamental to establish the microbial profile of a CF patient as to establish his/her genotype in order to understand the unique disease progression of each patient, particularly in respiratory sites. Although essentially based on DNA analysis, the microbiome provides the indispensable complement to interpret genotype: the phenotype. The microbiome comprises an extremely rich sum of data, enabling precise individual assessment, and is now an essential key to improving precision in CF management by providing prognostic and monitoring biomarkers, and possibly innovative therapeutic solutions. In the future, machine learning integrating data from the joint efforts of geneticists and microbiologists will be crucial for better understanding of this infectious genetic disease (Figure 1).

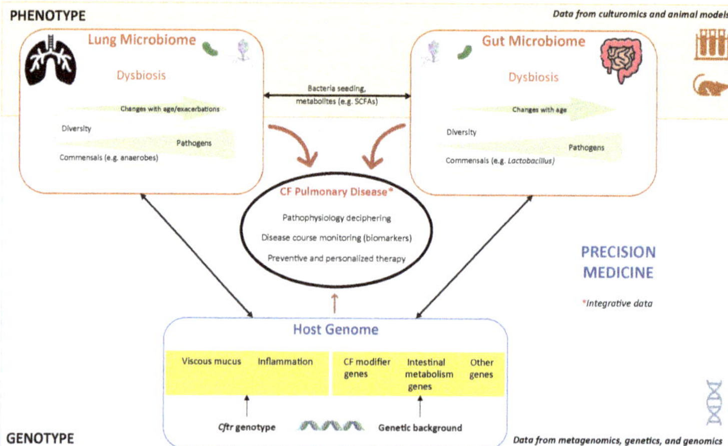

Figure 1. Contribution of microbiome science to cystic fibrosis (CF) research. This figure summarizes the interplay/complementarity between metagenomics and genetics in deciphering CF lung disease, and the combined tools in microbiome research. The genotype profile is stable and fixed since birth, whereas the phenotype provided by the microbiome profiles from both niches, lungs and gut changes with age. Both sets of data are necessary for precision medicine in CF.

Author Contributions: A.F. and G.H.-A. contributed equally to writing of the manuscript and design of the figure. All authors have read and agreed to the published version of the manuscript.

Funding: Work in the GGB Inserm Unit UMR1078-Microbiota axis is funded by by the French Ministry of Health (grant number PHRCI-2018/B/072), by Inserm Transfer, and by the associations Vaincre la Mucoviscidose (grant number RC20180502218) and Gaetan Saleün.

Acknowledgments: We thank Iain McGill for revision of the English manuscript.

Conflicts of Interest: The authors declare no conflict of interest.

References

1. Pranke, I.; Golec, A.; Hinzpeter, A.; Edelman, A.; Sermet-Gaudelus, I. Emerging therapeutic approaches for cystic fibrosis. from gene editing to personalized medicine. *Front. Pharm.* **2019**, *10*, 121. [CrossRef]

2. Corvol, H.; Thompson, K.E.; Tabary, O.; le Rouzic, P.; Guillot, L. Translating the genetics of cystic fibrosis to personalized medicine. *Transl. Res.* **2016**, *168*, 40–49. [CrossRef] [PubMed]

3. Travert, G.; Heeley, M.; Heeley, A. history of newborn screening for cystic fibrosis—The early years. *IJNS* **2020**, *6*, 8. [CrossRef]

4. O'Neal, W.K.; Knowles, M.R. Cystic fibrosis disease modifiers: Complex genetics defines the phenotypic diversity in a monogenic disease. *Annu. Rev. Genom. Hum. Genet.* **2018**, *19*, 201–222. [CrossRef] [PubMed]

5. Sosnay, P.R.; Raraigh, K.S.; Gibson, R.L. Molecular genetics of cystic fibrosis transmembrane conductance regulator. *Pedia. Clin. N. Am.* **2016**, *63*, 585–598. [CrossRef] [PubMed]

6. Brennan, M.-L.; Schrijver, I. Cystic Fibrosis. *J. Mol. Diagn.* **2016**, *18*, 3–14. [CrossRef]

7. Bell, S.C.; Mall, M.A.; Gutierrez, H.; Macek, M.; Madge, S.; Davies, J.C.; Burgel, P.-R.; Tullis, E.; Castaños, C.; Castellani, C.; et al. The future of cystic fibrosis care: A global perspective. *Lancet Respir. Med.* **2020**, *8*, 65–124. [CrossRef]

8. Hoen, A.G.; Li, J.; Moulton, L.A.; O'Toole, G.A.; Housman, M.L.; Koestler, D.C.; Guill, M.F.; Moore, J.H.; Hibberd, P.L.; Morrison, H.G.; et al. Associations between gut microbial colonization in early life and respiratory outcomes in cystic fibrosis. *J. Pediatrics* **2015**, *167*, 138–147.e3. [CrossRef]

9. Dayama, G.; Priya, S.; Niccum, D.E.; Khoruts, A.; Blekhman, R. Interactions between the gut microbiome and host gene regulation in cystic fibrosis. *Genome Med.* **2020**, *12*, 12. [CrossRef]

10. McCague, A.F.; Raraigh, K.S.; Pellicore, M.J.; Davis-Marcisak, E.F.; Evans, T.A.; Han, S.T.; Lu, Z.; Joynt, A.T.; Sharma, N.; Castellani, C.; et al. Correlating cystic fibrosis transmembrane conductance regulator function with clinical features to inform precision treatment of cystic fibrosis. *Am. J. Respir Crit Care Med.* **2019**, *199*, 1116–1126. [CrossRef]

11. Schippa, S.; Iebba, V.; Santangelo, F.; Gagliardi, A.; De Biase, R.V.; Stamato, A.; Bertasi, S.; Lucarelli, M.; Conte, M.P.; Quattrucci, S. Cystic fibrosis transmembrane conductance regulator (CFTR) allelic variants relate to shifts in faecal microbiota of cystic fibrosis patients. *PLoS ONE* **2013**, *8*, e61176. [CrossRef]

12. Vongthilath, R.; Richaud Thiriez, B.; Dehillotte, C.; Lemonnier, L.; Guillien, A.; Degano, B.; Dalphin, M.-L.; Dalphin, J.-C.; Plésiat, P. Clinical and microbiological characteristics of cystic fibrosis adults never colonized by *Pseudomonas aeruginosa*: Analysis of the French CF registry. *PLoS ONE* **2019**, *14*, e0210201. [CrossRef]

13. Elborn, J.S. Cystic fibrosis. *Lancet* **2016**, *388*, 2519–2531. [CrossRef]

14. Mekus, F.; Ballmann, M.; Bronsveld, I.; Bijman, J.; Veeze, H.; Tümmler, B. Categories of ΔF508 homozygous cystic fibrosis twin and sibling pairs with distinct phenotypic characteristics. *Twin Res.* **2000**, *3*, 277–293. [CrossRef] [PubMed]

15. Raynal, C.; Corvol, H. Variant classifications, databases and genotype-phenotype correlations. *Arch. Pédiatrie* **2020**, *27*, eS13–eS18. [CrossRef]

16. Marchesi, J.R.; Ravel, J. The vocabulary of microbiome research: A proposal. *Microbiome* **2015**, *3*, 31. [CrossRef] [PubMed]

17. Dickson, R.P.; Erb-Downward, J.R.; Martinez, F.J.; Huffnagle, G.B. The microbiome and the respiratory tract. *Annu. Rev. Physiol.* **2016**, *78*, 481–504. [CrossRef]

18. Cao, L.; Shcherbin, E.; Mohimani, H. A metabolome- and metagenome-wide association network reveals microbial natural products and microbial biotransformation products from the human microbiota. *mSystems* **2019**, *4*, e00387-19. [CrossRef]

19. Garg, N.; Wang, M.; Hyde, E.; da Silva, R.R.; Melnik, A.V.; Protsyuk, I.; Bouslimani, A.; Lim, Y.W.; Wong, R.; Humphrey, G.; et al. Three-dimensional microbiome and metabolome cartography of a diseased human lung. *Cell Host Microbe.* **2017**, *22*, 705–716.e4. [CrossRef]

20. Zemanick, E.T.; Wagner, B.D.; Robertson, C.E.; Ahrens, R.C.; Chmiel, J.F.; Clancy, J.P.; Gibson, R.L.; Harris, W.T.; Kurland, G.; Laguna, T.A.; et al. Airway microbiota across age and disease spectrum in cystic fibrosis. *Eur. Respir. J.* **2017**, *50*, 1700832. [CrossRef]

21. Frayman, K.B.; Wylie, K.M.; Armstrong, D.S.; Carzino, R.; Davis, S.D.; Ferkol, T.W.; Grimwood, K.; Storch, G.A.; Ranganathan, S.C. Differences in the lower airway microbiota of infants with and without cystic fibrosis. *J. Cyst. Fibros.* **2019**, *18*, 646–652. [CrossRef] [PubMed]

22. Frayman, K.B.; Armstrong, D.S.; Carzino, R.; Ferkol, T.W.; Grimwood, K.; Storch, G.A.; Teo, S.M.; Wylie, K.M.; Ranganathan, S.C. The lower airway microbiota in early cystic fibrosis lung disease: A longitudinal analysis. *Thorax* **2017**, *72*, 1104–1112. [CrossRef]

23. van der Gast, C.J.; Walker, A.W.; Stressmann, F.A.; Rogers, G.B.; Scott, P.; Daniels, T.W.; Carroll, M.P.; Parkhill, J.; Bruce, K.D. Partitioning core and satellite taxa from within cystic fibrosis lung bacterial communities. *ISME J.* **2011**, *5*, 780–791. [CrossRef] [PubMed]

24. Caruso, V.; Song, X.; Asquith, M.; Karstens, L. Performance of microbiome sequence inference methods in environments with varying biomass. *mSystems* **2019**, *4*, e00163-18. [CrossRef]

25. MetaHIT Consortium (additional members); Arumugam, M.; Raes, J.; Pelletier, E.; Le Paslier, D.; Yamada, T.; Mende, D.R.; Fernandes, G.R.; Tap, J.; Bruls, T.; et al. Enterotypes of the human gut microbiome. *Nature* **2011**, *473*, 174–180. [CrossRef]

26. Héry-Arnaud, G.; Boutin, S.; Cuthbertson, L.; Elborn, S.J.; Tunney, M.M. The lung and gut microbiome: What has to be taken into consideration for cystic fibrosis? *J. Cyst. Fibros.* **2019**, *18*, 13–21. [CrossRef] [PubMed]

27. Hogan, D.A.; Willger, S.D.; Dolben, E.L.; Hampton, T.H.; Stanton, B.A.; Morrison, H.G.; Sogin, M.L.; Czum, J.; Ashare, A. Analysis of lung microbiota in bronchoalveolar lavage, protected brush and sputum samples from subjects with mild-to-moderate cystic fibrosis lung disease. *PLoS ONE* **2016**, *11*, e0149998. [CrossRef] [PubMed]

28. Rogers, G.B.; Carroll, M.P.; Serisier, D.J.; Hockey, P.M.; Jones, G.; Kehagia, V.; Connett, G.J.; Bruce, K.D. Use of 16S rRNA gene profiling by terminal restriction fragment length polymorphism analysis to compare bacterial communities in sputum and mouthwash samples from patients with cystic fibrosis. *J. Clin. Microbiol.* **2006**, *44*, 2601–2604. [CrossRef] [PubMed]

29. Cuthbertson, L.; Walker, A.W.; Oliver, A.E.; Rogers, G.B.; Rivett, D.W.; Hampton, T.H.; Ashare, A.; Elborn, J.S.; De Soyza, A.; Carroll, M.P.; et al. Lung function and microbiota diversity in cystic fibrosis. *Microbiome* **2020**, *8*, 45. [CrossRef]

30. Ronchetti, K.; Tame, J.-D.; Paisey, C.; Thia, L.P.; Doull, I.; Howe, R.; Mahenthiralingam, E.; Forton, J.T. The CF-Sputum Induction Trial (CF-SpIT) to assess lower airway bacterial sampling in young children with cystic fibrosis: A prospective internally controlled interventional trial. *Lancet Respir. Med.* **2018**, *6*, 461–471. [CrossRef]

31. Klepac-Ceraj, V.; Lemon, K.P.; Martin, T.R.; Allgaier, M.; Kembel, S.W.; Knapp, A.A.; Lory, S.; Brodie, E.L.; Lynch, S.V.; Bohannan, B.J.M.; et al. Relationship between cystic fibrosis respiratory tract bacterial communities and age, genotype, antibiotics and Pseudomonas aeruginosa: Ecology of the cystic fibrosis respiratory tract bacterial community. *Environ. Microbiol.* **2010**, *12*, 1293–1303. [CrossRef] [PubMed]

32. Kim, D.; Hofstaedter, C.E.; Zhao, C.; Mattei, L.; Tanes, C.; Clarke, E.; Lauder, A.; Sherrill-Mix, S.; Chehoud, C.; Kelsen, J.; et al. Optimizing methods and dodging pitfalls in microbiome research. *Microbiome* **2017**, *5*, 52. [CrossRef] [PubMed]

33. Willger, S.D.; Grim, S.L.; Dolben, E.L.; Shipunova, A.; Hampton, T.H.; Morrison, H.G.; Filkins, L.M.; O'Toole, G.A.; Moulton, L.A.; Ashare, A.; et al. Characterization and quantification of the fungal microbiome in serial samples from individuals with cystic fibrosis. *Microbiome* **2014**, *2*, 40. [CrossRef] [PubMed]

34. Pausan, M.R.; Csorba, C.; Singer, G.; Till, H.; Schöpf, V.; Santigli, E.; Klug, B.; Högenauer, C.; Blohs, M.; Moissl-Eichinger, C. Exploring the archaeome: Detection of archaeal signatures in the human body. *Front. Microbiol.* **2019**, *10*, 2796. [CrossRef]

35. Billard, L.; Le Berre, R.; Pilorgé, L.; Payan, C.; Héry-Arnaud, G.; Vallet, S. Viruses in cystic fibrosis patients' airways. *Crit. Rev. Microbiol.* **2017**, *43*, 690–708. [CrossRef]

36. Wang, Z.; Liu, H.; Wang, F.; Yang, Y.; Wang, X.; Chen, B.; Stampfli, M.R.; Zhou, H.; Shu, W.; Brightling, C.E.; et al. A refined view of airway microbiome in chronic obstructive pulmonary disease at species and strain-levels. *Microbiology* **2020**. [CrossRef]

37. Pienkowska, K.; Wiehlmann, L.; Tümmler, B. Airway microbial metagenomics. *Microbes Infect.* **2018**, *20*, 536–542. [CrossRef]

38. Bacci, G.; Mengoni, A.; Fiscarelli, E.; Segata, N.; Taccetti, G.; Dolce, D.; Paganin, P.; Morelli, P.; Tuccio, V.; De Alessandri, A.; et al. A different microbiome gene repertoire in the airways of cystic fibrosis patients with severe lung disease. *IJMS* **2017**, *18*, 1654. [CrossRef]

39. Shi, X.; Gao, Z.; Lin, Q.; Zhao, L.; Ma, Q.; Kang, Y.; Yu, J. Meta-analysis reveals potential influence of oxidative stress on the airway microbiomes of cystic fibrosis patients. *Genom. Proteom. Bioinform.* **2020**, S1672022920300231. [CrossRef]

40. Twomey, K.B.; Alston, M.; An, S.-Q.; O'Connell, O.J.; McCarthy, Y.; Swarbreck, D.; Febrer, M.; Dow, J.M.; Plant, B.J.; Ryan, R.P. Microbiota and metabolite profiling reveal specific alterations in bacterial community structure and environment in the cystic fibrosis airway during exacerbation. *PLoS ONE* **2013**, *8*, e82432. [CrossRef]

41. Sharon, G.; Garg, N.; Debelius, J.; Knight, R.; Dorrestein, P.C.; Mazmanian, S.K. Specialized metabolites from the microbiome in health and disease. *Cell Metab.* **2014**, *20*, 719–730. [CrossRef] [PubMed]

42. Quinn, R.A.; Lim, Y.W.; Mak, T.D.; Whiteson, K.; Furlan, M.; Conrad, D.; Rohwer, F.; Dorrestein, P. Metabolomics of pulmonary exacerbations reveals the personalized nature of cystic fibrosis disease. *PeerJ* **2016**, *4*, e2174. [CrossRef] [PubMed]

43. Sokol, H.; Pigneur, B.; Watterlot, L.; Lakhdari, O.; Bermudez-Humaran, L.G.; Gratadoux, J.-J.; Blugeon, S.; Bridonneau, C.; Furet, J.-P.; Corthier, G.; et al. *Faecalibacterium prausnitzii* is an anti-inflammatory commensal bacterium identified by gut microbiota analysis of Crohn disease patients. *Proc. Natl. Acad. Sci. USA* **2008**, *105*, 16731–16736. [CrossRef] [PubMed]

44. Lamoureux, C.; Guilloux, C.-A.; Beauruelle, C.; Jolivet-Gougeon, A.; Héry-Arnaud, G. Anaerobes in cystic fibrosis patients' airways. *Crit. Rev. Microbiol.* **2019**, *45*, 103–117. [CrossRef] [PubMed]

45. Kirchner, S.; Fothergill, J.L.; Wright, E.A.; James, C.E.; Mowat, E.; Winstanley, C. Use of artificial sputum medium to test antibiotic efficacy against *Pseudomonas aeruginosa* in conditions more relevant to the cystic fibrosis lung. *JoVE* **2012**, 3857. [CrossRef] [PubMed]

46. Verhoeckx, K.; Cotter, P.; López-Expósito, I.; Kleiveland, C.; Lea, T.; Mackie, A.; Requena, T.; Swiatecka, D.; Wichers, H. (Eds.) *The Impact of Food Bioactives on Health*; Springer International Publishing: Cham, Switzerland, 2015; pp. 45–52.

47. Comstock, W.J.; Huh, E.; Weekes, R.; Watson, C.; Xu, T.; Dorrestein, P.C.; Quinn, R.A. The WinCF Model—An inexpensive and tractable microcosm of a mucus plugged bronchiole to study the microbiology of lung infections. *JoVE* **2017**, 55532. [CrossRef]

48. Lagier, J.-C.; Armougom, F.; Million, M.; Hugon, P.; Pagnier, I.; Robert, C.; Bittar, F.; Fournous, G.; Gimenez, G.; Maraninchi, M.; et al. Microbial culturomics: Paradigm shift in the human gut microbiome study. *Clin. Microbiol. Infect.* **2012**, *18*, 1185–1193. [CrossRef]

49. Vandeplassche, E.; Sass, A.; Lemarcq, A.; Dandekar, A.A.; Coenye, T.; Crabbé, A. In vitro evolution of *Pseudomonas aeruginosa* AA2 biofilms in the presence of cystic fibrosis lung microbiome members. *Sci. Rep.* **2019**, *9*, 12859. [CrossRef]

50. Scott, J.E.; O'Toole, G.A. The Yin and Yang of *Streptococcus* Lung infections in cystic fibrosis: A model for studying polymicrobial interactions. *J. Bacteriol.* **2019**, *201*, e00115-19. [CrossRef]

51. Lightly, T.J.; Phung, R.R.; Sorensen, J.L.; Cardona, S.T. Synthetic cystic fibrosis sputum medium diminishes *Burkholderia cenocepacia* antifungal activity against *Aspergillus fumigatus* independently of phenylacetic acid production. *Can. J. Microbiol.* **2017**, *63*, 427–438. [CrossRef]

52. Sibley, C.D.; Grinwis, M.E.; Field, T.R.; Eshaghurshan, C.S.; Faria, M.M.; Dowd, S.E.; Parkins, M.D.; Rabin, H.R.; Surette, M.G. Culture enriched molecular profiling of the cystic fibrosis airway microbiome. *PLoS ONE* **2011**, *6*, e22702. [CrossRef] [PubMed]

53. Dickson, R.P.; Erb-Downward, J.R.; Falkowski, N.R.; Hunter, E.M.; Ashley, S.L.; Huffnagle, G.B. The lung microbiota of healthy mice are highly variable, cluster by environment, and reflect variation in baseline lung innate immunity. *Am. J. Respir. Crit Care Med.* **2018**, *198*, 497–508. [CrossRef] [PubMed]

54. Laukens, D.; Brinkman, B.M.; Raes, J.; De Vos, M.; Vandenabeele, P. Heterogeneity of the gut microbiome in mice: Guidelines for optimizing experimental design. *FEMS Microbiol. Rev.* **2016**, *40*, 117–132. [CrossRef] [PubMed]

55. McCarron, A.; Donnelley, M.; Parsons, D. Airway disease phenotypes in animal models of cystic fibrosis. *Respir. Res.* **2018**, *19*, 54. [CrossRef]

56. Fiorotto, R.; Amenduni, M.; Mariotti, V.; Cadamuro, M.; Fabris, L.; Spirli, C.; Strazzabosco, M. Animal models for cystic fibrosis liver disease (CFLD). *Biochim. Biophys. Acta (BBA) Mol. Basis Dis.* **2019**, *1865*, 965–969. [CrossRef] [PubMed]

57. Sun, X.; Olivier, A.K.; Liang, B.; Yi, Y.; Sui, H.; Evans, T.I.; Zhang, Y.; Zhou, W.; Tyler, S.R.; Fisher, J.T.; et al. Gastrointestinal pathology in juvenile and adult cystic fibrosis transmembrane conductance regulator-knockout ferrets. *Am. J.Respir. Cell. Mol. Biol.* **2014**, *50*, 502–512. [CrossRef] [PubMed]

58. Cho, D.-Y.; Mackey, C.; Van Der Pol, W.J.; Skinner, D.; Morrow, C.D.; Schoeb, T.R.; Rowe, S.M.; Swords, W.E.; Tearney, G.J.; Woodworth, B.A. Sinus microanatomy and microbiota in a rabbit model of rhinosinusitis. *Front. Cell. Infect. Microbiol.* **2018**, *7*, 540. [CrossRef]

59. Stoltz, D.A.; Meyerholz, D.K.; Welsh, M.J. Origins of cystic fibrosis lung disease. *N. Engl. J. Med.* **2015**, *372*, 351–362. [CrossRef]

60. Fan, Z.; Perisse, I.V.; Cotton, C.U.; Regouski, M.; Meng, Q.; Domb, C.; Van Wettere, A.J.; Wang, Z.; Harris, A.; White, K.L.; et al. A sheep model of cystic fibrosis generated by CRISPR/Cas9 disruption of the *CFTR* gene. *JCI Insight* **2018**, *3*, e123529. [CrossRef]

61. Birket, S.E.; Davis, J.M.; Fernandez, C.M.; Tuggle, K.L.; Oden, A.M.; Chu, K.K.; Tearney, G.J.; Fanucchi, M.V.; Sorscher, E.J.; Rowe, S.M. Development of an airway mucus defect in the cystic fibrosis rat. *JCI Insight* **2018**, *3*, e97199. [CrossRef]

62. Norkina, O.; Burnett, T.G.; De Lisle, R.C. Bacterial overgrowth in the cystic fibrosis transmembrane conductance regulator null mouse small intestine. *Infect. Immun.* **2004**, *72*, 6040–6049. [CrossRef] [PubMed]

63. Bazett, M.; Bergeron, M.-E.; Haston, C.K. Streptomycin treatment alters the intestinal microbiome, pulmonary T cell profile and airway hyperresponsiveness in a cystic fibrosis mouse model. *Sci. Rep.* **2016**, *6*, 19189. [CrossRef] [PubMed]

64. Bazett, M.; Honeyman, L.; Stefanov, A.N.; Pope, C.E.; Hoffman, L.R.; Haston, C.K. Cystic fibrosis mouse model-dependent intestinal structure and gut microbiome. *Mamm Genome* **2015**, *26*, 222–234. [CrossRef] [PubMed]

65. Lynch, S.V.; Goldfarb, K.C.; Wild, Y.K.; Kong, W.; De Lisle, R.C.; Brodie, E.L. Cystic fibrosis transmembrane conductance regulator knockout mice exhibit aberrant gastrointestinal microbiota. *Gut Microbes* **2013**, *4*, 41–47. [CrossRef]

66. Meeker, S.M.; Mears, K.S.; Sangwan, N.; Brittnacher, M.J.; Weiss, E.J.; Treuting, P.M.; Tolley, N.; Pope, C.E.; Hager, K.R.; Vo, A.T.; et al. CFTR dysregulation drives active selection of the gut microbiome. *PLoS Pathog.* **2020**, *16*, e1008251. [CrossRef] [PubMed]

67. Debray, D.; El Mourabit, H.; Merabtene, F.; Brot, L.; Ulveling, D.; Chrétien, Y.; Rainteau, D.; Moszer, I.; Wendum, D.; Sokol, H.; et al. Diet-induced dysbiosis and genetic background synergize with cystic fibrosis transmembrane conductance regulator deficiency to promote cholangiopathy in mice. *Hepatol. Commun.* **2018**, *2*, 1533–1549. [CrossRef] [PubMed]

68. Millette, G.; Langlois, J.-P.; Brouillette, E.; Frost, E.H.; Cantin, A.M.; Malouin, F. Despite antagonism *in vitro, Pseudomonas aeruginosa* enhances *Staphylococcus aureus* colonization in a murine lung infection model. *Front. Microbiol.* **2019**, *10*, 2880. [CrossRef]

69. Marsland, B.J.; Gollwitzer, E.S. Host–microorganism interactions in lung diseases. *Nat. Rev Immunol.* **2014**, *14*, 827–835. [CrossRef]

70. Esther, C.R.; Muhlebach, M.S.; Ehre, C.; Hill, D.B.; Wolfgang, M.C.; Kesimer, M.; Ramsey, K.A.; Markovetz, M.R.; Garbarine, I.C.; Forest, M.G.; et al. Mucus accumulation in the lungs precedes structural changes and infection in children with cystic fibrosis. *Sci. Transl. Med.* **2019**, *11*, eaav3488. [CrossRef]

71. Mika, M.; Korten, I.; Qi, W.; Regamey, N.; Frey, U.; Casaulta, C.; Latzin, P.; Hilty, M. The nasal microbiota in infants with cystic fibrosis in the first year of life: A prospective cohort study. *Lancet Respir. Med.* **2016**, *4*, 627–635. [CrossRef]

72. Moran Losada, P.; Chouvarine, P.; Dorda, M.; Hedtfeld, S.; Mielke, S.; Schulz, A.; Wiehlmann, L.; Tümmler, B. The cystic fibrosis lower airways microbial metagenome. *ERJ Open Res.* **2016**, *2*, 00096–02015. [CrossRef] [PubMed]

73. Charlson, E.S.; Bittinger, K.; Haas, A.R.; Fitzgerald, A.S.; Frank, I.; Yadav, A.; Bushman, F.D.; Collman, R.G. Topographical continuity of bacterial populations in the healthy human respiratory tract. *Am. J. Respir Crit Care Med.* **2011**, *184*, 957–963. [CrossRef] [PubMed]

74. Boutin, S.; Graeber, S.Y.; Weitnauer, M.; Panitz, J.; Stahl, M.; Clausznitzer, D.; Kaderali, L.; Einarsson, G.; Tunney, M.M.; Elborn, J.S.; et al. Comparison of microbiomes from different niches of upper and lower airways in children and adolescents with cystic fibrosis. *PLoS ONE* **2015**, *10*, e0116029. [CrossRef] [PubMed]

75. Prevaes, S.M.P.J.; de Steenhuijsen Piters, W.A.A.; de Winter-de Groot, K.M.; Janssens, H.M.; Tramper-Stranders, G.A.; Chu, M.L.J.N.; Tiddens, H.A.; van Westreenen, M.; van der Ent, C.K.; Sanders, E.A.M.; et al. Concordance between upper and lower airway microbiota in infants with cystic fibrosis. *Eur. Respir. J.* **2017**, *49*, 1602235. [CrossRef] [PubMed]

76. Bernarde, C.; Keravec, M.; Mounier, J.; Gouriou, S.; Rault, G.; Férec, C.; Barbier, G.; Héry-Arnaud, G. Impact of the CFTR-potentiator ivacaftor on airway microbiota in cystic fibrosis patients carrying a G551D mutation. *PLoS ONE* **2015**, *10*, e0124124. [CrossRef] [PubMed]

77. Keravec, M.; Mounier, J.; Prestat, E.; Vallet, S.; Jansson, J.K.; Burgaud, G.; Rosec, S.; Gouriou, S.; Rault, G.; Coton, E.; et al. Insights into the respiratory tract microbiota of patients with cystic fibrosis during early *Pseudomonas aeruginosa* colonization. *SpringerPlus* **2015**, *4*, 405. [CrossRef]

78. Keravec, M.; Mounier, J.; Guilloux, C.-A.; Fangous, M.-S.; Mondot, S.; Vallet, S.; Gouriou, S.; Le Berre, R.; Rault, G.; Férec, C.; et al. *Porphyromonas*, a potential predictive biomarker of *Pseudomonas aeruginosa* pulmonary infection in cystic fibrosis. *BMJ Open Resp. Res.* **2019**, *6*, e000374. [CrossRef]

79. Ruppé, E.; Ghozlane, A.; Tap, J.; Pons, N.; Alvarez, A.-S.; Maziers, N.; Cuesta, T.; Hernando-Amado, S.; Clares, I.; Martínez, J.L.; et al. Prediction of the intestinal resistome by a three-dimensional structure-based method. *Nat. Microbiol.* **2019**, *4*, 112–123. [CrossRef]

80. Jankauskaitė, L.; Misevičienė, V.; Vaidelienė, L.; Kėvalas, R. Lower airway virology in health and disease—From invaders to symbionts. *Medicina* **2018**, *54*, 72. [CrossRef]

81. Rolain, J.M.; Fancello, L.; Desnues, C.; Raoult, D. Bacteriophages as vehicles of the resistome in cystic fibrosis. *J. Antimicrob. Chemother.* **2011**, *66*, 2444–2447. [CrossRef]

82. Kramer, R.; Sauer-Heilborn, A.; Welte, T.; Guzman, C.A.; Abraham, W.-R.; Höfle, M.G. Cohort study of airway mycobiome in adult cystic fibrosis patients: Differences in community structure between fungi and bacteria reveal predominance of transient fungal elements. *J. Clin. Microbiol.* **2015**, *53*, 2900–2907. [CrossRef] [PubMed]

83. Delhaes, L.; Monchy, S.; Fréalle, E.; Hubans, C.; Salleron, J.; Leroy, S.; Prevotat, A.; Wallet, F.; Wallaert, B.; Dei-Cas, E.; et al. The airway microbiota in cystic fibrosis: A complex fungal and bacterial community—Implications for therapeutic management. *PLoS ONE* **2012**, *7*, e36313. [CrossRef] [PubMed]

84. The Mucofong Investigation Group; Soret, P.; Vandenborght, L.-E.; Francis, F.; Coron, N.; Enaud, R.; Avalos, M.; Schaeverbeke, T.; Berger, P.; Fayon, M.; et al. Respiratory mycobiome and suggestion of inter-kingdom network during acute pulmonary exacerbation in cystic fibrosis. *Sci. Rep.* **2020**, *10*, 3589. [CrossRef]

85. Koskinen, K.; Pausan, M.R.; Perras, A.K.; Beck, M.; Bang, C.; Mora, M.; Schilhabel, A.; Schmitz, R.; Moissl-Eichinger, C. First insights into the diverse human archaeome: Specific detection of archaea in the gastrointestinal tract, lung, and nose and on skin. *mBio* **2017**, *8*, e00824-17. [CrossRef]

86. Cox, M.J.; Allgaier, M.; Taylor, B.; Baek, M.S.; Huang, Y.J.; Daly, R.A.; Karaoz, U.; Andersen, G.L.; Brown, R.; Fujimura, K.E.; et al. Airway microbiota and pathogen abundance in age-stratified cystic fibrosis patients. *PLoS ONE* **2010**, *5*, e11044. [CrossRef]

87. Zhao, J.; Schloss, P.D.; Kalikin, L.M.; Carmody, L.A.; Foster, B.K.; Petrosino, J.F.; Cavalcoli, J.D.; VanDevanter, D.R.; Murray, S.; Li, J.Z.; et al. Decade-long bacterial community dynamics in cystic fibrosis airways. *Proc. Natl. Acad. Sci. USA* **2012**, *109*, 5809–5814. [CrossRef]

88. Jorth, P.; Ehsan, Z.; Rezayat, A.; Caldwell, E.; Pope, C.; Brewington, J.J.; Goss, C.H.; Benscoter, D.; Clancy, J.P.; Singh, P.K. Direct lung sampling indicates that established pathogens dominate early infections in children with cystic fibrosis. *Cell Rep.* **2019**, *27*, 1190–1204.e3. [CrossRef]

89. De Koff, E.M.; de Groot, K.M.W.; Bogaert, D. Development of the respiratory tract microbiota in cystic fibrosis. *Curr. Opin. Pulm. Med.* **2016**, *22*, 623–628. [CrossRef]

90. Zemanick, E.T.; Harris, J.K.; Wagner, B.D.; Robertson, C.E.; Sagel, S.D.; Stevens, M.J.; Accurso, F.J.; Laguna, T.A. Inflammation and airway microbiota during cystic fibrosis pulmonary exacerbations. *PLoS ONE* **2013**, *8*, e62917. [CrossRef]

91. Cuthbertson, L.; Rogers, G.B.; Walker, A.W.; Oliver, A.; Green, L.E.; Daniels, T.W.V.; Carroll, M.P.; Parkhill, J.; Bruce, K.D.; van der Gast, C.J. Respiratory microbiota resistance and resilience to pulmonary exacerbation and subsequent antimicrobial intervention. *ISME J.* **2016**, *10*, 1081–1091. [CrossRef]

92. Li, J.; Hao, C.; Ren, L.; Xiao, Y.; Wang, J.; Qin, X. Data mining of lung microbiota in cystic fibrosis patients. *PLoS ONE* **2016**, *11*, e0164510. [CrossRef] [PubMed]

93. Anand, S.; Mande, S.S. Diet, microbiota and gut-lung connection. *Front. Microbiol.* **2018**, *9*, 2147. [CrossRef] [PubMed]

94. Zhang, D.; Li, S.; Wang, N.; Tan, H.-Y.; Zhang, Z.; Feng, Y. The cross-talk between gut microbiota and lungs in common lung diseases. *Front. Microbiol.* **2020**, *11*, 301. [CrossRef]

95. Nielsen, S.; Needham, B.; Leach, S.T.; Day, A.S.; Jaffe, A.; Thomas, T.; Ooi, C.Y. Disrupted progression of the intestinal microbiota with age in children with cystic fibrosis. *Sci. Rep.* **2016**, *6*, 24857. [CrossRef] [PubMed]

96. Goodrich, J.K.; Davenport, E.R.; Clark, A.G.; Ley, R.E. The relationship between the human genome and microbiome comes into view. *Annu. Rev. Genet.* **2017**, *51*, 413–433. [CrossRef] [PubMed]

97. Goodrich, J.K.; Waters, J.L.; Poole, A.C.; Sutter, J.L.; Koren, O.; Blekhman, R.; Beaumont, M.; Van Treuren, W.; Knight, R.; Bell, J.T.; et al. Human genetics shape the gut microbiome. *Cell* **2014**, *159*, 789–799. [CrossRef]

98. Vernocchi, P.; Del Chierico, F.; Quagliariello, A.; Ercolini, D.; Lucidi, V.; Putignani, L. A Metagenomic and in silico functional prediction of gut microbiota profiles may concur in discovering new cystic fibrosis patient-targeted probiotics. *Nutrients* **2017**, *9*, 1342. [CrossRef]

99. Muhlebach, M.S.; Hatch, J.E.; Einarsson, G.G.; McGrath, S.J.; Gilipin, D.F.; Lavelle, G.; Mirkovic, B.; Murray, M.A.; McNally, P.; Gotman, N.; et al. Anaerobic bacteria cultured from cystic fibrosis airways correlate to milder disease: A multisite study. *Eur. Respir. J.* **2018**, *52*, 1800242. [CrossRef]

100. Miragoli, F.; Federici, S.; Ferrari, S.; Minuti, A.; Rebecchi, A.; Bruzzese, E.; Buccigrossi, V.; Guarino, A.; Callegari, M.L. Impact of cystic fibrosis disease on archaea and bacteria composition of gut microbiota. *FEMS Microbiol. Ecol.* **2017**, *93*, fiw230. [CrossRef]

101. Ikpa, P.T.; Meijsen, K.F.; Nieuwenhuijze, N.D.A.; Dulla, K.; de Jonge, H.R.; Bijvelds, M.J.C. Transcriptome analysis of the distal small intestine of Cftr null mice. *Genomics* **2020**, *112*, 1139–1150. [CrossRef]
102. Rogers, G.B.; Taylor, S.L.; Hoffman, L.R.; Burr, L.D. The impact of CFTR modulator therapies on CF airway microbiology. *J. Cyst. Fibros.* **2019**, S156919931930829X. [CrossRef] [PubMed]
103. Ooi, C.Y.; Syed, S.A.; Rossi, L.; Garg, M.; Needham, B.; Avolio, J.; Young, K.; Surette, M.G.; Gonska, T. Impact of CFTR modulation with ivacaftor on gut microbiota and intestinal inflammation. *Sci. Rep.* **2018**, *8*, 17834. [CrossRef] [PubMed]
104. Rowe, S.M.; Heltshe, S.L.; Gonska, T.; Donaldson, S.H.; Borowitz, D.; Gelfond, D.; Sagel, S.D.; Khan, U.; Mayer-Hamblett, N.; Van Dalfsen, J.M.; et al. Clinical mechanism of the cystic fibrosis transmembrane conductance regulator potentiator ivacaftor in G551D-mediated cystic fibrosis. *Am. J. Respir Crit Care Med.* **2014**, *190*, 175–184. [CrossRef] [PubMed]
105. Peleg, A.Y.; Choo, J.M.; Langan, K.M.; Edgeworth, D.; Keating, D.; Wilson, J.; Rogers, G.B.; Kotsimbos, T. Antibiotic exposure and interpersonal variance mask the effect of ivacaftor on respiratory microbiota composition. *J. Cyst. Fibros.* **2018**, *17*, 50–56. [CrossRef]
106. Harris, J.K.; Wagner, B.D.; Zemanick, E.T.; Robertson, C.E.; Stevens, M.J.; Heltshe, S.L.; Rowe, S.M.; Sagel, S.D. Changes in airway microbiome and inflammation with ivacaftor treatment in patients with cystic fibrosis and the G551D mutation. *Ann. ATS* **2020**, *17*, 212–220. [CrossRef]
107. Duytschaever, G.; Huys, G.; Bekaert, M.; Boulanger, L.; De Boeck, K.; Vandamme, P. Dysbiosis of bifidobacteria and *Clostridium* cluster XIVa in the cystic fibrosis fecal microbiota. *J. Cyst. Fibros.* **2013**, *12*, 206–215. [CrossRef]
108. Muhlebach, M.S.; Zorn, B.T.; Esther, C.R.; Hatch, J.E.; Murray, C.P.; Turkovic, L.; Ranganathan, S.C.; Boucher, R.C.; Stick, S.M.; Wolfgang, M.C. Initial acquisition and succession of the cystic fibrosis lung microbiome is associated with disease progression in infants and preschool children. *PLoS Pathog.* **2018**, *14*, e1006798. [CrossRef]
109. Acosta, N.; Heirali, A.; Somayaji, R.; Surette, M.G.; Workentine, M.L.; Sibley, C.D.; Rabin, H.R.; Parkins, M.D. Sputum microbiota is predictive of long-term clinical outcomes in young adults with cystic fibrosis. *Thorax* **2018**, *73*, 1016–1025. [CrossRef]
110. Sherrard, L.J.; Bell, S.C. Lower airway microbiota for 'biomarker' measurements of cystic fibrosis disease progression? *Thorax* **2018**, *73*, 1001–1003. [CrossRef]
111. Cobián Güemes, A.G.; Lim, Y.W.; Quinn, R.A.; Conrad, D.J.; Benler, S.; Maughan, H.; Edwards, R.; Brettin, T.; Cantú, V.A.; Cuevas, D.; et al. Cystic fibrosis rapid response: Translating multi-omics data into clinically relevant information. *mBio* **2019**, *10*, e00431-19. [CrossRef]
112. Heirali, A.A.; Acosta, N.; Storey, D.G.; Workentine, M.L.; Somayaji, R.; Laforest-Lapointe, I.; Leung, W.; Quon, B.S.; Berthiaume, Y.; Rabin, H.R.; et al. The effects of cycled inhaled aztreonam on the cystic fibrosis (CF) lung microbiome. *J. Cyst. Fibros.* **2019**, *18*, 829–837. [CrossRef] [PubMed]
113. Alexandre, Y.; Le Blay, G.; Boisramé-Gastrin, S.; Le Gall, F.; Héry-Arnaud, G.; Gouriou, S.; Vallet, S.; Le Berre, R. Probiotics: A new way to fight bacterial pulmonary infections? *Méd. Mal. Infect.* **2014**, *44*, 9–17. [CrossRef] [PubMed]
114. Cho, D.; Skinner, D.; Lim, D.J.; Mclemore, J.G.; Koch, C.G.; Zhang, S.; Swords, W.E.; Hunter, R.; Crossman, D.K.; Crowley, M.R.; et al. The impact of *Lactococcus lactis* (probiotic nasal rinse) co-culture on growth of patient-derived strains of *Pseudomonas aeruginosa*. *Int. Forum. Allergy Rhinol.* **2020**, alr.22521. [CrossRef] [PubMed]
115. Antosca, K.M.; Chernikova, D.A.; Price, C.E.; Ruoff, K.L.; Li, K.; Guill, M.F.; Sontag, N.R.; Morrison, H.G.; Hao, S.; Drumm, M.L.; et al. Altered stool microbiota of infants with cystic fibrosis shows a reduction in genera associated with immune programming from birth. *J. Bacteriol.* **2019**, *201*, e00274-19. [CrossRef]
116. Alvarez, S.; Herrero, C.; Bru, E.; Perdigon, G. Effect of Lactobacillus casei and Yogurt Administration on Prevention of *Pseudomonas aeruginosa* Infection in Young Mice. *J. Food Prot.* **2001**, *64*, 1768–1774. [CrossRef]
117. Tan, H.; Wang, C.; Zhang, Q.; Tang, X.; Zhao, J.; Zhang, H.; Zhai, Q.; Chen, W. Preliminary safety assessment of a new *Bacteroides fragilis* isolate. *Food Chem. Toxicol.* **2020**, *135*, 110934. [CrossRef]
118. Butler, R. Non-invasive tests in animal models and humans: A new paradigm for assessing efficacy of biologics including prebiotics and probiotics. *CPD* **2008**, *14*, 1341–1350. [CrossRef]
119. Portal, C.; Gouyer, V.; Léonard, R.; Husson, M.-O.; Gottrand, F.; Desseyn, J.-L. Long-term dietary (n-3) polyunsaturated fatty acids show benefits to the lungs of Cftr F508del mice. *PLoS ONE* **2018**, *13*, e0197808. [CrossRef]

120. Paoli, A.; Mancin, L.; Bianco, A.; Thomas, E.; Mota, J.F.; Piccini, F. Ketogenic diet and microbiota: Friends or enemies? *Genes* **2019**, *10*, 534. [CrossRef]
121. Kanhere, M.; Chassaing, B.; Gewirtz, A.T.; Tangpricha, V. Role of vitamin D on gut microbiota in cystic fibrosis. *J. Steroid Biochem. Mol. Biol.* **2018**, *175*, 82–87. [CrossRef]

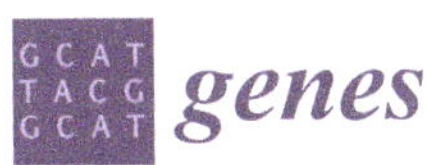 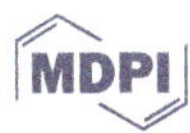

Review

The Impact of the CFTR Gene Discovery on Cystic Fibrosis Diagnosis, Counseling, and Preventive Therapy

Philip M. Farrell [1],*, Michael J. Rock [2] and Mei W. Baker [2,3]

[1] Departments of Pediatrics and Population Health Sciences, University of Wisconsin School of Medicine and Public Health, 600 Highland Madison, WI 53792, USA

[2] Department of Pediatrics, University of Wisconsin School of Medicine and Public Health, 600 Highland Ave, Madison, WI 53792, USA; mjrock@pediatrics.wisc.edu (M.J.R.); mwbaker@wisc.edu (M.W.B.)

[3] Newborn Screening Laboratory, Wisconsin State Laboratory of Hygiene, University of Wisconsin–Madison, 465 Henry Mall, Madison, WI 53706, USA

* Correspondence: pmfarrell@wisc.edu; Tel.: +1-608-345-2308

Received: 27 March 2020; Accepted: 7 April 2020; Published: 8 April 2020

Abstract: Discovery of the cystic fibrosis transmembrane conductance regulator (*CFTR*) gene was the long-awaited scientific advance that dramatically improved the diagnosis and treatment of cystic fibrosis (CF). The combination of a first-tier biomarker, immunoreactive trypsinogen (IRT), and, if high, DNA analysis for CF-causing variants, has enabled regions where CF is prevalent to screen neonates and achieve diagnoses within 1–2 weeks of birth when most patients are asymptomatic. In addition, IRT/DNA (*CFTR*) screening protocols simultaneously contribute important genetic data to determine genotype, prognosticate, and plan preventive therapies such as CFTR modulator selection. As the genomics era proceeds with affordable biotechnologies, the potential added value of whole genome sequencing will probably enhance personalized, precision care that can begin during infancy. Issues remain, however, about the optimal size of *CFTR* panels in genetically diverse regions and how best to deal with incidental findings. Because prospects for a primary DNA screening test are on the horizon, the debate about detecting heterozygote carriers will likely intensify, especially as we learn more about this relatively common genotype. Perhaps, at that time, concerns about CF heterozygote carrier detection will subside, and it will become recognized as beneficial. We share new perspectives on that issue in this article.

Keywords: cystic fibrosis; newborn screening; trypsinogen; *CFTR* gene; next generation sequencing; health policy

---

1. Introduction

Every physician's first duty is to diagnose—accurately and promptly—because diagnosis is the first step of treatment. In the case of cystic fibrosis (CF), accurate and prompt diagnosis was impossible before the newborn screening (NBS) era for the majority of patients [1]. In fact, children with CF typically experienced a diagnostic odyssey [2] and suffered irreversible malnutrition [3] and/or lung disease [4] before they had their diagnoses established through sweat chloride tests. Others, perhaps 5%–10% and certainly at least 1% [5], died undiagnosed; those unfortunate patients would have had fatal hyponatremic/hypochloremic dehydration, protein-energy malnutrition, or catastrophic lung disease [3,4]. It is likely that these tragic fatalities continue in some regions of the world where CF NBS has not yet been implemented [1]. The advantages of early diagnosis are not only intuitive but were identified in clinical research as early as 1970, when Shwachman et al. [6] reported a classic study showing that survival was much better when diagnosis occurred before three months of age.

Early NBS attempts using meconium, however, failed feasibility assessment [7]. Fortunately, the use of dried blood spot screening, which was immediately successful for phenylketonuria [8], became attractive for CF when Crossley et al. [9] discovered in New Zealand that high immunoreactive trypsinogen (IRT) levels predicted a higher risk for CF. Because most regions had well-functioning systems in place for universal collection of dried blood spot specimens and their analysis in a central laboratory, the stage was set for CF NBS using IRT as an initial and, about two weeks later, a "recall" test to confirm hypertrypsinogenemia [10]. Skepticism remained, however, because of concerns about the IRT test per se, whether or not significant clinical benefits actually occurred with early diagnoses, and how much adverse impact was being imposed on parents of screened neonates, i.e., the degree of psychosocial harm [11]. In retrospect, the major issue that initially limited CF NBS acceptance concerned the IRT/IRT screening strategy (a protocol with relatively low sensitivity) using a biomarker with variable reliability [12,13]. Consequently, it became clear that more research was needed on all aspects of CF NBS and that the IRT method of screening needed to be improved. In fact, a decade after the report from New Zealand, there was still worldwide debate among health policy decision-makers whether or not CF NBS was worthwhile [1] and even doubt among organizations like the US Cystic Fibrosis Foundation (CFF)—expressed emphatically when it sponsored a negative but influential commentary [11]. Consequently, CF NBS implementation was slow in North America and Europe, and one country (France) even discontinued their national IRT-based program [1]. Suddenly, however, the situation changed dramatically, when the *CFTR* discovery was reported in September 1989 [14]. This major advance forever changed the landscape with regard to both diagnosis and treatment.

2. Development of the IRT/DNA Screening Strategy

Dans les champs de l'observation le hasard ne favorise que les esprits prepares (in the field of observation, chance favors only the prepared mind), emphasized Louis Pasteur during his lecture at the University of Lille on 7 December 1854. The story surrounding transformation from IRT/IRT to IRT/DNA in Wisconsin fulfills Pasteur's admonition. Beginning in April 1985, after securing grants from the CFF and NIH, Wisconsin's two CF Centers began a randomized clinical trial (RCT) of newborn screening that led to a conclusion by 1989 that the IRT/IRT test was good, but not good enough, for routine use by public health laboratories [15]. The results supporting that conclusion were in the process of being reported in *Pediatrics* at a time when the delay from manuscript acceptance (in this case, 3 July 1989) to publication was typically at least a few months. Under Conclusions, it was stated that the IRT test will not be adequate as a sole screening method but might be useful as an initial marker if followed by another tier as in the thyroxin/TSH combination for congenital hypothyroidism. However, as Rock et al. [15] awaited the page proofs, the discovery of the cystic fibrosis transmembrane conductance regulator (*CFTR*) gene and the p.Phe508del (c.1521_1523delCTT) variant was reported [14], and with the Editor's approval, the following comment was added under a new section, entitled Speculation and Relevance: *With advances in technology and the recent identification of one of the cystic fibrosis mutations and the identification of other mutations to soon follow, we believe that the strategy for cystic fibrosis newborn screening will need to evolve into a true two-tier screening test. The first tier would be the IRT assay; if the IRT assay is positive, the second tier would be performed on the same original blood spot, and it would be a probe for the cystic fibrosis mutations. The implementation of cystic fibrosis screening, however, should be delayed until a clear benefit of newborn screening has been identified.*

While the Rock et al. [15] article was still in press, and thanks to applicable NIH grant support, Farrell recruited an excellent molecular geneticist, Ronald Gregg, and early in 1990 a reliable but laborious method was developed [16–19] to incorporate into the RCT. In summary, using a method just described by Jinks et al. [20], DNA was isolated from a 5-mm blood-soaked filter paper circle obtained from a Guthrie card, denatured, PCR-amplified, and then analyzed on polyacrylamide gel with the genotype determined according to the "rapid" method of Rommens et al. [21]. Prior to implementation of the IRT /DNA screening protocol, a pilot phase was performed to evaluate the validity of the contemplated DNA testing procedure. The Wisconsin's team's main concern was the possibility of error due to sample cross-contamination because of the serial sample punching procedures used by the newborn screening laboratory. Some low-level cross-contamination seemed likely to occur, because the automated punches used to prepare samples from Guthrie cards cannot be decontaminated sufficiently to destroy DNA from previously punched cards. Consequently, we were concerned that the amount of contamination might be sufficient for detection by the PCR-based assay. Blinded dried blood samples obtained previously from 300 infants with an elevated IRT, including 43 CF patients, were analyzed for p.Phe508. All the p.Phe508 homozygotes detected were known to have CF. Repeat analysis on independently collected blood samples confirmed the original genotype. Therefore, it was concluded that the very low level of cross-contamination that might occur with serial punching of cards is insufficient to interfere with the DNA analysis [17].

Next, and soon thereafter, all definitively diagnosed CF patients followed in the Madison and Milwaukee Centers were studied to determine the prevalence of p.Phe508del. Fortunately, the predominance of this principal CF-causing variant was apparent immediately. The data on 547 patients revealed that 264 (48.3%) were homozygous, 220 (40.2%) were p.Phe508del compound heterozygotes, and only 63 (11.5%) had two other CFTR variants. Thus, a two-tier screening test with IRT/DNA(p.Phe508del), using lower levels of IRT as the cutoff for the second tier, was determined to be valuable and have much better sensitivity than the 75% identified with the IRT/IRT protocol [12,15]. In addition, there are many other advantages listed in Table 1. It was particularly comforting to find that IRT/DNA eliminated the problem Rock et al. [22] had reported previously: that IRT alone identified an inordinately high percentage of premature and African American infants who were not at increased risk for CF but likely to have false positive IRT levels in initial dried blood spot testing.

Table 1. Advantages of IRT/DNA(CFTR) newborn screening compared to IRT/IRT.

1.	Increased sensitivity → improved validity
2.	Accelerated screening test completion by 5–7 days → 2-week diagnoses
3.	Enables simultaneous determination of genotype
a.	Allowing prediction of pancreatic functional status
b.	Facilitating selection of CFTR modulator for preventive therapy
4.	Eliminates 2-week recall specimen collection (avoid loss of infants to follow up)
5.	Avoid problem of rapidly decreasing IRT as infants "age"
6.	Provides presumptive (genetic) diagnosis in at least 75% of cases
7.	Facilitates planning for follow-up of IRT/DNA positive infants
a.	With 2 mutations, the parents' knowledge of probable CF prior to the sweat test facilitates immediate education and treatment
b.	Facilitates rapid interpretation of intermediate sweat chloride levels
c.	With 1 mutation, there is a low (~3%) residual risk or probability of CF
8.	Eliminates low APGAR false IRT positive problems due to perinatal stress, particularly in premature infants with low APGAR scores
9.	Reduces or eliminates the problems associated with higher IRT levels in African American babies
10.	Identifies heterozygote carrier families for the genetic counseling benefit

Consequently, the Wisconsin RCT incorporated IRT/DNA as the screening test in 1991, and the project was expanded to a comprehensive epidemiologic study of childhood CF [23]. By 1991, IRT/DNA was also successfully implemented for routine screening in South Australia by Ranieri et al. [24] and soon thereafter in other regions [1], such as Brittany, where the molecular genetics expertise of Claude Férec's laboratory was readily applied to two-tier CF NBS [25]. In retrospect, the discovery that about 90% of Europeans and Europe-derived CF populations have at least one p.Phe508del variant greatly facilitated widespread implementation of the world's first DNA-based population screening test—the IRT/DNA(p.Phe508del) method. Its advantages and demonstration of benefits [15,26] outweighing the inevitable harms of any screening test set the stage for the Centers for Disease Control and Prevention (CDC) and the US CFF to advocate for universal CF NBS in 2004 [2] and 2005 [27], respectively. The delay in approvals by these organizations can be attributed to the fact that such advocacy was unprecedented, and both the CDC and CFF were concerned that the potential harm could outweigh the benefits [2,11,27]. These actions stimulated nationwide screening of 4 million American babies annually in less than 5 years and now worldwide screening programs, as shown in Figure 1. Moreover, a complete transformation of the care strategy for children with CF [23,28–30] emerged as routine early diagnosis facilitated preventive therapies, reflecting the view that prevention is far better than intervention for chronic, potentially irreversible disease.

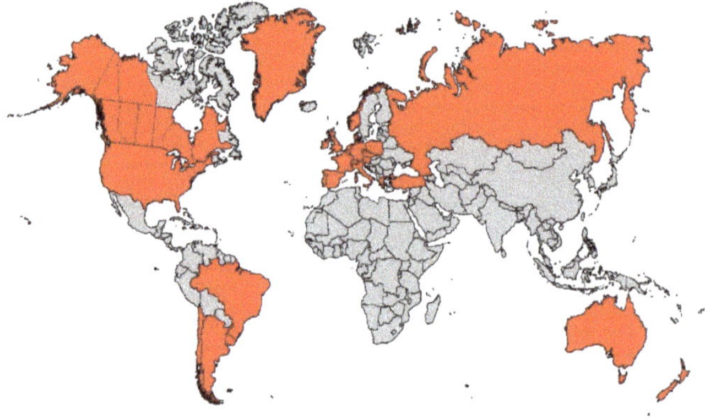

Figure 1. Cystic fibrosis newborn screening in 2020 around the world where the disease is prevalent.

3. Improvements in IRT/DNA Screening Protocols

Although the two-tier screening test with IRT/DNA and the p.Phe508del variant only using lower cutoff levels of IRT was advantageous [12,17], and needed to be continued for the RCT, the Wisconsin team decided to change the protocol when randomization ended on 30 June 1994 after NBS-derived nutritional benefits were becoming evident [15,26]. Thus, the Wisconsin State Laboratory of Hygiene, led by Ron Laessig and Gary Hoffman, recognized that routine CF NBS should be introduced with two improvements in the screening algorithm. First, it had become clear during the RCT that the biomarker IRT was a very challenging analyte with regard to setting reliable, stable cutoff values. In fact, there were both seasonal and kit-related variations that prevented equitable use of IRT and mitigation of false negative results [12,31]. This recognition led to the floating IRT cutoff value tactic, in which the highest 4%–5% of the daily specimens were reflexed to the DNA tier [12].

In addition, recognizing the important contribution of Comeau et al. [32], many regions expanded the DNA tier to a *CFTR* multimutation panel and a sensitivity of >95% was achieved routinely (in some years, 100% sensitivity) [18]. In addition, the quality of screening improved significantly by not only allowing test completion on the initial dried blood spot specimen, thus improving timeliness, but providing valuable information on most patients' *CFTR* variants. It was quickly learned with IRT/DNA(*CFTR*) that the vast majority of CF cases can be presumptively (genetically) diagnosed within a week of birth from the initial blood specimen and valuable genetic data obtained to predict pancreatic functional status [33]. Later, the rapid genotyping capability of IRT/DNA (*CFTR*) screening also provided guidance for selection of CFTR modulators which can now be used to achieve organ preservation if begun early [34]. On the other hand, the *CFTR* multi-mutation tactic increases the number of incidental findings, particularly detection of CF heterozygote carriers, an increasingly important topic that is discussed in detail subsequently, and identification of those with CRMS/CFSPID (cystic fibrosis transmembrane conductance regulator-related metabolic syndrome/cystic fibrosis screen positive, inconclusive diagnosis) [35,36], which is well reviewed elsewhere [37] and beyond the scope of this article.

Concerns about the higher costs of DNA/*CFTR* analyses and increased carrier detection have led to another change in regions wedded to collecting two dried blood specimens, namely the IRT/IRT/DNA protocol [38]. This algorithm modification achieves those two objectives (lower costs and fewer carriers detected) but delays diagnoses and does not improve sensitivity [39]. In view of the early risks of CF in infants such as potentially fatal hyponatremic/hypochloremic dehydration [40], and the likelihood of early malnutrition [41], it has become clear that timeliness in diagnosing the disease is an imperative. Thus, more research is needed on comparing the impact of IRT/DNA with IRT/IRT/DNA protocols. Similarly, algorithms employing pancreatitis-associated protein (PAP) and other supplemental tests need to be investigated further [1,35]. These algorithms may add potential advantages such as providing a "safety net" [35].

4. Application of Next Generation Sequencing

Despite its great advantages and popularity, there are many imperfections of IRT/DNA screening. One of the biggest challenges is a lower-than-ideal positive predictive value (PPV), resulting in as many as 10 heterozygote infant carriers (i.e., those with high IRT levels and single identified *CFTR* variants) for every CF case diagnosed after follow-up sweat testing. Although a 10:1 ratio may be disconcerting, other NBS tests lead to a higher proportion of false positive results such as screening for congenital adrenal hyperplasia [42]. In CF, however, the situation is exacerbated by the need for confirmatory sweat testing aa well as the occurrence of an insufficient quantity of sweat collected or an inconclusive sweat test outcome in at least 10% of the screen-positive infants. In addition, the *CFTR* panels in general use during the past two decades have had insufficient CF-causing variants to allow the detection of minority populations in many regions where uncommon CF-causing variants occur such as M1101K (c.3302T>A), found in Hutterite populations [43], and H199Y (c.595C>T) or S492F (c.1475C>T) seen in Hispanic populations [44]. As the genetic diversity of populations increases, the panels used for IRT/DNA screening will not adequately meet the goal of avoiding inequities, because missed cases are more likely among non-Caucasians. These challenges led CF NBS laboratories [45,46] to consider biotechnologies that would greatly expand the *CFTR* panel after two major advances that facilitated such a change—the advent of next generation sequencing (NGS) [47] and the knowledge gained from the CFTR2 project [48,49].

NGS, a deep, high-throughput, massive parallel DNA sequencing technology, has become popular during the past decade for genetic and genomic sequencing. Rapid progress in NGS chemistry and instrumentation coupled to the simultaneous development of advanced bioinformatics methods makes NGS feasible in public health laboratories that are responsible for NBS. Baker et al. [45] reported their successful experience with using NGS to increase the detection capability of *CFTR* pathogenic variants using DNA isolated from routine dried blood spot specimens. The NGS assay was designed to sequence all the coding regions, intron/exon boundaries, and selected intronic regions. The data analysis software was designed to mask much of the sequence data and reveal only the predetermined CF-causing variants in the *CFTR* gene as characterized by the CFTR2 project [48,49]. The significance of this study includes: (1) it was the first report from a public health NBS laboratory regarding the technical feasibility of applying NGS in routine NBS practice; and (2) the reported laboratory-developed DNA isolation method in this study is applicable to other molecular testing currently used in public health NBS laboratories, such as multiplexing real-time PCR assays to screen for severe combined immunodeficiency (SCID) [50] and spinal muscular atrophy (SMA) [51,52].

Built on the technical feasibility of applying NGS in routine NBS practice, the Wisconsin NBS program has, since April, 2016, further implemented the NGS *CFTR* variant panel as the routine second-tier testing method following first-tier IRT testing. Any newborn with one or more CF-causing variants identified is referred for a follow-up sweat chloride test as confirmatory testing. Recently, NGS data were reanalyzed on the infants with sweat chloride concentrations greater than 30 mmol/L after one CF-causing variant was identified through a regular NBS screening protocol. The NGS data reanalysis was performed by removing preset panel restrictions and viewing all variants. NGS data reanalysis is a cost-effective practice for identifying a second pathogenic or likely pathogenic *CFTR* variant in infants with a likely CF or CRMS/ CFSPID diagnosis [37]. When a single, second *CFTR* variant is detected with sequencing via NGS in a patient with a positive sweat test and/or symptoms of CF, it is quite likely to be pathogenic. Moreover, mutations in some classes like a Class I premature termination codon (PTC) can be assumed to be pathogenic; as Sosnay et al. state, "the assumption that variants predicted to introduce a PTC are deleterious is commonly accepted practice" [48]. The current *CFTR* variant panel in Wisconsin includes 328 CF-causing variants and the most common deletions (exon 2–3 deletion and exon 22–23 deletion) but not one deep intronic variant and other large deletions and duplications; this may be increased further in the future as the more CF-causing variants are added to the CFTR2 website. The State of New York also uses NGS and includes a third-tier *CFTR* sequence step before reporting all pathogenic and probable pathogenic variants prior to sweat testing, i.e., an "IRT/DNA/SEQ" algorithm [46], that markedly improves PPV.

5. The Potentially Added Value of Genomic Sequencing

The not-too-distant future holds many more opportunities for discovery of CF gene modifiers … *whole-genome sequencing will expand GWAS-type studies to rare variant analyses* [53]. NGS has made whole genome sequencing (WGS) feasible and affordable with platforms that are commercially available and proven reliable. Compared to whole exome sequencing, WGS is preferable, because the former only covers about 1.4% of the genome and will miss loci of potential clinical importance. Additionally, the modest cost of WGS now available is compelling. In fact, the cost of WGS is already similar to what many hospitals charge for bilateral sweat chloride tests. Clinical applications have therefore become attractive. Its use for diagnoses in critically ill newborns has already been established so that it will eventually become routine in neonatal intensive care units [54,55].

Although improvements in the diagnosis and treatment of CF have led to better outcomes for the majority of patients, the impact of pancreatic insufficiency, causing malnutrition and the occurrence of early obstructive lung disease with recurrent respiratory infections, can make identifying appropriate therapies challenging in many patients. In fact, some children labeled "non-responders" do not respond well to early GI/nutritional treatment, and they also have worse lung disease [56,57]. These observations underscore a gap in our understanding of what else will be needed to ensure successful therapeutic strategies, especially preventive care. Although the development of CFTR modulators has begun to revolutionize the treatment of CF patients, variable responses to these expensive modalities has created another important gap that needs to be addressed. With universal NBS for CF identifying presymptomatic patients, better opportunities have emerged for closing these gaps. Thus, Wisconsin recently launched a project entitled "Assessing the Added Value of Whole Genome Sequencing in Cystic Fibrosis Newborn Screening" to address the hypothesis that identifying non-*CFTR* genetic variants in individual patients could enlighten therapeutic decision-making [58]. Particular attention is being given to potential genetic modifiers of lung disease and nutrigenomic/pharmacogenomic variants related to common medications.

Exploring nutrigenomic and pharmacogenomic variants that are CF-relevant and can be readily identified with WGS appears to be fruitful according to our preliminary data [58,59]. A recently published study of siblings with different lung disease manifestations but an identical *CFTR* genotype predicting severe disease (p.Phe508del/CFTRdele2,3) generated WGS data that were informative [58]. The patients' variable phenotypes were accompanied by a surprising degree of differences in both genetic modifier and pharmacogenomics variants. In addition, in another study designed to gain insights about the variable response of CF patients to vitamin D supplements, WGS data were obtained and analyzed in 20 children whose 25-hydroxycholecalciferol levels varied during 4–24 months of treatment. Using a polygenic score technique to assess six informative loci, Lai et al. [59] found a significant nutrigenomic correlation. This study is currently being expanded with inclusion of more children and also adults with CF. Further research will be needed and is likely to be completed in the near future to determine if genomics added to DNA-based screening/genotyping will be valuable.

6. Prospects for a Primary DNA Screening Test

Many regions have implemented NBS for CF using the IRT/DNA two-tier protocol with a limited panel of variants [1]. According to 14 years of Wisconsin screening data, this protocol has had approximately 97% sensitivity, and the false negatives were due mainly to low IRT levels [31]. To avoid the false negative results caused by low IRT levels, a primary DNA-based screening test could be a potential solution. From the technical perspective, DNA-based assays as primary screening tests have been done routinely in screening for SCID [50] and SMA [51,52]. For SCID, although measuring T-cell receptor excision circles (TRECs) uses molecular techniques, it does not provide specific genetic information about the individual. TRECs are small circles of DNA created in T cells during their maturation in the thymus. Their presence indicates maturation of T cells; TRECs are reduced in SCID [50]. For SMA, the screening assays are designed to assess for deletions in the survival of motor neuron 1 (SMN1) gene. Undetectable SMN1 by real-time PCR indicates a high risk for SMA due to homozygous deletion of exon 7. This condition was recently added to the US Recommended Uniform Screening Panel (RUSP) [52]. The screening test for SMA is genetic testing, but the strategy of only targeting *SMN1* absence makes it possible to avoid SMA carrier identification in newborns. Success with SMA primary DNA-based screening, however, has created interest in applying the same strategy for CF NBS when analytical biotechnology advances enough to enable fast, affordable complete *CFTR* analysis for CF-causing variants, as it inevitably will and perhaps not very far into the future. Even if/when a primary DNA screening test for CF becomes technically feasible, unavoidable CF carrier identification will continue to be a challenging situation.

7. Incidental Findings and Implications of Emerging Data for Genetic Counseling

An important impact of the *CFTR* gene discovery relates to CF heterozygote carriers who are now being identified in countless numbers through prenatal and neonatal screening. One of the concerns about expanding *CFTR* panels beyond the previously common 23 CF-causing variants [60] has been the increase in incidental findings, particularly heterozygous infants, i.e., false positives with high IRT levels, one *CFTR* variant, and negative sweat tests. The PPV of the IRT/DNA test ranges from about 10% to 63% depending on the algorithm and the number of CFTR variants in the panel [61]. Detecting up to 10 carriers for every CF case diagnosed has been disconcerting for some, while others consider this an added benefit of CF NBS. Those in the former camp argue that that the purpose of CF NBS is identification of affected CF patients, and some have suggested that only more severely affected children should be the target population [62]. On the other hand, CF specialists who readily tolerate, or even advocate for, carrier detection as a byproduct of NBS can point out the many parents who have regarded that outcome as beneficial and appreciated the genetic counseling. In rare instances, an older sibling with CF has also been found in association with a false positive NBS result, and in most cases better informed reproductive planning has ensued from the genetic counseling. With greatly expanded *CFTR* panels and the prospects of a primary DNA/*CFTR* screening test, the issue of detecting infants who are carriers takes on greater importance and deserves detailed consideration.

There has been relatively little research done on the CF heterozygote carrier and no previous review of the published data and their implications. In a recent international study, it was determined that the p.Phe508del variant arose in Western Europe at least 5000 years ago [63,64]. Data on the time to the most recent common ancestor also revealed that it spread from west to east during the *longue durée* of the Bronze Age [65] and into the Iron Age and beyond [64]. Hazardous environmental exposures were numerous over that period [65]. Linking the p.Phe508del/wild type individual to a selective advantage has not yet been possible, despite some efforts [66], but there can be no doubt that CF heterozygotes must have had a selective advantage [67]. The high prevalence of p.Phe508del among native Europeans implies that the p.Phe508del/wild-type individual has a heretofore undiscovered health, survival, or fertility advantage. However, when parents ask questions in false-positive cases about what CF carrier status might mean for their baby, we have lacked answers. Nevertheless, this situation seems to be changing, as some research has focused on the CF carrier.

Certainly, it has been known for many years that IRT levels in infants who prove to be carriers are higher than the general population of screened babies [68,69]. This manifestation of *CFTR* variant/wild type status was initially surprising but is now well accepted. It agrees with earlier observations that CF carriers have higher sweat chloride levels than normal [70,71]. As long ago as 1962, a study by di Sant'Agnese and Powell [70] revealed an impressive difference between 97 obligate CF carriers (parents of patients with CF) and 117 "unselected adult controls" (mean sweat chloride values of 32 and 17 mmol/L, respectively; $p < 0.01$), suggesting that the sweat electrolyte abnormality should be considered a subclinical phenotypic manifestation in the CF heterozygote. In addition, taking advantage of NBS follow up data, Farrell and Koscik [72] showed conclusively that, after controlling the age factor, CF heterozygote carriers with the p.Phe508del variant have significantly increased sweat electrolyte concentrations, although they were not high enough to be in the range diagnostic of the disease. In retrospect, this should not be surprising since as Miller et al. [73] point out "carriers have ~50% as much CFTR anion channel activity as controls... and in some epithelia, anion transport is known to be reduced in carriers."

With regard to symptoms and disease risk, Wang et al. [74] reported that adult obligate CF heterozygotes have a much higher prevalence of chronic rhinosinusitis than the general population. Others have reported a higher incidence of pancreatitis in genetically proven CF carrier adults [75,76]. When disorders such as chronic pancreatitis occur in these patients, they might be better classified as having a CFTR-related disorder (CFTR-RD) [77], rather than simply being labeled CF carriers, but recent observations [73,75,78] may stimulate reassessment of terminology. In addition to chronic sinusitis, three phenotypes are included in the CFTR-RD category: CBAVD (congenital bilateral absence of the vas deferens) causing male infertility, acute recurrent or chronic pancreatitis, and bronchiectasis [77]. The prevalence of these and other conditions in CF carriers is surprisingly high as discussed below.

In 2011, Tluczek et al. [78] first identified a higher risk of disease in CF carriers. Specifically, based on evaluating children with a high IRT plus one CF-causing variant and a negative sweat test, Tluzcek et al. [78] observed that these carriers have more health system encounters for documented illnesses during their first year than healthy infants with negative NBS results. More recently, Miller et al. [73] published a provocative study involving 18,902 carriers matched with controls and reported that those with one *CFTR* variant have a significantly increased risk for 57 of 59 CF-related diagnostic conditions based on odds ratio analyses. The relative risks were increased for some conditions previously associated with CF carriers (e.g., pancreatitis, male infertility, and bronchiectasis), but others were not previously suspected, such as diabetes, constipation and cholelithiasis. Although the clinical significance of their findings remains to be determined, being identified as a CF carrier may promote attention to avoiding other disease-risk factors (e.g., the importance of avoiding heavy alcohol consumption in those who are intrinsically susceptible to pancreatitis). Moreover, Miller et al. [73] pointed out that identifying CF carriers may provide rational treatment options in the future for symptomatic carriers using drugs designed to enhance CFTR function. On the other hand, when applying these results to genetic counseling, it is important to keep in mind the differences between relative and absolute risk. As Miller et al. [73] point out, the relative risk for chronic pancreatitis is high with an odds ratio of 6.76 [95% CI, 4.87–9.39] but the absolute risk is less than 1% (only 0.429 per 100 carriers). However, when all the CFTR-RD conditions [74,77] are considered in male carriers based on the data of Miller et al. [73], the cumulative absolute risk is 19.07 per 100 CF heterozygotes—not a trivial prevalence.

Thus, in addition to having a probable health benefit that explains their high frequency, CF carriers appear to be at increased risk for some diseases because of their partial CFTR dysfunction.

To place this situation in perspective and learn from previous experiences, we need to consider the situation with sickle hemoglobin heterozygotes—individuals labeled as SCT for sickle cell trait. For more than a half-century, they have been identified in a variety of screening programs. After NBS for hemoglobinopathies via cellulose acetate electrophoresis became routine in the US during the late 1970s [79], numerous follow-up system problems occurred initially, particularly among African-American families. These included confusion, inappropriate labeling, stigmatization, and mistreatment. Over time, however, better follow-up communication practices have improved outcomes. Now, with data that clearly show serious health risks of SCT and benefits of early recognition, the advantages of heterozygote detection are generally accepted [80,81]. Thus, recognizing that SCT is actionable, health care systems have learned more about how to manage SCT-related communications and ensure effective, timely counseling [82]. Because the severe risks are delayed beyond childhood, when precipitating factors may supervene, such as dehydration during strenuous athletic events [80,81], counseling for SCT risks that occurs immediately after NBS must be repeated and target the heterozygous individual at an appropriate time [82]. The benefits are undeniable, however, especially the prevention of sudden death by simple hydration [80–83].

When considered collectively, the observations reviewed above suggest that we should not be describing CF carriers as completely healthy. Although providers who argue against incidental CF carrier detection do not recognize its advantages and regard these CF NBS incidental findings as "unwanted," the benefits of counseling parents of infant carriers are clear [84,85]. As more information is learned about the CF heterozygote condition, we suggest that attitudes and practices may need to change and ensure truthful education and effective communications about the implications of CF carrier status. Although the initial genetic counseling may eventually need to include the possibility that heterozygote infants have a higher risk of CFTR-RD conditions [73–77], incidental detection of carrier status in false-positive infants does not yet seem actionable for the child because of the low absolute risks and thus the expectation that most CF heterozygotes will be healthy—at least until later in life. Consequently, as with SCT, the counseling will have to be timed appropriately and target the carrier when risk factor mitigation could be valuable and CFTR modulators potentially useful for severe disorders like pancreatitis [75,76].

8. The Opportunities for Preventive Therapies

Management of CF disease has traditionally relied on symptom-based treatments [86]. Thus, a "one size fits all" philosophy has been common for many years, in which a plethora of drugs are being used in standard doses. Malnutrition and growth faltering, obstructive lung disease with suppurative respiratory infections, and unresponsive pulmonary exacerbations are challenging to treat, especially in "non-responders [56,57]. Thus, preventive therapies are increasingly attractive and feasible. There are four problems in CF that are amenable to prophylactic strategies, namely: (1) salt loss in sweat that can cause fatal hyponatremic/hypochloremic dehydration; (2) pancreatic insufficiency; (3) malnutrition; and (4) chronic obstructive lung disease with recurrent infections [4]. Although excessive salt loss may seem minor and can be readily prevented with salt supplements, CF patients still die from this problem, and the breast-fed infant is especially vulnerable in hot weather. Treatment with a lifetime of daily salt supplements is effective and essential, even when a patient is taking CFTR modulators [28]. Pancreatic insufficiency and its sequelae (risk of malnutrition, recurrent pancreatitis, and diabetes mellitus) have always been considered a permanent component of CF for the majority of patients with susceptible genotypes. To most CF specialists' surprise, however, CFTR modulator therapy has been associated with at least partial preservation of pancreatic function in recent studies examining this issue [34,84–86]. In fact, the weight gains of CF patients in the original trials of ivacaftor suggested its potential to reduce the detrimental impact of pancreatic insufficiency [28], and subsequent observations support this hypothesis [87–89]. Prevention of malnutrition in most children with CF diagnosed early in the Wisconsin RCT was achieved with an aggressive approach to nutritional management, emphasizing the combination of pancreatic enzyme replacement therapy, high caloric intake, and supplements of fat soluble vitamins plus essential fatty acid supplements [30,90]. On the other hand, some children were found to be "non-responders" to this regimen [56,57,91], and this has led to more research [59]. Lastly, the most important target for preventive therapy is the respiratory system, because the quality and quantity of life in individual patients' experience usually depends on the severity of lung disease. Thus, the most exciting aspect of CFTR modulator therapy is its potential for ameliorating lung disease as discussed in detail elsewhere [28,88,89]. For CF patients, therefore, the transformation from intervention to prevention, associated with early diagnosis and novel treatments, is clearly the most impactful result of the discovery of the *CFTR* gene.

9. Conclusions

The discovery of the *CFTR* gene was the scientific advance that improved our ability to diagnose CF rapidly, genotype patients simultaneously, predict pancreatic functional status immediately, and then plan preventive care. The era of genetic/genomic medicine has brightened the outlook for all patients with CF and especially children, who are now in most cases diagnosed while still asymptomatic.

Author Contributions: All three authors contributed substantially to the research and views reported herein. All authors have read and agreed to the published version of the manuscript.

Funding: Our research has been funded by the National Institutes of Health (DK34108), the Cystic Fibrosis Foundation, and The Legacy of Angels Foundation.

Acknowledgments: We thank the late Ron Laessig, Gary Hoffman and Ronald Gregg for their essential contributions to the development of the Wisconsin CF newborn screening program and Anita Laxova for coordinating the Wisconsin RCT of CF newborn screening. We are also grateful to Elinor Langfelder-Schwind, Karen Raraigh, and Michael Farrell for their review, revisions, and advice regarding Section 7 on incidental findings and to Erin Ryan for her help with the manuscript preparation.

Conflicts of Interest: The authors declare no conflict of interest.

References

1. Scotet, V.; Gutierrez, H.; Farrell, P.M. Newborn Screening for CF across the Globe—Where Is It Worthwhile? *Int. J. Neonatal Screen.* **2020**, *6*, 18. [CrossRef]

2. Grosse, S.D.; Boyle, C.A.; Botkin, J.R.; Comeau, A.M.; Kharrazi, M.; Rosenfeld, M.; Wilfond, B.S. Newborn Screening for Cystic Fibrosis: Evaluation of Benefits and Risks and Recommendations for State Newborn Screening Programs. In *MMWR. Recommendations and Reports: Morbidity and Mortality Weekly Report. Recommendations and Reports*; Centers for Disease Control and Prevention: Antlanta, GA, USA, 2004; Volume Voume 53, pp. 1–36.

3. Farrell, P.; Gilbert-Barness, E.; Bell, J.; Gregg, R.; Mischler, E.; Odell, G.; Shahidi, N.; Robertson, I.; Evans, J. Progressive Malnutrition, Severe Anemia, Hepatic Dysfunction, and Respiratory Failure in a Three-Month-Old White Girl. *Am. J. Med. Genet.* **1993**, *45*, 725–738. [CrossRef] [PubMed]

4. Accurso, F.J.; Sontag, M.K.; Wagener, J.S. Complications Associated with Symptomatic Diagnosis in Infants with Cystic Fibrosis. *J. Pediatr.* **2005**, *147*, S37–S41. [CrossRef] [PubMed]

5. Kharrazi, M.; Yang, J.; Bishop, T.; Lessing, S.; Young, S.; Graham, S.; Pearl, M.; Chow, H.; Ho, T.; Currier, R.; et al. Newborn Screening for Cystic Fibrosis in California. *Pediatrics* **2015**, *136*, 1062–1072. [CrossRef]

6. Shwachman, H.; Kulczycki, L.L. Long-Term Study of One Hundred Five Patients with Cystic Fibrosis: Studies Made Over a Five- to Fourteen-Year Period. *AMA J. Dis. Child.* **1958**, *96*, 6–15. [CrossRef]

7. Bruns, W.T.; Connell, T.R.; Lacey, J.A.; Whisler, K.E. Test Strip Meconium Screening for Cystic Fibrosis. *Am. J. Dis. Child.* **1977**, *131*, 71–73. [CrossRef]

8. Guthrie, R.; Susi, A. A Simple Phenylalanne Method for Detecting Phenylketonuria in Large Populations of Newborn Infants. *Pediatrics* **1963**, *32*, 338–343.

9. Crossley, J.R.; Elliott, R.B.; Smith, P.A. Dried-Blood Spot Screening for Cystic Fibrosis in the Newborn. *Lancet (Lond. Engl.)* **1979**, *1*, 472–474. [CrossRef]

10. Hammond, K.B.; Abman, S.H.; Sokol, R.J.; Accurso, F.J. Efficacy of Statewide Neonatal Screening for Cystic Fibrosis by Assay of Trypsinogen Concentrations. *N. Engl. J. Med.* **1991**, *325*, 769–774. [CrossRef]

11. Taussig, L.M.; Boat, T.F.; Dayton, D.; Fost, N.; Hammond, K.; Holtzman, N.; Johnson, W.; Kaback, M.M.; Kennel, J.; Rosenstein, B.J.; et al. Neonatal Screening for Cystic Fibrosis: Position Paper. *Pediatrics* **1983**, *72*, 741–745.

12. Kloosterboer, M.; Hoffman, G.; Rock, M.; Gershan, W.; Laxova, A.; Li, Z.; Farrell, P.M. Clarification of Laboratory and Clinical Variables That Influence Cystic Fibrosis Newborn Screening with Initial Analysis of Immunoreactive Trypsinogen. *Pediatrics* **2009**, *123*, e338–e346. [CrossRef] [PubMed]

13. Therrell, B.L.; Hannon, W.H.; Hoffman, G.; Ojodu, J.; Farrell, P.M. Immunoreactive Trypsinogen (IRT) as a Biomarker for Cystic Fibrosis: Challenges in Newborn Dried Blood Spot Screening. *Mol. Genet. Metab.* **2012**, *106*, 1–6. [CrossRef] [PubMed]

14. Kerem, B.S.; Rommens, J.M.; Buchanan, J.A.; Markiewicz, D.; Cox, T.K.; Chakravarti, A.; Buchwald, M.; Tsui, L.C. Identification of the Cystic Fibrosis Gene: Genetic Analysis. *Science* **1989**, *245*, 1073–1080. [CrossRef] [PubMed]

15. Farrell, P.M.; Kosorok, M.R.; Rock, M.J.; Laxova, A.; Zeng, L.; Lai, H.C.; Hoffman, G.; Laessig, R.H.; Splaingard, M.L. Early Diagnosis of Cystic Fibrosis through Neonatal Screening Prevents Severe Malnutrition and Improves Long-Term Growth. *Pediatrics* **2001**, *107*, 1–13. [CrossRef]

16. Wilfond, B.; Gregg, R.G.; Laxova, A.; Hassemer, D.; Mischler, E.F.P. Mutation Analysis for CF Newborn Screening: A Two-Tiered Approach. *Pediatr. Pulmonol. Suppl.* **1991**, *6*, 238.

17. Gregg, R.G.; Wilfond, B.S.; Farrell, P.M.; Laxova, A.; Hassemer, D.; Mischler, E.H. Application of DNA Analysis in a Population-Screening Program for Neonatal Diagnosis of Cystic Fibrosis (CF): Comparison of Screening Protocols. *Am. J. Hum. Genet.* **1993**, *52*, 616–626.

18. Gregg, R.G.; Simantel, A.; Farrell, P.M.; Koscik, R.; Kosorok, M.R.; Laxova, A.; Laessig, R.; Hoffman, G.; Hassemer, D.; Mischler, E.H.; et al. Newborn Screening for Cystic Fibrosis in Wisconsin: Comparison of Biochemical and Molecular Methods. *Pediatrics* **1997**, *99*, 819–824. [CrossRef]

19. Farrell, P.M.; Mischler, E.H.; Fost, N.C.; Wilfond, B.S.; Tluczek, A.; Gregg, R.G.; Bruns, W.T.; Hassemer, D.J.; Laessig, R.H. Current Issues in Neonatal Screening for Cystic Fibrosis and Implications of the CF Gene Discovery. *Pediatr. Pulmonol.* **1991**, *11* (Suppl. 7), 11–18. [CrossRef]

20. Jinks, D.C.; Minter, M.; Tarver, D.A.; Vanderford, M.; Hejtmancik, J.F.; McCabe, E.R.B. Molecular Genetic Diagnosis of Sickle Cell Disease Using Dried Blood Specimens on Blotters Used for Newborn Screening. *Hum. Genet.* **1989**, *81*, 363–366. [CrossRef]

21. Rommens, J.; Kerem, B.S.; Greer, W.; Chang, P.; Tsui, L.C.; Ray, P. Rapid Nonradioactive Detection of the Major Cystic Fibrosis Mutation. *Am. J. Hum. Genet.* **1990**, *46*, 395–396.

22. Rock, M.J.; Mischler, E.H.; Farrell, P.M.; Wei, L.J.; Bruns, W.T.; Hassemer, D.J.; Laessig, R.H. Newborn Screening for Cystic Fibrosis Is Complicated by Age-Related Decline in Immunoreactive Trypsinogen Levels. *Pediatrics* **1990**, *85*, 1001–1007. [CrossRef] [PubMed]

23. Farrell, P.M. Improving the Health of Patients with Cystic Fibrosis through Newborn Screening. Wisconsin Cystic Fibrosis Neonatal Screening Study Group. *Adv. Pediatr.* **2000**, *47*, 79–115. [PubMed]

24. Ranieri, E.; Ryall, R.G.; Morris, C.P.; Nelson, P.V.; Carey, W.F.; Pollard, A.C.; Robertson, E.F. Neonatal Screening Strategy for Cystic Fibrosis Using Immunoreactive Trypsinogen and Direct Gene Anylysis. *Br. Med. J.* **1991**, *302*, 1237–1240. [CrossRef] [PubMed]

25. Férec, C.; Verlingue, C.; Parent, P.; Morin, J.F.; Codet, J.P.; Rault, G.; Dagorne, M.; Lemoigne, A.; Journel, H.; Roussey, M. Neonatal Screening for Cystic Fibrosis: Result of a Pilot Study Using Both Immunoreactive Trypsinogen and Cystic Fibrosis Gene Mutation Analyses. *Hum. Genet.* **1995**, *96*, 542–548. [CrossRef]

26. Farrell, P.M.; Lai, H.C.J.; Li, Z.; Kosorok, M.R.; Laxova, A.; Green, C.G.; Collins, J.; Hoffman, G.; Laessig, R.; Rock, M.J.; et al. Evidence on Improved Outcomes with Early Diagnosis of Cystic Fibrosis through Neonatal Screening: Enough Is Enough! *J. Pediatr.* **2005**, *147*, S30–S36. [CrossRef]

27. Campbell, P.W.; White, T.B. Newborn Screening for Cystic Fibrosis: An Opportunity to Improve Care and Outcomes. *J. Pediatr.* **2005**, *147*, S2–S5. [CrossRef]

28. Ramsey, B.W.; Davies, J.; McElvaney, N.G.; Tullis, E.; Bell, S.C.; Dřevínek, P.; Griese, M.; McKone, E.F.; Wainwright, C.E.; Konstan, M.W.; et al. A CFTR Potentiator in Patients with Cystic Fibrosis and the G551D Mutation. *N. Engl. J. Med.* **2011**, *365*, 1663–1672. [CrossRef]

29. Middleton, P.G.; Mall, M.A.; Dřevínek, P.; Lands, L.C.; McKone, E.F.; Polineni, D.; Ramsey, B.W.; Taylor-Cousar, J.L.; Tullis, E.; Vermeulen, F.; et al. Elexacaftor-Tezacaftor-Ivacaftor for Cystic Fibrosis with a Single Phe508del Allele. *N. Engl. J. Med.* **2019**, *381*, 1809–1819. [CrossRef]

30. Borowitz, D.; Robinson, K.A.; Rosenfeld, M.; Davis, S.D.; Sabadosa, K.A.; Spear, S.L.; Michel, S.H.; Parad, R.B.; White, T.B.; Farrell, P.M.; et al. Cystic Fibrosis Foundation Evidence-Based Guidelines for Management of Infants with Cystic Fibrosis. *J. Pediatr.* **2009**, *155* (Suppl. 6), S73–S93. [CrossRef]

31. Rock, M.J.; Levy, H.; Zaleski, C.; Farrell, P.M. Factors Accounting for a Missed Diagnosis of Cystic Fibrosis after Newborn Screening. *Pediatr. Pulmonol.* **2011**, *46*, 1166–1174. [CrossRef]

32. Comeau, A.M.; Parad, R.B.; Dorkin, H.L.; Dovey, M.; Gerstle, R.; Haver, K.; Lapey, A.; O'Sullivan, B.P.; Waltz, D.A.; Zwerdling, R.G.; et al. Population-Based Newborn Screening for Genetic Disorders When Multiple Mutation DNA Testing Is Incorporated: A Cystic Fibrosis Newborn Screening Model Demonstrating Increased Sensitivity but More Carrier Detections. *Pediatrics* **2004**, *113*, 1573–1581. [CrossRef] [PubMed]

33. Kerem, E.; Kerem, B. Genotype-phenotype Correlations in Cystic Fibrosis. *Pediatr. Pulmonol.* **1996**, *22*, 387–395. [CrossRef]

34. De Boeck, K. Cystic Fibrosis in the Year 2020: A Disease with a New Face. In *Acta Paediatrica, International Journal of Paediatrics*; Blackwell Publishing Ltd.: Oxford, UK, 2020. [CrossRef]

35. Sommerburg, O.; Hammermann, J.; Lindner, M.; Stahl, M.; Muckenthaler, M.; Kohlmueller, D.; Happich, M.; Kulozik, A.E.; Stopsack, M.; Gahr, M.; et al. Five Years of Experience with Biochemical Cystic Fibrosis Newborn Screening Based on IRT/PAP in Germany. *Pediatr. Pulmonol.* **2015**, *50*, 655–664. [CrossRef] [PubMed]

36. Munck, A.; Mayell, S.J.; Winters, V.; Shawcross, A.; Derichs, N.; Parad, R.; Barben, J.; Southern, K.W. Cystic Fibrosis Screen Positive, Inconclusive Diagnosis (CFSPID): A New Designation and Management Recommendations for Infants with an Inconclusive Diagnosis Following Newborn Screening. *J. Cyst. Fibros.* **2015**, *14*, 706–713. [CrossRef]

37. Ren, C.L.; Borowitz, D.S.; Gonska, T.; Howenstine, M.S.; Levy, H.; Massie, J.; Milla, C.; Munck, A.; Southern, K.W. Cystic Fibrosis Transmembrane Conductance Regulator-Related Metabolic Syndrome and Cystic Fibrosis Screen Positive, Inconclusive Diagnosis. *J. Pediatr.* **2017**, *181*, S45–S51.e1. [CrossRef]

38. Sontag, M.K.; Wright, D.; Beebe, J.; Accurso, F.J.; Sagel, S.D. A New Cystic Fibrosis Newborn Screening Algorithm: IRT/IRT1↑/DNA. *J. Pediatr.* **2009**, *155*, 618–622. [CrossRef]

39. CLSI. *Newborn Screening for Cystic Fibrosis*, 2nd ed.; CLSI guideline NBS05; Clinical and Laboratory Standards Institute: Wayne, PA, USA, 2019.

40. Di Sant'Agnese, P.A. Neonatal and General Aspects of Cystic Fibrosis. In *Current Topics in Clinical Chemistry-Clinical Biochemistry of the Neonate*; Young, D.C., Hicks, J.M., Eds.; John Wiley and Sons Inc.: New York, NY, USA, 1976.

41. Reardon, M.C.; Hammond, K.B.; Accurso, F.J.; Fisher, C.D.; McCabe, E.R.B.; Cotton, E.K.; Bowman, C.M. Nutritional Deficits Exist before 2 Months of Age in Some Infants with Cystic Fibrosis Identified by Screening Test. *J. Pediatr.* **1984**, *105*, 271–274. [CrossRef]

42. Allen, D.B.; Farrell, P.M. Newborn Screening: Principles and Practice. *Adv. Pediatr.* **1996**, *43*, 231–270.

43. Zielenski, J.; Fujiwara, T.M.; Markiewicz, D.; Paradis, A.J.; Anacleto, A.I.; Richards, B.; Schwartz, R.H.; Klinger, K.W.; Tsui, L.C.; Morgan, K. Identification of the M1101K Mutation in the Cystic Fibrosis Transmembrane Conductance Regulator (CFTR) Gene and Complete Detection of Cystic Fibrosis Mutations in the Hutterite Population. *Am. J. Hum. Genet.* **1993**, *52*, 609–615.

44. Watts, K.D.; Layne, B.; Harris, A.; McColley, S.A. Hispanic Infants with Cystic Fibrosis Show Low CFTR Mutation Detection Rates in the Illinois Newborn Screening Program. *J. Genet. Couns.* **2012**, *21*, 671–675. [CrossRef]

45. Baker, M.W.; Atkins, A.E.; Cordovado, S.K.; Hendrix, M.; Earley, M.C.; Farrell, P.M. Improving Newborn Screening for Cystic Fibrosis Using Next-Generation Sequencing Technology: A Technical Feasibility Study. *Genet. Med.* **2016**, *18*, 231–238. [CrossRef] [PubMed]

46. Hughes, E.E.; Stevens, C.F.; Saavedra-Matiz, C.A.; Tavakoli, N.P.; Krein, L.M.; Parker, A.; Zhang, Z.; Maloney, B.; Vogel, B.; DeCelie-Germana, J.; et al. Clinical Sensitivity of Cystic Fibrosis Mutation Panels in a Diverse Population. *Hum. Mutat.* **2016**, *37*, 201–208. [CrossRef] [PubMed]

47. Metzker, M.L. Sequencing Technologies the next Generation. *Nat. Rev. Genet.* **2010**, 31–46. [CrossRef] [PubMed]

48. Sosnay, P.R.; Siklosi, K.R.; Van Goor, F.; Kaniecki, K.; Yu, H.; Sharma, N.; Ramalho, A.S.; Amaral, M.D.; Dorfman, R.; Zielenski, J.; et al. Defining the Disease Liability of Variants in the Cystic Fibrosis Transmembrane Conductance Regulator Gene. *Nat. Genet.* **2013**, *45*, 1160–1167. [CrossRef] [PubMed]

49. Sosnay, P.R.; Salinas, D.B.; White, T.B.; Ren, C.L.; Farrell, P.M.; Raraigh, K.S.; Girodon, E.; Castellani, C. Applying Cystic Fibrosis Transmembrane Conductance Regulator Genetics and CFTR2 Data to Facilitate Diagnoses. *J. Pediatr.* **2017**, *181*, S27.e1–S32.e1. [CrossRef]

50. Baker, M.W.; Grossman, W.J.; Laessig, R.H.; Hoffman, G.L.; Brokopp, C.D.; Kurtycz, D.F.; Cogley, M.F.; Litsheim, T.J.; Katcher, M.L.; Routes, J.M. Development of a Routine Newborn Screening Protocol for Severe Combined Immunodeficiency. *J. Allergy Clin. Immunol.* **2009**, *124*, 522–527. [CrossRef]

51. Vill, K.; Kölbel, H.; Schwartz, O.; Blaschek, A.; Olgemöller, B.; Harms, E.; Burggraf, S.; Röschinger, W.; Durner, J.; Gläser, D.; et al. One Year of Newborn Screening for SMA – Results of a German Pilot Project. *J. Neuromuscul. Dis.* **2019**, *6*, 503–515. [CrossRef]

52. Fabie, N.A.V.; Pappas, K.B.; Feldman, G.L. The Current State of Newborn Screening in the United States. In *Pediatric Clinics of North America*; W.B. Saunders: Philadelphia, PA, USA, 2019; pp. 369–386. [CrossRef]

53. O'Neal, W.K.; Knowles, M.R. Cystic Fibrosis Disease Modifiers: Complex Genetics Defines the Phenotypic Diversity in a Monogenic Disease. *Annu. Rev. Genomics Hum. Genet.* **2018**, *19*, 201–222. [CrossRef]

54. Petrikin, J.E.; Willig, L.K.; Smith, L.D.; Kingsmore, S.F. Rapid Whole Genome Sequencing and Precision Neonatology. In *Seminars in Perinatology*; W.B. Saunders: Philadelphia, PA, USA, 2015; pp. 623–631. [CrossRef]

55. Willig, L.K.; Petrikin, J.E.; Smith, L.D.; Saunders, C.J.; Thiffault, I.; Miller, N.A.; Soden, S.E.; Cakici, J.A.; Herd, S.M.; Twist, G.; et al. Whole-Genome Sequencing for Identification of Mendelian Disorders in Critically Ill Infants: A Retrospective Analysis of Diagnostic and Clinical Findings. *Lancet Respir. Med.* **2015**, *3*, 377–387. [CrossRef]

56. Lai, H.J.; Shoff, S.M.; Farrell, P.M. Recovery of Birth Weight z Score within 2 Years of Diagnosis Is Positively Associated with Pulmonary Status at 6 Years of Age in Children with Cystic Fibrosis. *Pediatrics* **2009**, *123*, 714–722. [CrossRef]

57. Sanders, D.B.; Zhang, Z.; Farrell, P.M.; Lai, H.C.J. Early Life Growth Patterns Persist for 12 years and Impact Pulmonary Outcomes in Cystic Fibrosis. *J. Cyst. Fibros.* **2018**, *17*, 528–535. [CrossRef] [PubMed]

58. Wilk, M.A.; Braun, A.T.; Farrell, P.M.; Laxova, A.; Brown, D.M.; Holt, J.M.; Birch, C.L.; Sosonkina, N.; Wilk, B.M.; Worthey, E.A. Applying Whole-Genome Sequencing in Relation to Phenotype and Outcomes in Siblings with Cystic Fibrosis. *Cold Spring Harb. Mol. Case Stud.* **2020**, *6*. [CrossRef] [PubMed]

59. Lai, H.J.; Lu, Q.; Chin, L.H.; Wilk, M.; Worthey, E.; the FIRST Study Group. Whole-Genome Sequencing Reveals That Genetic Variations Predict Effectiveness of Vitamin D Supplemntation in Young Children with CF. *Cyst. Fibros. Suppl.* **2019**, *18*, S47. [CrossRef]

60. Watson, M.S.; Cutting, G.R.; Desnick, R.J.; Driscoll, D.A.; Klinger, K.; Mennuti, M.; Palomaki, G.E.; Popovich, B.W.; Pratt, V.M.; Rohlfs, E.M.; et al. Cystic Fibrosis Population Carrier Screening: 2004 Revision of American College of Medical Genetics Mutation Panel. *Genet. Med.* **2004**, 387–391. [CrossRef]

61. Dankert-Roelse, J.E.; Bouva, M.J.; Jakobs, B.S.; Janssens, H.M.; de Winter-de Groot, K.M.; Schönbeck, Y.; Gille, J.J.P.; Gulmans, V.A.M.; Verschoof-Puite, R.K.; Schielen, P.C.J.I.; et al. Newborn Blood Spot Screening for Cystic Fibrosis with a Four-Step Screening Strategy in The Netherlands. *J. Cyst. Fibros.* **2019**, *18*, 54–63. [CrossRef]

62. Scotet, V.; Audrézet, M.P.; Roussey, M.; Rault, G.; Dirou-Prigent, A.; Journel, H.; Moisan-Petit, V.; Storni, V.; Férec, C. Immunoreactive Trypsin/DNA Newborn Screening for Cystic Fibrosis: Should the R117H Variant Be Included in CFTR Mutation Panels? *Pediatrics* **2006**, *118*, e1523–e1529. [CrossRef]

63. Serre, J.L.; Simon-Bouy, B.; Mornet, E.; Jaume-Roig, B.; Balassopoulou, A.; Schwartz, M.; Taillandier, A.; Boué, J.; Boué, A. Studies of RFLP Closely Linked to the Cystic Fibrosis Locus throughout Europe Lead to New Considerations in Populations Genetics. *Hum. Genet.* **1990**, *84*, 449–454. [CrossRef]

64. Farrell, P.; Férec, C.; Macek, M.; Frischer, T.; Renner, S.; Riss, K.; Barton, D.; Repetto, T.; Tzetis, M.; Giteau, K.; et al. Estimating the Age of p.(Phe508del) with Family Studies of Geographically Distinct European Populations and the Early Spread of Cystic Fibrosis. *Eur. J. Hum. Genet.* **2018**, *26*, 1832–1839. [CrossRef]

65. Poolman, E.M.; Galvani, A.P. Evaluating Candidate Agents of Selective Pressure for Cystic Fibrosis. *J. R. Soc. Interface* **2007**, *4*, 91–98. [CrossRef]

66. Price, T. *Europe before Rome*; Oxford University Press: New York, NY, USA, 2013.

67. Romeo, G.; Devoto, M.; Galietta, L.J. Why Is the Cystic Fibrosis Gene so Frequent? *Hum. Genet.* **1989**, *84*, 1–5. [CrossRef]

68. Scotet, V.; De Braekeleer, M.; Audrézet, M.P.; Lodé, L.; Verlingue, C.; Quéré, I.; Mercier, B.; Duguépéroux, I.; Codet, J.P.; Moineau, M.P.; et al. Prevalence of CFTR Mutations in Hypertrypsinaemia Detected through Neonatal Screening for Cystic Fibrosis. *Clin. Genet.* **2001**, *59*, 42–47. [CrossRef] [PubMed]

69. Castellani, C.; Picci, L.; Scarpa, M.; Dechecchi, M.C.; Zanolla, L.; Assael, B.M.; Zacchello, F. Cystic Fibrosis Carriers Have Higher Neonatal Immunoreactive Trypsinogen Values than Non-Carriers. *Am. J. Med. Genet.* **2005**, *135 A*, 142–144. [CrossRef]

70. Sant'Agnese, P.A.; Powell, G.F. The Eccrine Sweat Defect in Cystic Fibrosis of the Pancrease (mucoviscidosis). *Ann. N. Y. Acad. Sci.* **1962**, *93*, 555–599. [CrossRef]

71. Sproul, A.; Huang, N. Diagnosis of Heterozygosity for Cystic Fibrosis by Discriminatory Analysis of Sweat Chloride Distribution. *J. Pediatr.* **1966**, *69*, 759–770. [CrossRef]

72. Farrell, P.M.; Koscik, R.E. Sweat Chloride Concentrations in Infants Homozygous or Heterozygous for F508 Cystic Fibrosis. *Pediatrics* **1996**, *97*, 524–528. [PubMed]

73. Miller, A.C.; Comellas, A.P.; Hornick, D.B.; Stoltz, D.A.; Cavanaugh, J.E.; Gerke, A.K.; Welsh, M.J.; Zabner, J.; Polgreen, P.M. Cystic Fibrosis Carriers Are at Increased Risk for a Wide Range of Cystic Fibrosis-Related Conditions. *Proc. Natl. Acad. Sci. USA* **2020**, *117*, 1621–1627. [CrossRef]

74. Wang, X.J.; Kim, J.; McWilliams, R.; Cutting, G.R. Increased Prevalence of Chronic Rhinosinusitis in Carriers of a Cystic Fibrosis Mutation. *Arch. Otolaryngol.-Head Neck Surg.* **2005**, *131*, 237–240. [CrossRef]

75. Cohn, J.A.; Neoptolemos, J.P.; Feng, J.; Yan, J.; Jiang, Z.; Greenhalf, W.; McFaul, C.; Mountford, R.; Sommer, S.S. Increased Risk of Idiopathic Chronic Pancreatitis in Cystic Fibrosis Carriers. *Hum. Mutat.* **2005**, *26*, 303–307. [CrossRef]

76. Sharer, N.; Schwarz, M.; Malone, G.; Howarth, A.; Painter, J.; Super, M.; Braganza, J. Mutations of the Cystic Fibrosis Gene in Patients with Chronic Pancreatitis. *N. Engl. J. Med.* **1998**, *339*, 645–652. [CrossRef]

77. Bombieri, C.; Claustres, M.; De Boeck, K.; Derichs, N.; Dodge, J.; Girodon, E.; Sermet, I.; Schwarz, M.; Tzetis, M.; Wilschanski, M.; et al. Recommendations for the Classification of Diseases as CFTR-Related Disorders. *J. Cyst. Fibros.* **2011**, *10* (Suppl. 2), S86–S102. [CrossRef]

78. Tluczek, A.; McKechnie, A.C.; Brown, R.L. Factors Associated with Parental Perception of Child Vulnerability 12 Months after Abnormal Newborn Screening Results. *Res. Nurs. Heal.* **2011**, *34*, 389–400. [CrossRef] [PubMed]

79. Schmidt, R.M.; Brosious, E.M.; Holland, S.; Wright, J.M.; Serjeant, G.R. Use of Blood Specimens Collected on Filter Paper in Screening for Abnormal Hemoglobins. *Clin. Chem.* **1976**, *22*, 685–687. [CrossRef] [PubMed]

80. Naik, R.P.; Smith-Whitley, K.; Hassell, K.L.; Umeh, N.I.; De Montalembert, M.; Sahota, P.; Haywood, C.; Jenkins, J.; Lloyd-Puryear, M.A.; Joiner, C.H.; et al. Clinical Outcomes Associated with Sickle Cell Trait: A Systematic Review. *Ann. Intern. Med.* **2018**, 619–627. [CrossRef] [PubMed]

81. Podduturi, V.; Guileyardo, J.M. Sickle Cell Trait as a Contributory Cause of Death in Natural Disease. *J. Forens. Sci.* **2015**, *60*, 807–811. [CrossRef]

82. Pecker, L.H.; Naik, R.P. The Current State of Sickle Cell Trait: Implications for Reproductive and Genetic Counseling. *Blood* **2018**, 2331–2338. [CrossRef]

83. Shephard, R.J. Sickle Cell Trait: What Are the Costs and Benefits of Screening? In *Journal of Sports Medicine and Physical Fitness*; Edizioni Minerva Medica: Turin, Italy, 2016; pp. 1562–1573.

84. Wheeler, P.G.; Smith, R.; Dorkin, H.; Parad, R.B.; Comeau, A.M.; Bianchi, D.W. Genetic Counseling after Implementation of Statewide Cystic Fibrosis Newborn Screening: Two Years' Experience in One Medical Center. *Genet. Med.* **2001**, *3*, 411–415. [CrossRef]

85. Cavanagh, L.; Compton, C.J.; Tluczek, A.; Brown, R.L.; Farrell, P.M. Long-Term Evaluation of Genetic Counseling Following False-Positive Newborn Screen for Cystic Fibrosis. *J. Genet. Couns.* **2010**, *19*, 199–210. [CrossRef]

86. Clancy, J.P.; Cotton, C.U.; Donaldson, S.H.; Solomon, G.M.; VanDevanter, D.R.; Boyle, M.P.; Gentzsch, M.; Nick, J.A.; Illek, B.; Wallenburg, J.C.; et al. CFTR Modulator Theratyping: Current Status, Gaps and Future Directions. *J. Cyst. Fibrosis* **2019**, 22–34. [CrossRef]

87. Bellin, M.D.; Laguna, T.; Leschyshyn, J.; Regelmann, W.; Dunitz, J.; Billings, J.; Moran, A. Insulin Secretion Improves in Cystic Fibrosis Following Ivacaftor Correction of CFTR: A Small Pilot Study. *Pediatr. Diabetes* **2013**, *14*, 417–421. [CrossRef]

88. Rosenfeld, M.; Wainwright, C.E.; Higgins, M.; Wang, L.T.; McKee, C.; Campbell, D.; Tian, S.; Schneider, J.; Cunningham, S.; Davies, J.C.; et al. Ivacaftor Treatment of Cystic Fibrosis in Children Aged 12 to <24 Months and with a CFTR Gating Mutation (ARRIVAL): A Phase 3 Single-Arm Study. *Lancet Respir. Med.* **2018**, *6*, 545–553. [CrossRef]

89. Rosenfeld, M.; Cunningham, S.; Harris, W.T.; Lapey, A.; Regelmann, W.E.; Sawicki, G.S.; Southern, K.W.; Chilvers, M.; Higgins, M.; Tian, S.; et al. An Open-Label Extension Study of Ivacaftor in Children with CF and a CFTR Gating Mutation Initiating Treatment at Age 2–5 years (KLIMB). *J. Cyst. Fibros.* **2019**, *18*, 838–843. [CrossRef] [PubMed]

90. Stallings, V.A.; Stark, L.J.; Robinson, K.A.; Feranchak, A.P.; Quinton, H. Evidence-Based Practice Recommendations for Nutrition-Related Management of Children and Adults with Cystic Fibrosis and Pancreatic Insufficiency: Results of a Systematic Review. *J. Am. Diet. Assoc.* **2008**, *108*, 832–839. [CrossRef] [PubMed]

91. Shoff, S.M.; Ahn, H.Y.; Davis, L.; Lai, H.C.; Douglas, J.; Fost, N.; Green, C.; Gregg, R.; Kosorok, M.; Laessig, R.; et al. Temporal Associations among Energy Intake, Plasma Linoleic Acid, and Growth Improvement in Response to Treatment Initiation after Diagnosis of Cystic Fibrosis. *Pediatrics* **2006**, *117*, 391–400. [CrossRef] [PubMed]

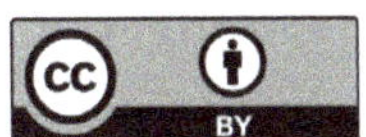

MDPI

St. Alban-Anlage 66

4052 Basel

Switzerland

Tel. +41 61 683 77 34

Fax +41 61 302 89 18

www.mdpi.com

Genes Editorial Office

E-mail: genes@mdpi.com

www.mdpi.com/journal/genes